RETRANSPLANTATION

Transplantation and Clinical Immunology
Symposia Fondation Marcel Mérieux

VOLUME 29

Retransplantation

Proceedings of the 29th Conference on Transplantation and Clinical Immunology, 9–11 June, 1997

Edited by

J.L. Touraine
J. Traeger
H. Bétuel
J.M. Dubernard
J.P. Revillard
C. Dupuy

SPRINGER-SCIENCE+BUSINESS MEDIA, B.V.

A C.I.P. Catalogue record for this book is available from the Library of Congress

ISBN 978-94-017-4110-1 ISBN 978-0-585-38142-8 (eBook)
DOI 10.1007/978-0-585-38142-8

Printed on acid-free paper

Table of contents

Part 9: Oral communications

List of contributors

R. ARNOLD
University of Pittsburgh
Center for Medical Ethics
Division of General Internal Medicine
200 Lothrop Street – MUH, Suite W-919
Pittsburgh, PA 15213-2582
USA

M.A. BELGER
UKTSSA
Fox Den Road
Stoke Gifford
Bristol BS12 5RR
UK

F. BERTHOUX
Service de Nephrologie et
Transplantation Renale
Hopital Nord
F-42055 Saint Etienne Cedex 2
France

C. BURILLON
Hopital Edouard Herriot
Pavillion C – Ophtalmologie
5, Place d'Arsonval
69437 Lyon Cedex 03
France

B. CHARPENTIER
CHU Bicetre
Service de Nephrologie
78, rue du General Leclerc
F-94275 Le Kremlin Bicetre Cedex
France

F.H.J. CLAAS
Academish Zienkenhuis Leiden
Dept. of immunohematology and Blood
Bank
Rinjsburgerweg 10
Postbus 9600
Leiden
The Netherlands

Y.W. CHO
UCLA School of Medicine
Tissue Typing Laboratory
950 Veteran Avenue
Los Angeles, CA 90095-1652
USA

P. COCHAT
Hopital Edouard Herriot
Pavillon S
5, Place d'Arsonval
F-69437 Lyon Cedex 3
France

B. CUZIN
Hopital Edouard Herriot
Pavillon V
5, Place d'Arsonval
F-69437 Lyon Cedex 3
France

J.H. DAUBER
Pulmonary Transplant Medicine Service
University of Pittsburgh Medical Center
440 Scaife Hall
3550 Terrace Street
Pittsburgh, PA 15261
USA

C. DUCERF
Hopital de la Croix Rousse
Service de Chirurgie
103, Grand Rue de la Croix Rousse
F-69137 Lyon Cedex 04
France

P.A. DYER
Central Manchester Healthcare NHS
Trust
Tissue Typing Laboratory
St Mary's Hospital
Hathersage Road
Manchester M13 0JH
UK

R.W. EVANS
Mayo Clinic
Department of Health Sciences Research
Section of Health Services Evaluation
Rochester, MN 55905
USA

J.A. HANSEN
Fred Hutchinson Cancer Research Center
1124 Columbia Street
Seattle, WA 98104-2092
USA

C. HOLMBERG
Children's Hospital
University of Helsinki
Stenbackinkatu 11
F-00290 Helsinki
Finland

D. HOUSSIN
Etablissement Francais des Greffes
28, rue de Charenton
F-75012 Paris
France

S.H. HUNT
Clinical Professor of Medicine
Stanford University School of Medicine
Falk Cardiovascular Research Center
Department of Cardiothoracic Surgery
Stanford, CA 94305-5247
USA

R.H. KERMAN
The University of Texas
Histocompatibility and Immune Evaluation Laboratories
6431 Fannin – Suite 6 240
Houston, TX 77030
USA

J.W. KUPIEC-WEGLINSKI
Surgical Research Laboratories
Harvard Medical School
260 Longwood Avenue
Boston, MA 02115
USA

D. LOISANCE
Hopital Henry Mondor
51, Avenue du Marechal de Lattre de Tassigny
F-94010 Creteil Cedex
France

B. MIRANDA
Organization Nacional de Transplantes
Sinesio Delgado, 8
E-28029 Madrid
Spain

P.J. MORRIS
Nuffield Department of Surgery
Oxford Transplant Centre
Churchill Hospital
Headington, Oxford OX3 7LJ
UK

G. OPELZ
Department of Transplantation Immunology
Institute of Immunology
University of Heidelberg
Im Neuenheimer Feld 305
D-69120 Heidelberg
Germany

F. OPPENHEIMER
Hospital Clinic
Renal Transplant Unit
Provincial de Barcelona
Villarroel, 170
0836 Barcelona
Spain

L.C. PAUL
St Michael's Hospital
30, Bond Street
Toronto, Ontario M6B 1W8
Canada

I. PENN
Department of Surgery
Transplantation Division
University of Cincinnati Medical Center
231 Bethesda Avenue
Cincinnati, OH 45267-0558
USA

Y. PIRSON
Universite Catholique de Louvain
Cliniques Universitaires Saint Luc
Service de Nephrologie
Avenue Hippocrate 10 UCL 10/18 52
B-1200 Bruxelles
Belgium

E. REED
College of Physicians
Surgeons of Columbia University
Department of Pathology
630 West - 168th Street
New York, NY 10032
USA

J.-P. REVILLARD
Hopital Edouard Herriot
Pavillon P
5, Place d'Arsonval
F-69437 Lyon Cedex 03
France

D. SAMUEL
Hopital Paul Brousse
Centre-Hepato-Biliaire
12, Avenue Paul Vaillant Couturier
F-94804 Villejuif
France

E.A. SANTIAGO-DELPIN
Sociedad Espanola de Auxillio Mytuo y Beneficencia de P.R.
Apartado 1227
00919-1227 Hato Rey
Puerto Rico

S. SARNACKI
Hopital des Enfants Malades
Service de Chirurgie Pédiatrique
149, rue de Sèvres
F-75743 Paris Cedex 15
France

A SECCHI
Fondazione Centro S. Raffaeme del Monte Tabor
Direzione Scientifica Ricerca Clinica
Via Olgettina 60
20132 Milano
Italy

J.-P. SOULILLOU
ITERT
CHU Hotel Dieu
30, Boulevard Jean Monnet
B.P. 1005
F-44035 Nantes Cedex 01
France

D.E.R. SUTHERLAND
University of Minnesota
Department of Surgery
Box 280
420 Delaware Street S.E.
Minneapolis, MN 55455
USA

J. VANHAECKE
Service de Cardiologie
Hopital Universitaire Gasthuisberg
Herestraat 49
B-3000 Leuven
Belgium

K.J. WOOD
The University of Oxford
Nuffield Department of Surgery
Level 6
The John Radcliffe Hospital
Oxford OX3 9DU
UK

Introduction

With a long practice of organ transplantation, retransplantation has become a major goal in patients with long-term failure of their first transplant (chronic rejection, exhaustion of the transplant, recurrence of the initial disease, etc.). In addition, retransplantation can be necessary in the initial period, due to severe acute rejection, a non-functioning organ, or surgical complication.

Immunological and non-immunological factors affecting the success of a second transplant are described in this volume, together with alternatives to retransplantation.

It is hoped that in the future retransplants will be less frequent, as a result of improved prevention of transplant failure.

J.L. Touraine et al. (eds.), Retransplantation, xvii.

PART ONE

Present results of retransplantation

1. Current results of organ retransplantation

GERHARD OPELZ & THOMAS WUJCIAK
For the Collaborative Transplant Study

Although organ transplant success rates have improved in recent years due to improved patient management and the availability of more effective immunosuppressive drugs, immunological rejection remains an important problem. Patients who reject a transplant become candidates for retransplantation. The situation is fundamentally different for kidney transplant recipients, who usually return to dialysis after rejection and can be retransplanted electively, and heart and liver recipients for whom life saving machine support is not routinely available. Therefore, kidney retransplants are performed at a much higher rate than heart or liver retransplants.

Figures 1 and 2 show the evolution from 1989 to 1995 of kidney transplant waiting lists in North America and Western Europe. Whereas the numbers of patients awaiting retransplantation increased from 1989 to 1995, the numbers of patients awaiting first transplants increased even more. It is therefore not surprising that, although there was an increase in the absolute numbers of retransplants performed, the fraction of retransplants remained stable throughout

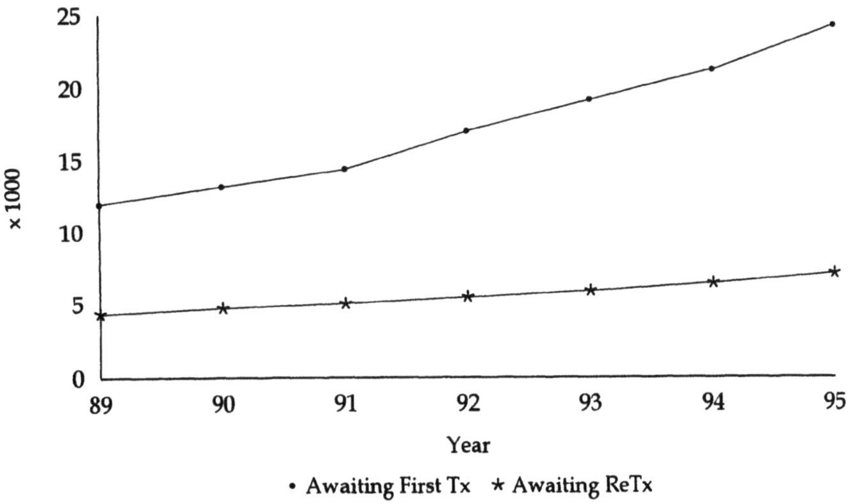

Fig. 1. Evolution of kidney transplant waiting list from 1989 to 1995 in North America. Source: UNOS.

J.L. Touraine et al. (eds.), Retransplantation, 3–14.

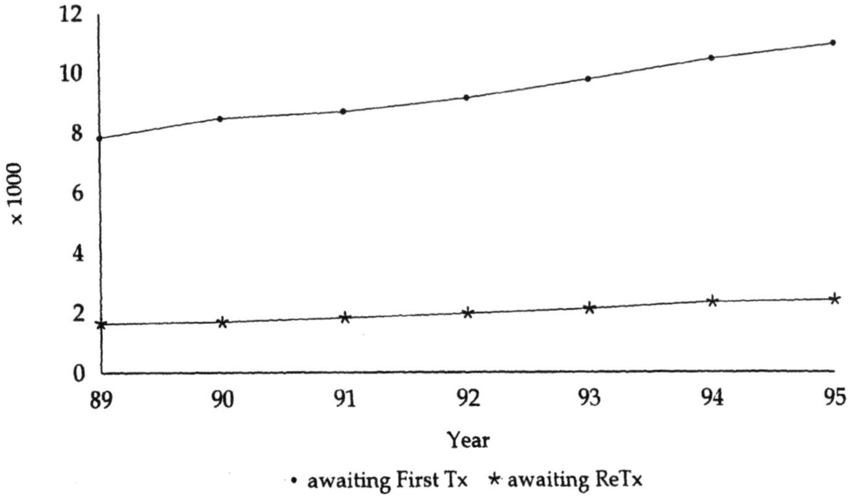

Fig. 2. Evolution of kidney transplant waiting list in Western Europe. Source: Eurotransplant Leiden. The data are representative for the Benelux countries, Australia and Germany.

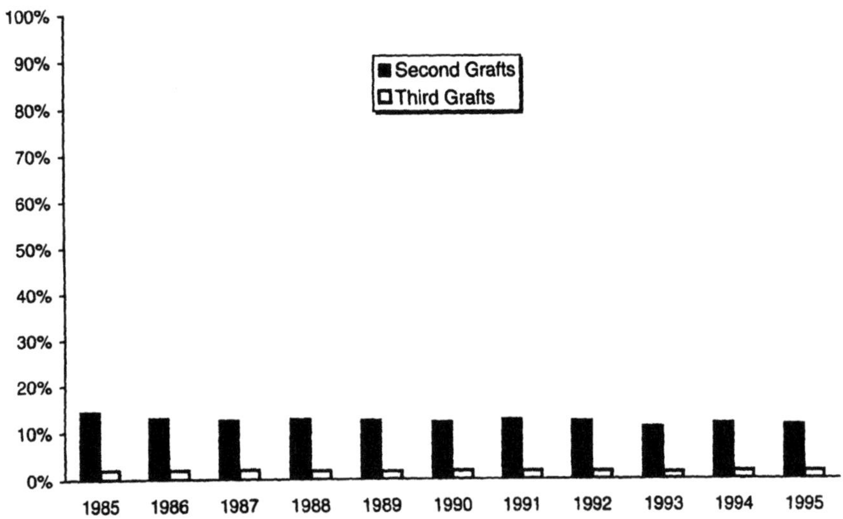

Fig. 3. Fraction of second and third cadaver kidney transplants reported to the Collaborative Transplant Study from 1985 to 1995.

the years. Figure 3 shows that approximately 15% of all cadavar kidney transplants reported to the Collaborative Transplant Study from 1985 to 1995 were retransplants. The rates at which retransplants were performed in North America and Europe were very similar (Figures 4 and 5).

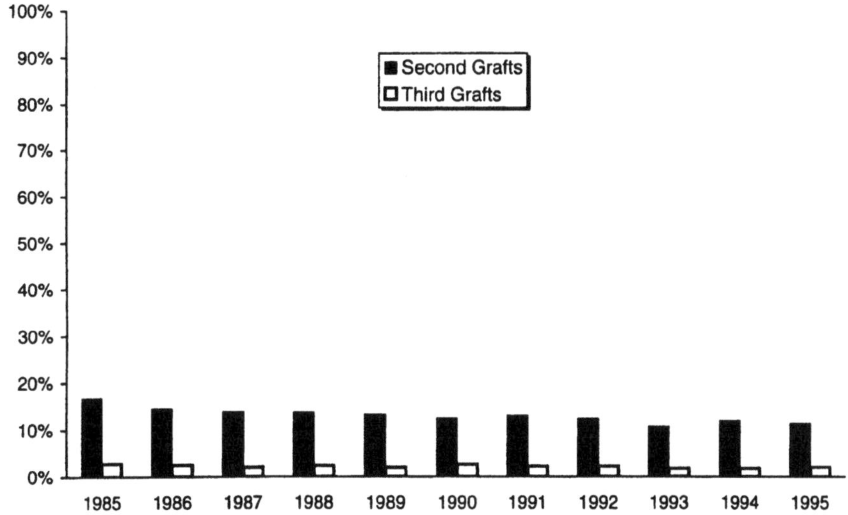

Fig. 4. Fraction of second and third cadaver kidney transplants reported to the Collaborative Transplant Study from North America.

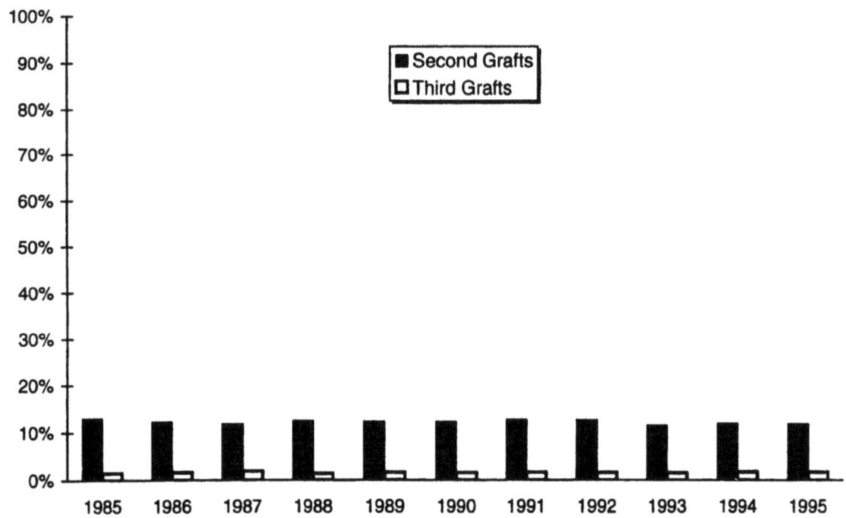

Fig. 5. Fraction of second and third cadaver kidney transplants reported to the Collaborative Transplant Study from Europe.

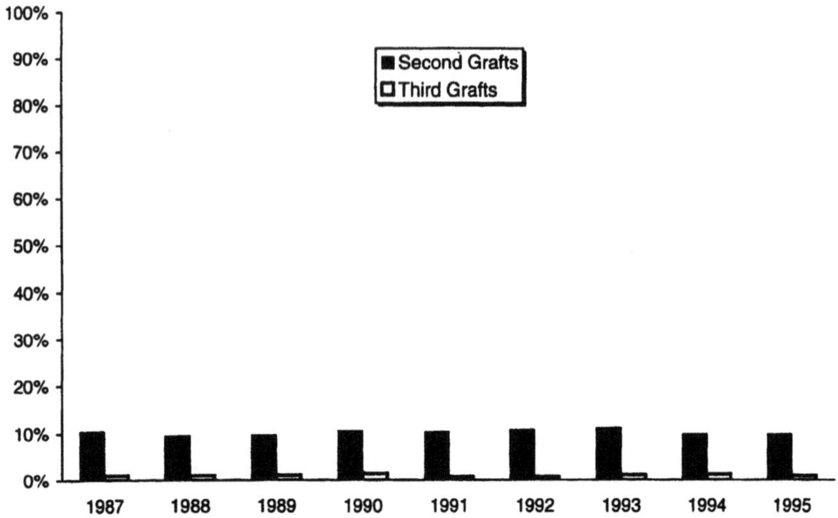

Fig. 6. Fraction of second and third liver transplants reported to the Collaborative Transplant Study from 1987 to 1995.

Liver retransplants also were performed at a fairly stable frequency which was approximately 10% of the total (Figure 6). In contrast, heart retransplants were performed much less commonly, at an average rate of approximately 3% (Figure 7).

One would expect that rejection of a previous graft would sensitize a patient and thereby lead to a reduced likelihood of success for a retransplant. That such sensitization in all likelihood is directed against HLA antigens is suggested by the results shown in Figure 8. Transplants from HLA-identical sibling donors do not show a decreased success rate when first, second or third grafts are compared. A modest decline in the success rate is noticeable in HLA 1-haplotype matched related donor grafts. The most pronounced progressive decrease in the success rates of first, second and third grafts is evident in cadaver kidney grafts.

It was noted many years ago that second kidney grafts did very poorly if the first graft was rejected within a few weeks, whereas second grafts did quite well if the first graft had lasted for a year or longer [1]. The large data material of the Collaborative Transplant Study allows a more detailed analysis. Interestingly, second graft survival becomes progressively better the longer the first graft functioned (Figure 9). A notable exception are grafts that functioned for <1 month, probably because this group includes technical failures which did not result in immunological sensitization.

Figure 10 shows that a similar relationship exists between the success rate of third kidney transplants and the duration of function of second grafts.

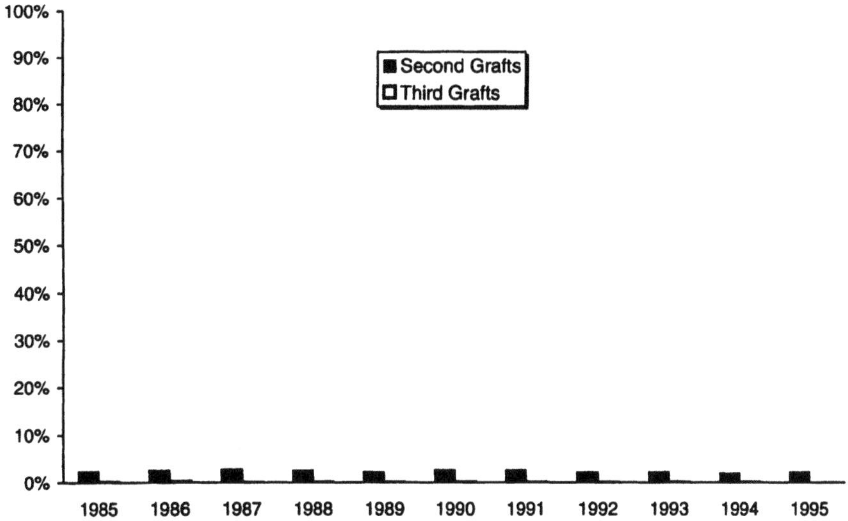

Fig. 7. Fraction of second and third heart transplants reported to the Collaborative Transplant Study from 1985 to 1995.

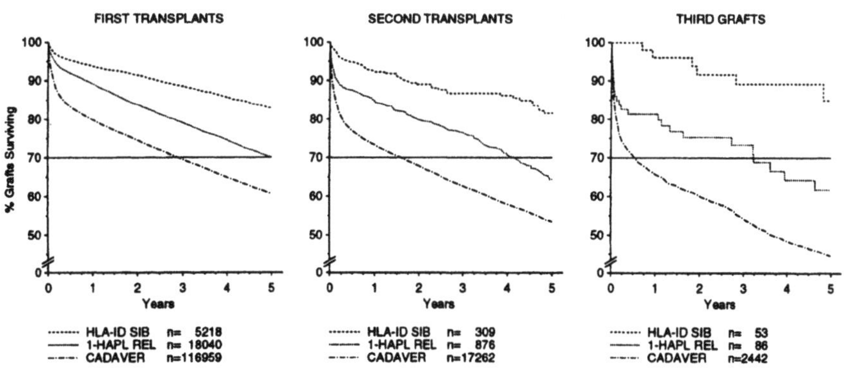

Fig. 8. 5-year graft survival rates for first, second and third kidney grafts from HLA-identical sibling donors, HLA 1-haplotype matched related donors, and cadaver donors. The horizontal line at 70% was drawn for reference. Numbers of patients analyzed are indicated.

Figure 11 shows the influence of HLA matching on cadaver kidney retransplants with a previous graft duration of <1 year or >1 year. While the effect of matching is stronger in grafts with a shorter duration of previous graft function, the matching effect is highly significant in both patient subgroups. In other words, prolonged previous graft function does not eliminate the influence of HLA matching. This is enforced impressively in an analysis of retransplants with a previous graft function of >3 years. Even in this patient subset, the

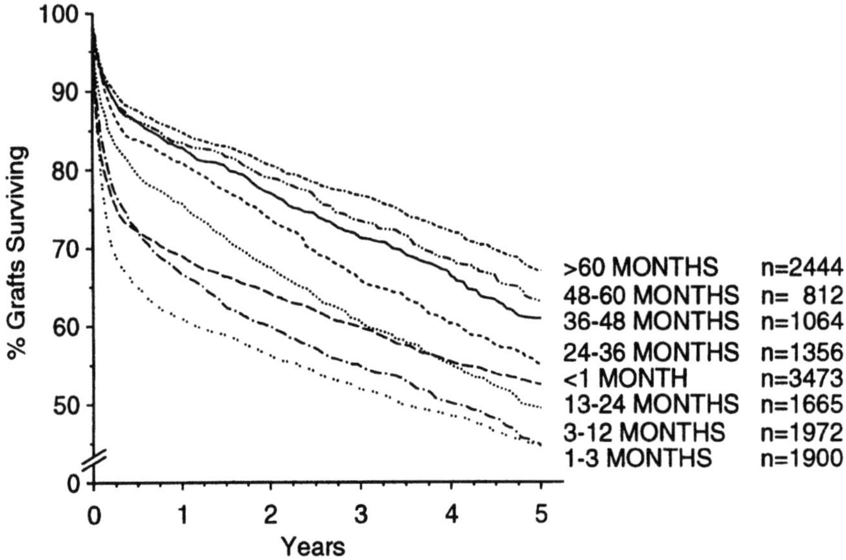

Fig. 9. Graft survival rates of second cadaver kidney transplants according to the duration of first graft function. The number of months that the first graft functioned and the number of patients studied is indicated for each group. Regression: $p < 0.0001$.

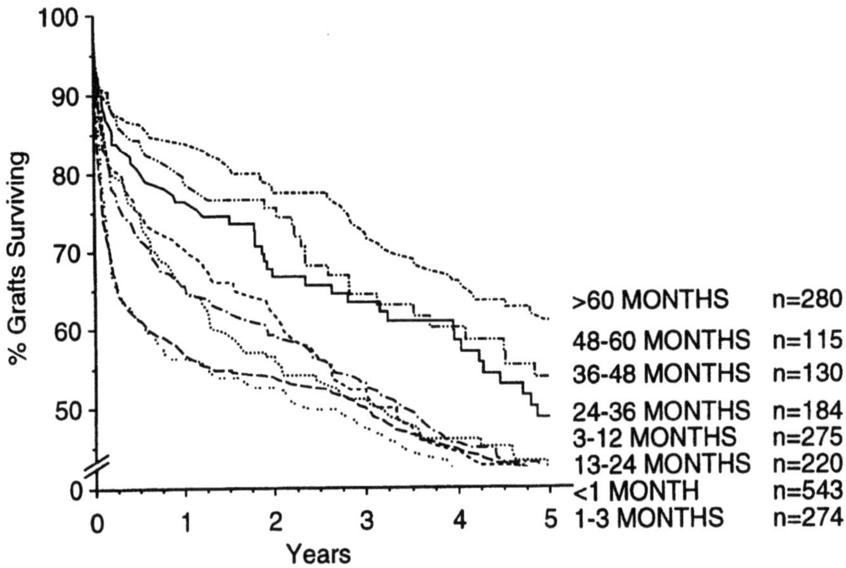

Fig. 10. Success rate of third cadaver kidney transplants in relation to the duration of function of second grafts.

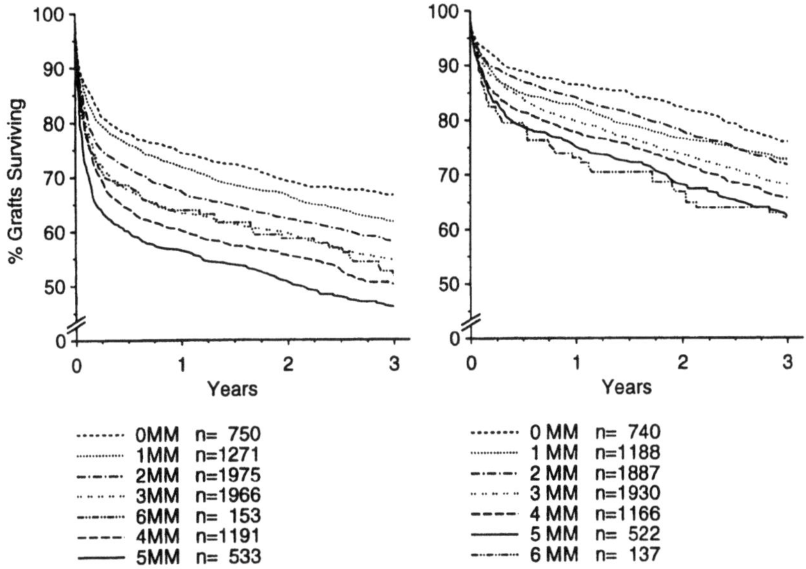

Fig. 11. Influence of HLA-matching on outcome of cadaver retransplants. The transplants were separated according to the duration of previous graft function: <1 year (left half) or >1 year (right half). The numbers of HLA−A+B+DR mismatches and numbers of patients studied are indicated. Regression $p < 0.001$ for both subsets.

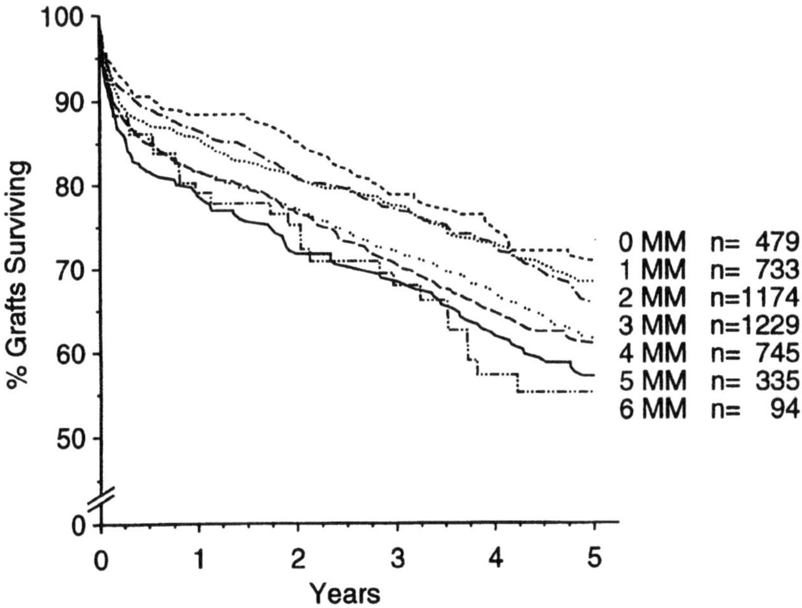

Fig. 12. Effect of HLA matching on outcome of cadaver retransplants with a previous graft duration of >3 years. The effect of matching was highly significant (regression $p < 0.001$).

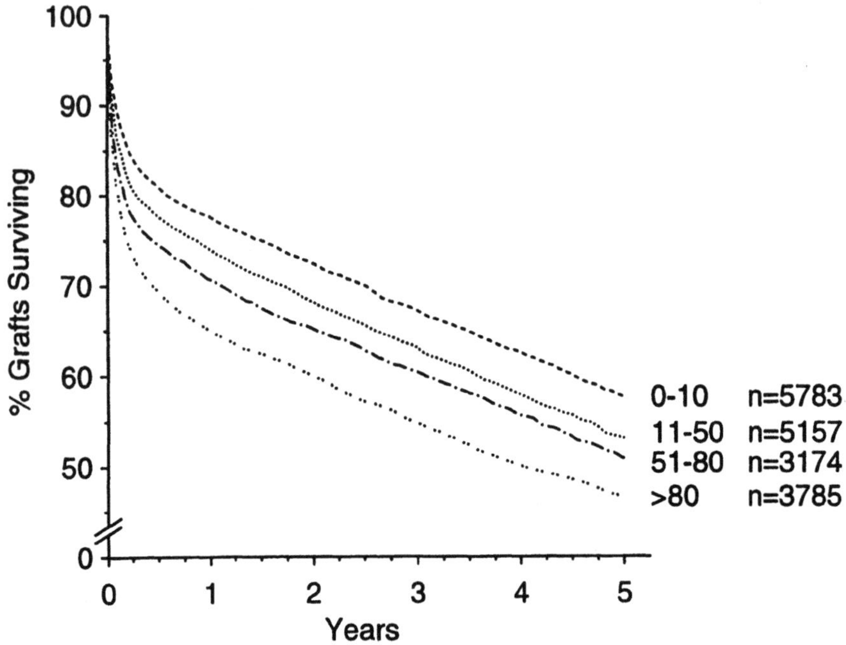

Fig. 13. Influence of preformed lymphocytotoxic antibodies on outcome of cadaver retransplants. Percentage panel reactivity in percent and numbers of patients studied are indicated. Regression $p < 0.0001$.

influence of HLA matching on graft survival is highly statistically significant (Figure 12).

Figure 13 depicts the influence of preformed lymphocytotoxic antibodies on the survival rate of cadaver kidney retransplants. In spite of the fact that all pretransplant crossmatches were reported as negative (no antibody reactivity against donor cells), there was a highly significant association of graft survival with the percentage of panel reactivity. Importantly, the effect of HLA matching is pronounced in retransplants with highly reactive preformed antibodies. Whereas matching is strongly influential also in first graft recipients with high antibody reactivity, the effect is particularly impressive in retransplants (Figure 14).

Figure 15 shows that a positive B-cell crossmatch has an impact on graft survival that is nearly twice as strong in retransplants as compared to first transplants.

Figure 16 depicts the results of first and repeat heart transplants. Whereas first kidney and heart transplants have similar survival rates, the success rate of heart retransplants is strikingly lower than that of kidney regrafts. However, as shown in Figure 17, the association of retransplant success rate with the duration of previous graft function, which was shown above for kidney

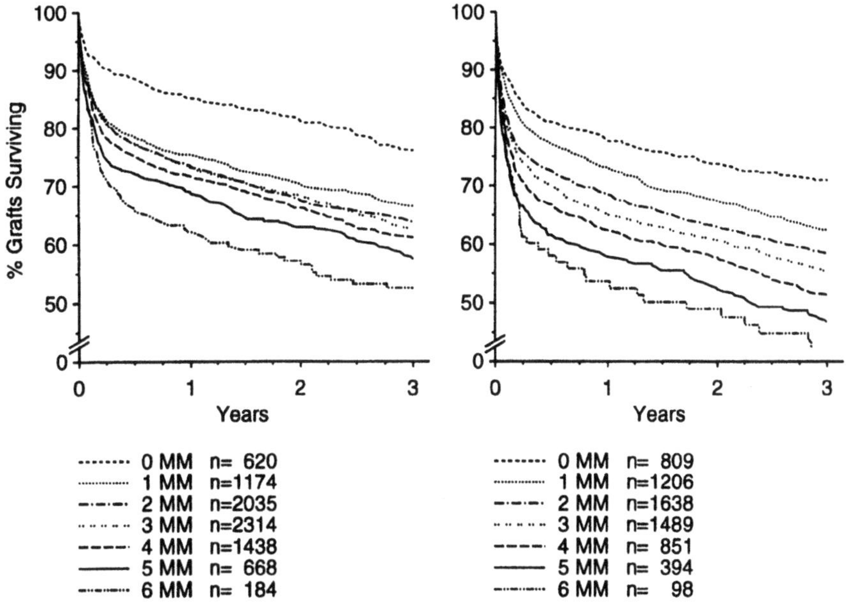

Fig. 14. Effect of matching for HLA−A+B+DR in patients with >50% antibody reactivity. Matching had a highly significant influence both in first transplants (left half) and retransplants (right half): Regression $p < 0.0001$.

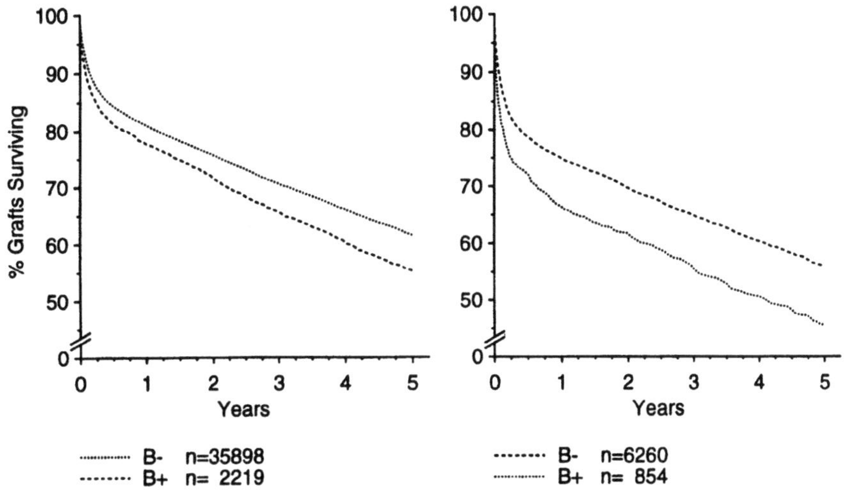

Fig. 15. Effect of positive B-cell crossmatch on outcome of first cadaver kidney transplants (left half) and cadaver retransplants (right half). Log rank $p < 0.001$.

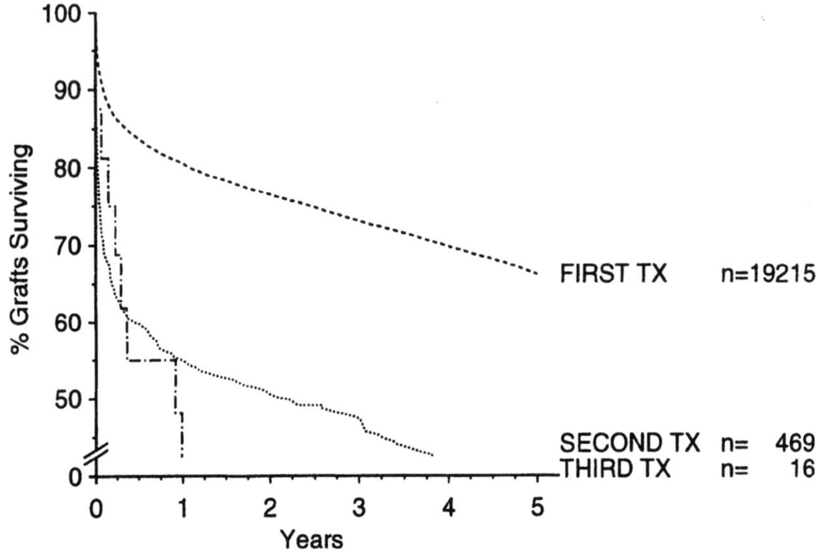

Fig. 16. Success rates of first, second and third orthotopic heart transplants. Numbers of patients analyzed are indicated.

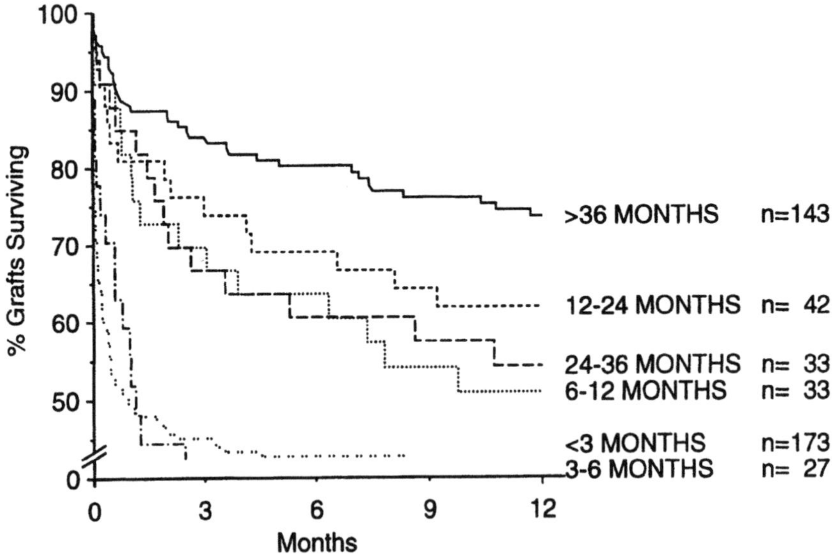

Fig. 17. Outcome of second heart transplants in relation to the duration of first graft function. Note the excellent survival of second grafts in patients whose first grafts functioned for >36 months.

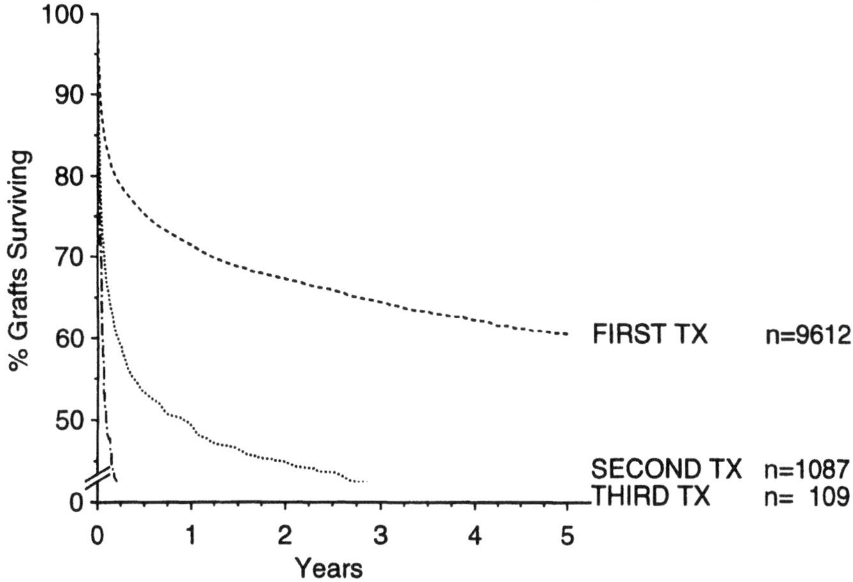

Fig. 18. Success rates of first, second and third liver transplants performed from 1988 to 1996.

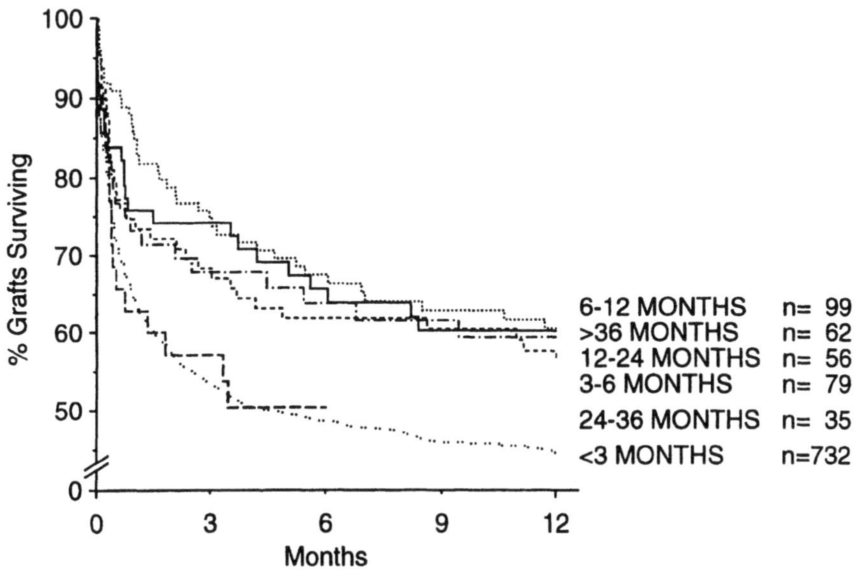

Fig. 19. Outcome of second liver transplants in relation to the duration of previous graft function. The vast majority of liver retransplants were performed after a short first graft duration of <3 months.

transplants, also applies to heart transplants. Patients who received a second heart transplant after a first graft function of more than three years had an excellent outcome.

The results of liver retransplantation are inferior to those of first grafts (Figure 18). The relationship between duration of first graft function with the outcome of second grafts is not as clear as that shown for kidneys and hearts. Notably, the vast majority of second liver grafts were performed after a first graft duration of <3 months and this group showed a particularly poor success rate (Figure 19).

Acknowledgment

The generous contributions of kidney-, heart- and liver transplant programs participating in the Collaborative Transplant Study are gratefully acknowledged.

Reference

1. Opelz G, Mickey MR, Terasaki PI. Prolonged survival of second human kidney transplants. Science 1972; 178: 617–619.

2. Five-year follow-up of organ retransplantation

M. A. BELGER

Objective

A review of organ retransplantation in the UK and Republic of Ireland over the past 10 years, and identifying the factors which influence the outcome of second and subsequent transplants.

Data sources

Data held on the National Transplant Database, for transplant units in the UK and Republic of Ireland during the ten years 1987–1996. Over which time there have been 2732 kidney and 624 liver retransplants, and 142 cardiothoracic retransplants reported.

Study selection

Trends in solid organ retransplantation over the 10 years (1987–1996) have been undertaken for all transplant types. Due to the relatively small numbers of liver and cardiothoracic retransplants, multi-factorial analysis has been confined to kidneys. A multi-factorial analysis of factors influencing five year transplant survival for kidney retransplants, has been undertaken on 1265 recipients from 22 centres with 97.5% follow-up at five years.

Results

The multi-factorial analysis has highlighted year of transplant ($p < 0.01$), donor age ($p = 0.01$), recipient age ($p < 0.01$) and number of A, B and DR HLA mismatches ($p < 0.01$) as having an influence on the survival of retransplants in kidney recipients, comparisons with the factors which influence the outcome of first grafts are similar. During the past 10 years, 34% of kidney retransplants were for beneficially matched recipients (000, 100 or 010 A, B, DR mismatches) compared with 22% of first transplants. In addition, the mean age of recipients was lower for retransplants in kidney recipients, 37.5 (retransplants) compared to 42.9 first transplants. Both of these factors have an advantageous effect on transplant outcome, and could in part explain the similarities in five year survival estimates for first and second transplants.

J.L. Touraine et al. (eds.), Retransplantation, 15–16.

Conclusions

In the UK and Republic of Ireland almost 3500 solid organ retransplants have been performed over the past 10 years. The majority of these have been in kidney recipients. The outcome of these transplants are influenced by similar factors to those found in first transplants. Kidney retransplant recipients are younger and better HLA matched than those receiving a first transplant, which may explain the small differences in five year survival estimates between the two groups of recipients.

3. Retransplantation of marrow and hematopoietic stem cells from normal donors

JOHN A. HANSEN, JERALD P. RADICH, EFFIE PETERSDORF,
PAUL J. MARTIN & CLAUDIO ANASETTI

Introduction

Transplantation of marrow or hematopoietic stem cells (HSC) from a normal donor requires high-dose marrow ablative conditioning in order to achieve full and sustained engraftment [1]. Graft failure is an uncommon problem following transplantation of marrow from an HLA identical sibling, but occurs more frequently in recipients of marrow from an HLA incompatible donor [2]. Graft failure can have catastrophic consequences, and prolonged pancytopenia may place the patient at high risk of infection or hemorrhage. Although severe graft failure is often fatal, autologous recovery of hematopoiesis can occur in some patients. The absence of donor cells and presence of host lymphoid cells suggests rejection as the cause of graft failure. Severe graft failure refractory to treatment with hematopoietic growth factors is a primary indication for retransplantation. Retransplantation may also be necessitated by recurrence of hematological malignancy. Additional immune suppression is usually necessary before retransplantation, and patients are usually very sensitive to the toxicity of additional conditioning therapy, especially if the time interval after initial transplantation is short. The feasibility of retransplantation and the optimal method depend on the primary disease and the condition of the patient.

Causes of graft failure

Failure to achieve sustained engraftment can occur because of the transplantation of an insufficient number of HSC or immune mediated graft rejection. The number of stem cells present in aspirated marrow, umbilical cord blood or growth factor mobilized peripheral blood can vary greatly. The rate of engraftment correlates with the dose of HSC transplanted [3, 4], and patients receiving a low marrow cell dose or a low number of umbilical cord blood cells are more likely to experience graft failure [5–7]. T cells of host origin can be detected in patients with graft failure, and lymphocytes harvested from graft failure patients can be shown to be cytolytic to donor cells [8]. Efforts to increase the marrow cell dose by conventional aspiration methods are limited by anesthesia time and other safety considerations. Recently, however a new

J.L. Touraine et al. (eds.), Retransplantation, 17–23.

technology has been developed for mobilizing and then collecting relatively large numbers of HSC from peripheral blood (PBSC) by administration of recombinant hematopoietic growth factor, usually for five days followed by apheresis [4].

The relationship between engraftment and cell dose is complex. Multiple factors, including the patient's primary disease, history alloimmunization by pregnancy or blood transfusion, and the immunosuppressive effect of prior radiation and chemotherapy, may modulate the patient's immune response capacity and thereby alter the potential for graft rejection. Host resistance to engraftment can be overcome by increasing the intensity of the pretransplant conditioning regimen [9]. Alkylating agents such as busulfan (BU), cyclophosphamide (CY) and thiotepa (TP) given together or in combination with total body irradiation (TBI) are effective in causing potent immune suppression. However, these drugs can be very toxic to vital organs such as the liver, heart, lungs and kidneys when given at the required doses. Cyclosporine (CSP) or FK506 given in combination with methotrexate (MTX) as prophylaxis for graft-versus-host disease (GVHD) can also facilitate engraftment, presumably by suppressing residual alloreactive host cells [10]. Depletion of T cells from donor marrow prior to transplantation, is an effective alternative approach to GVHD prevention, however donor T cells play an important role in facilitating engraftment, and transplantation of T cell-depleted marrow is associated with an increased risk of graft failure [11].

The risk of graft failure is very high in patients presensitized to the donor with graft failure occurring in 70% of patients who have a positive anti-donor serum crossmatch [10]. In the absence of a donor-specific positive crossmatch, the presence of anti-HLA antibodies to random donors does not appear to increase the risk of graft failure. Lacking effective means for overcoming donor-specific presensitization, we regard a positive crossmatch a contraindication to transplantation.

Management of graft failure

Patients with graft failure can be relatively stable or critically ill depending on the degree of residual hematopoietic function. Severe neutropenia is usually the most serious problem, but thrombocytopenia in an alloimmunized platelet transfusion-refractory patient can also be life threatening. The standard evaluation of graft failure includes marrow aspiration and biopsy, and an analysis of chimerism in both marrow and peripheral blood. In patients transplanted for a hematological malignancy, cytogenetic studies may be helpful in detecting relapse if there is a known clonal marker for the malignant cells. Informative genomic polymorphisms can be identified by DNA amplification using primers that flank variable number tandem repeats (VNTR) [12]. If the donor and recipient are mismatched for gender, X and Y chromosomes in marrow and peripheral blood cells can be identified by fluorescent *in situ* hybridization

[13]. Cells can be separated into T cell, B cell and myeloid subsets before analysis to determine the extent of donor chimerism in different lineages.

Approaches to second transplants for patients with graft failure

If possible, retransplantation for graft failure should utilize a different donor than the initial transplant for at least two reasons. First, the patient may have primed T cells directed to unique major or minor histocompatibility antigens expressed by the initial donor, and it may be possible to select a second donor who does not share these specific alloantigenic differences with the first donor. Second, second marrow donation from the same donor usually yields a cell dose lower than that obtained in the original marrow harvest [14]. The problem of a lower cell yield at second harvest may be avoided by the use of growth factor mobilized PBSC.

Retransplantation following graft rejection requires additional immune suppression therapy to neutralize residual donor-reactive immunity especially in the presence of persistent host-derived T cells. Risk of graft failure increases in patients transplanted from an HLA incompatible related donor [2], and graft failure also occurs more frequently following transplants from unrelated donors, despite phenotypic matching for HLA-A, B and DR [6, 10]. An analysis of transplants in 269 patients with a hematological maligancy who received a marrow graft from an HLA haploidentical donor variably incompatible for the HLA-A, B and DR antigens of the nonshared haplotype identified 33 cases (12%) of severe graft failure [10]. Seventeen of the graft failure patients died with pancytopenia 15 to 64 (median 27) days without receiving a second marrow infusion, and a second marrow transplant from the same donor was attempted in 15 patients. Six patients received an infusion of donor marrow without additional immune suppression therapy 30 to 73 days after the first transplant, and all 6 died within 5 to 35 (median 15) days without evidence of engraftment. Nine patients received an infusion of donor marrow following conditioning with CY (50 mg/kg/day over 4 days) with or without antithymocyte globulin (ATG) 31 to 81 (median 35) days after the first transplant. Five patients survived at least 14 days, 3 with evidence of transient engraftment (ANC > 500/μl), but all 5 died of either refractory graft failure or infection. Only one of the original group of 33 graft failure patients survives. This patient received an infusion of autologous marrow cells that had been cryopreserved prior to the initial transplant.

Graft failure patients tolerate cytotoxic agents such as cyclophosphamide or irradiation very poorly. To minimize the hazards of retransplantation, we have developed a relatively non-toxic and non-myeloablative conditioning regimen for immune suppression utilizing high dose glucocorticoids and an anti-CD3 monoclonal antibody. We selected the non-mitogenic anti-CD3 murine IgG2b antibody BC3 based on a prior clinical trial in which BC3 was used as therapy for patients with cyclosporine and steroid-resistant GVHD. In this trial, BC3 was shown to be an active and relatively well tolerated agent [15]. Fifteen graft rejection patients with severe marrow aplasia, an absolute neutrophil count (ANC) < 100/μl, and no detectable donor cells have been given BC3 and high dose corticosteroids followed by HSC from the original donor as previously described [16]. The graft consisted of donor marrow cells in 9 cases and G-CSF mobilized PBSC in 6 cases. Ten of 15 patients survive, 9 with sustained donor engraftment. One patient died on day 2 after second transplant, one died on day 14 with evidence of early engraftment, one had no engraftment and 2 had transient engraftment. One of the latter survives with autologous HSC recovery. The 9 remaining patients achieved an ANC 500/μl between post-transplant day 7 and 15 (median, 9.5 days). Sustained donor cell engraftment was demonstrated for up to one year from second transplant by chimerism testing. Six of the 9 engrafted patients are surviving. Two have died from GVHD and one from a fungal pneumonia without GVHD 50 days after second transplant. These results represent an improvement from our historical experience. The approach is especially encouraging because it suggests that significant immune suppression is possible without the risks associated with more toxic and myeloablative regimens.

Recurrence of hematological malignancy following transplantation from a normal donor

Relapse of a hematological malignancy following transplantation almost always occurs in host cells. Leukemic cells can suppress normal hematopoiesis and relapse may present initially as graft failure. The normal T cells present in a relapse patient, however are usually of donor origin. Options for managing post-transplant relapse have been limited, especially if relapse occurs within one year after transplantation. The toxicity threshold to conventional anti-tumor therapy is low when administered early after transplantation, and early relapse implies a very resistant malignancy. A longer interval time between the initial transplant and relapse is associated with a better prognosis for the second transplant.

Retransplantation of allogeneic marrow for patients with recurrent malignancy

We have previously reported the outcome of second marrow transplants for 77 consecutive patients aged 2–51 years (median 25 years) who relapsed subsequent to allogeneic marrow grafting following high-dose chemotherapy and TBI [17]. These patients received their first transplant for treatment of acute lymphoblastic leukemia (ALL, $n = 15$), acute myelogenous leukemia (AML, $n = 32$), chronic myeloid leukemia (CML, $n = 28$) and lymphoma ($n = 2$). The same donor was used for the first and second transplant. Since TBI was included in the conditioning regimen administered prior to the first transplant, a high-dose chemotherapy regimen without TBI was selected for the second transplant. The regimen for the second transplant consisted of BU and CY, or CY, carmustine (BCNU) and eptoside (VP-16). No GVHD prophylaxis was given for 8 patients, T cell depletion was performed for 36 patients and combinations of CSP, MTX and ATG were used for 33 patients. Engraftment occurred in each of 74 evaluable patients. Severe veno-oclusive disease (VOD) was the most common cause of grade III–IV regimen-related toxicity, occurring in 20 patients. The probability of death by day 100 from non-leukemia causes was 36%. We have recently updated the experience of this cohort. The cumulative incidence of relapse was 47%, and the probability of disease-free survival (DFS) was 9% at 9 years. The DFS rates for ALL, AML and CML were 6%, 6% and 14% respectively. Multivariable analysis showed that risk of relapse was inversely associated with the occurrence of acute GVHD ($RR = 0.2$, $p < 0.001$). The hazard of treatment failure was reduced in the presence of acute GVHD ($RR = 0.5$, $p = 0.008$), but increased in patients 10 years of age ($RR = 2.5$, $p = 0.034$) and in the presence of severe VOD ($RR = 10.6$, $p < 0.001$). The association of GVHD with a lower probability of relapse demonstrates a graft-versus-leukemia (GVL) effect that can occur following transplantation of normal HSC, presumably mediated by donor T cells [18, 19]. The overall poor DFS results and the high rate of relapse are explained primarily by the presence of refractory disease no longer responsive to chemotherapy. The high incidence of VOD and non-relapse mortality indicates that the toxicity of the conditioning regimen was excessive for this group of second transplant patients. Unfortunately, these patients are very sensitive to the toxicities of currently available anti-cancer agents.

We have also performed second marrow transplants for 15 patients aged 1–58 years (median 4 years) who relapsed subsequent to allogeneic marrow ($n = 14$) or autologous ($n = 1$) transplant following a high-dose BU/CY preparative regimen. These patients received their first transplant for treatment of ALL ($n = 1$), AML ($n = 11$), CML ($n = 2$) and multiple myeloma ($n = 1$). The same donor was used for the first and second transplant in nine cases. In six cases a mismatched sib or parent was used as the donor for the second transplant. CY and TBI was used as the preparative regimen for the second transplant. Non-leukemic deaths occurred in 4 patients. Six patients relapsed (cumulative incidence, 40%), and 4 survive disease-free at a median of nearly 6 years ($DFS = 27\%$). Given the small sample size it is impossible to discern whether this relative favorable outcome compared to the 77 patients noted above is due to the sequence of the TBI and chemo-only preparative regimens, the difference in the age distributions of the two cohorts, or other factors.

Alternate approaches to treating posttransplant relapse

A repeat high dose conditioning regimen may not always be necessary for patients who relapse following a HCS allograft. If the patients is receiving immune suppression therapy for GVHD prophylaxis and relapse occurs, tumor cells can disappear following withdrawal of immune suppression [20]. Unfortunately, withdrawal of immune suppression may also result in uncontrolled GVHD. In patients without active GVHD recurrent malignancy may respond to an infusion of T lymphocytes from the marrow donor. With this approach, remission can be induced in more than 50% of patients with CML, but GVHD and transient marrow aplasia are significant complications [21]. Attempts are underway to improve the safety of donor lymphocyte infusions by using appropriate numbers of selected T cells capable of inducing GVL but not GVHD [22] or by infusing cultured donor T cells that react preferentially with host leukemic cells.

Summary

Graft failure following high-dose myeloablative therapy and HSC grafting occurs infrequently when an adequate number of HLA-identical stem cells are given. Graft failure is a significant problem for patients with certain diseases especially when the only available donor is HLA-incompatible. Transplants should be avoided when the donor lymphocyte crossmatch is positive. Retransplantation is feasible, and results appear to be better when relatively noncytotoxic immune suppression is used rather than conventional conditioning regimens with high-dose alkylating agents or irradiation. Recurrence of malignancy is a more frequent indication for retransplantation, but results have been discouraging because of the toxicity associated with the conditioning regimen and the resistance of the malignancy to chemotherapy. Alternative strategies based on immune modulation and enhancing the anti-tumor effect of donor T cells are promising.

Acknowledgments

This work was supported by grants from the National Institutes of Health, AI33484, CA15704 and CA18029. We thank Alison Sell for assistance in preparing the manuscript.

References

1. Thomas E, Storb R, Clift RA et al. Bone marrow transplantation. N. Engl. J. Med. 1975; 292: 832–843.
2. Anasetti C, Amos D, Beatty PG et al. Effect of HLA compatibility on engraftment of bone marrow transplants in patients with leukemia or lymphoma. N. Engl. J. Med. 1989; 320: 197–204.
3. Sierra J, Storer B, Hansen JA et al. Transplantation of marrow cells from unrelated donors for treatment of high-risk acute leukemia: the effect of leukemic burden, donor HLA-matching, and marrow cell dose. Blood 1995; 89: 4226–4235.
4. Bensinger WI, Clift R, Martin P et al. Allogeneic peripheral blood stem cell transplantation in patients with advanced hematologic malignancies: a retrospective comparison with marrow transplantation. Blood 1996; 88: 2794–2800.

5. Storb R, Prentice RL, Thomas ED. Marrow transplantation for treatment of aplastic anemia. An analysis of factors associated with graft rejection. N. Engl. J. Med. 1977; 296: 61–66.
6. Petersdorf EW, Longton GM, Anasetti C et al. Association of HLA-C disparity with graft failure after marrow transplantation from unrelated donors. Blood 1997; 89: 1818–1823.
7. Rubinstein P, Carrier C, Adamson, et al. New York Blood Center's program for unrelated placental/umbilical cord blood (PBC) transplantation: 243 transplant in the first 3 years. Blood 1996; 88: 557: 142a.
8. Fleischhauer K, Kernan NA, O'Reilly RJ, Dupont B, Yang SY. Bone marrow-allograft rejection by T lymphocytes recognizing a single amino acid difference in HLA-B44. N. Engl. J. Med. 1990; 323: 1818–1822.
9. Martin PJ, Hansen JA, Torok-Storb B et al. Graft failure in patients receiving T cell-depleted HLA-identical allogeneic marrow transplants. Bone Marrow Transplant. 1988; 3: 445–456.
10. Anasetti C, Hansen JA. Effect of HLA incompatibility in marrow transplantation from unrelated and HLA-mismatched related donors. Transfus. Sci. 1994; 15: 221–230.
11. Martin PJ, Hansen JA, Buckner CD et al. Effects of in vitro depletion of T cells in HLA-identical allogeneic marrow grafts. Blood 1985; 66: 664–672.
12. Scharf S. PCR amplification of VNTRs. In: Innis MA, Gelfand DH, Sninshy JJ (eds.), PCR Strategies. San Diego, Academic Press, 1995.
13. Hall JM, Lingenfelter P, Adams SL, Lasser D, Hansen JA, Bean MA. Detection of maternal cells in human umbilical cord blood using fluorescence *in situ* hybridization. Blood 1995; 86: 2892–2832.
14. Buckner CD, Clift RA, Sanders JE et al. Marrow harvesting from normal donors. Blood 1984; 64: 630–634.
15. Anasetti C, Martin PJ, Storb R et al. Treatment of acute graft-versus-host disease with a nonmitogenic anti-CD3 monoclonal antibody. Transplantation 1992; 54: 844–851.
16. Anasetti C, Martin PJ, Storb R, Hansen JA. Engraftment of allogeneic hematopoietic stem cells in patients conditioned only with anti-CD3 monoclonal antibody BC3 plus methylprednisolone. Blood 1994; 84: 980: 249a.
17. Radich JP, Sanders JE, Buckner CD et al. Second allogeneic marrow transplantation for patients with recurrent leukemia after initial transplant with total-body irradiation containing regimens. J. Clin. Oncol. 1993; 11: 304–313.
18. Weiden P, Flournoy N, Thomas ED et al. Antileukemic effect of graft-versus-host disease in human recipients of allogeneic marrow grafts. N. Engl. J. Med. 1979; 300: 1068–1073.
19. Horowtiz MM, Gale RP, Sondel PM et al. Graft-versus-leukemia reactions following bone marrow transplantation in humans. Blood 1990; 75: 555–562.
20. Higano CS, Brixey M, Bryant EM et al. Durable complete remission of acute nonlymphocytic leukemia associated with discontinuation of immunosuppression following relapse after allogeneic bone marrow transplantation. A case report of a probable graft-versus-leukemia effect. Transplantation 1990; 50: 175–177.
21. Kolb HJ, Mittermuller J, Clemm C et al. Donor leukocyte transfusions for treatment of recurrent chronic myelogenous leukemia in marrow transplant patients. Blood 1990; 76: 2462–2465.
22. Drobyski WR, Keever Ca, Roth MS et al. Salvage immunotherapy using donor leukocyte infusions as treatment for relapsed chronic myelogenous leukemia after allogeneic bone marrow transplantation: Efficacy and toxicity of a defined T-cell dose. Blood 1993; 82: 2310–2318.

4. Present status of cornea retransplantation and results

C. BURILLON

Objective

To identify the risk factors of graft failure and to evaluate the present status and the outcome of cornea retransplantation.

Methods

The results of 41 repeat penetrating keratoplasties over a 5 year period (1986–1991) are presented and are compared with previous published works on repeat corneal grafts.

Results

At the end of the study period, only 21 re-grafts were clear and 20 were opaque. Visual improvement occurred in 21 eyes, deterioration in 4, and 16 remained unchanged. Graft failure was mainly attributed to endothelial failure (in pseudophakic and aphakic bullous keratopathy and in Fuch's endothelial dystrophy) and to rejection (in herpes simplex keratitis). Vascularized recipient corneas and inflammatory conditions were predisposing factors for allograft reaction.

The most important problem is to clearly understand the pathogenesis of the graft failure and to define the preoperative management to avoid a second rejection.

Conclusion

These data are quite encouraging in terms of visual outcome and graft clarity in cases of repeat penetrating keratoplasty.

However, due to the lack of donors, specifically since 1992 in France, unfortunately the number of re-graft is decreasing.

J.L. Touraine et al. (eds.), Retransplantation, 25.

PART TWO

Risk factors in retransplantation

5. The fate of second kidney transplant after recurrence of glomerulonephritis in the first transplant

MARTINE DE MEYER, CLAIRE POUTEIL-NOBLE, JACQUES PEETERS, JEAN-PIERRE COSYNS, BRIGITTE McGREGOR, YVES VANRENTERGHEM, JEAN-LOUIS TOURAINE, JEAN-PAUL SQUIFFLET & YVES PIRSON

Introduction

Though recurrent primary glomerulonephritis (PG) currently accounts for only less than 2% of all graft failures in the adult [1–4], this rate is expected to increase with both the improvement of patient and graft survivals and the ineffectiveness of most attempts at recurrence treatment. The patient who has lost a first graft to PG recurrence expectedly wishes proper information on the risk of recurrence in a further graft. Except for focal glomerulosclerosis (FGS) [5–7], there is very scarce data on this issue in the literature. We thus decided to review our experience with the fate of a second transplant in patients who had recurrence of PG in their first transplant.

Patients and methods

We reviewed the charts of patients transplanted twice in our three institutions and in whom recurrence of PG in the first graft was documented. Patients with glomerulonephritis accompanying systemic diseases were excluded.

Recurrence of PG was defined by (1) histologically proven diagnosis of PG in native kidneys, (2) demonstration of both the same histologic picture in the first graft and appearance of proteinuria >1 g/24 h (in all varieties of PGN) with microscopic haematuria (in case of membrano-proliferative glomerulonephritis or IgA nephropathy). The only possible exception concerned FSG for which recurrence in the first graft was also admitted on the basis of recurrent nephrotic syndrome within the first 3 months with optically normal glomeruli.

We were able to collect 18 cases meeting the above-mentioned criteria: 5 with FSG, 10 with membrano-proliferative glomerulonephritis type I (MPG), 2 with membranous nephropathy (MN) and 1 with IgA nephropathy (IgAN). We recorded demographic characteristics, hepatitis B and C status, source of the grafts, type of immunosuppressive regimen and other therapeutic manoeuvres,

J.L. Touraine et al. (eds.), Retransplantation, 29–38.

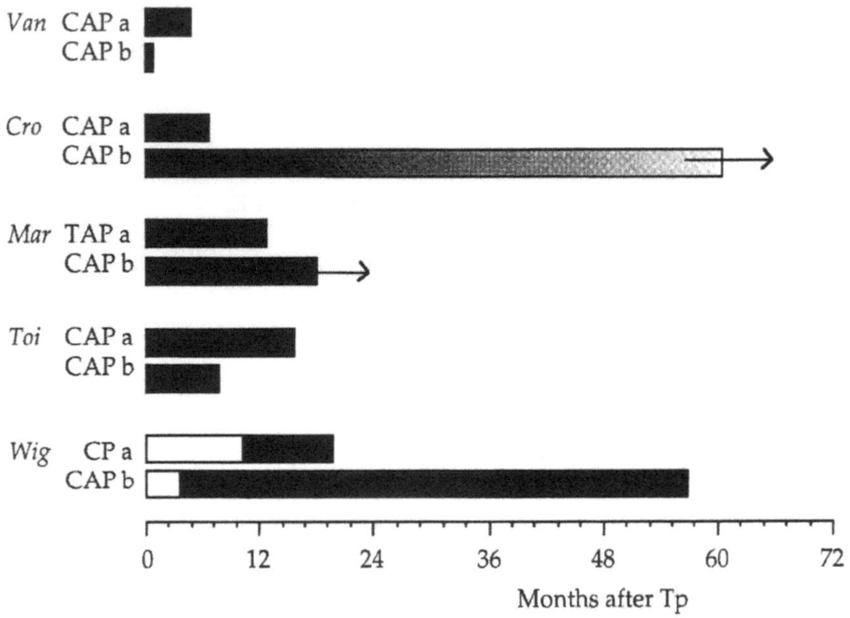

Fig. 1. Outcome of second graft in 5 patients who lost their first graft from FSG recurrence. C: cyclosporine; A: azathioprine; P: prednisone; T: tacrolimus. a: first graft; b: second graft. □ proteinuria <1 g/24 h; ■ proteinuria >1 g/24 h; closed rectangles: graft lost; rectangles with arrow: functioning graft.

course of clinical and histologic recurrence in the first graft and outcome of second graft.

Results

Focal segmental glomerulosclerosis (Figure 1)

Five men with documented FSG in their native kidneys received a first cadaver transplantation (Tp) at a mean age of 22 (range 13–43) years. HBs antigen, anti-HCV antibodies and anti-HIV antibodies were absent in all tested patients (5/5, 4/4 and 5/5, respectively). Binephrectomy was performed at the time of first Tp in one patient (Wig) and 3 months after first Tp in another patient (Cro). All were given cyclosporine ($n = 4$) or tacrolimus ($n = 1$) based double ($n = 1$) or triple ($n = 4$) therapy. In all patients, nephrotic syndrome developed (within the first month in 4 patients and at 9 months in 1 patient) and FSG was histologically demonstrated 1–10 (mean 5) months after Tp, leading to graft loss 5–20 months after Tp. Late substitution of azathioprine for cyclophosphamide in two of them had no effect on the course of recurrence.

These 5 patients received a second cadaver Tp 6–70 (mean 29) months after first Tp failure. All were given cyclosporine–azathioprine–prednisolone. Nephrotic syndrome recurred in all patients, within the first month in the 4 patients who had recurrence in the same time interval after first Tp, and at 3 months in the patient who had recurrence 9 months after first Tp. In 4 patients, nephrotic syndrome did not remit (despite substitution of cyclosporine for tacrolimus in one patient), leading to graft loss in 3 of them 1–57 months after second Tp. In the remaining patient (Cro), early treatment with plasma exchanges, intravenous immunoglobulins and oral cyclophosphamide reversed nephrotic syndrome; at follow-up (60 months after 2nd Tp) proteinuria is 0.5 g/24 h and graft function is normal.

Membrano-proliferative glomerulonephritis (Figure 2)

Ten patients (7 men, 3 women) with biopsy-proven membrano-proliferative glomerulonephritis (MPG) type I in their native kidneys received a first Tp (4 from a cadaveric donor and 6 from a living donor) at a mean age of 25 (range 11–41) years. Pretransplant binephrectomy was performed in only one patient (Mos). HBs antigen and anti-HCV antibodies were positive in 3/10 and 2/8 tested patients, respectively (2 were coinfected with HBV and HCV); anti-HIV antibodies were absent in all patients. Five patients were given cyclosporine-based double ($n = 2$) or triple ($n = 3$) therapy; the 5 remaining patients were given azathioprine-steroids. In all patients, the first manifestation of recurrence was microscopic haematuria, occurring within the first year (mean 4 months; range 1–10) in 6 patients and later (mean 60 months; range 15–156) in the 4 others. Graft was lost 4–48 (mean 29) months after Tp in the 6 patients with early recurrence and 77–165 (mean 123) months post-Tp in the 4 patients with late recurrence. Substitution of azathioprine for cyclophosphamide in two patients did not affect the course of recurrence.

Two patients received a second Tp (one from a living donor and one from a cadaver donor) at the stage of preterminal graft failure, whereas the 8 others received a second cadaver Tp 6–48 (mean 28) months after resumption of dialysis. Eight patients were given cyclosporine ($n = 7$) or tacrolimus ($n = 1$) tritherapy and the two others azathioprine-steroids. All 6 patients who had had early recurrence in their first Tp again had recurrence in the second Tp within 1–10 months after Tp, with subsequent graft loss in 4 of them (17–144 months after second Tp) and persistent nephritic syndrome in the two others (follow-up 9 and 23 months). By contrast, none of the 4 patients with late recurrence in the first graft have manifested so far signs of recurrence in the second graft (mean follow-up 78 months; range 8–191). It is however to note that in 2 of them, current follow-up has not yet reached the time at which recurrence had appeared in the first graft. No serological or histological characteristics was found to be clearly associated with repeated recurrence (Table 1).

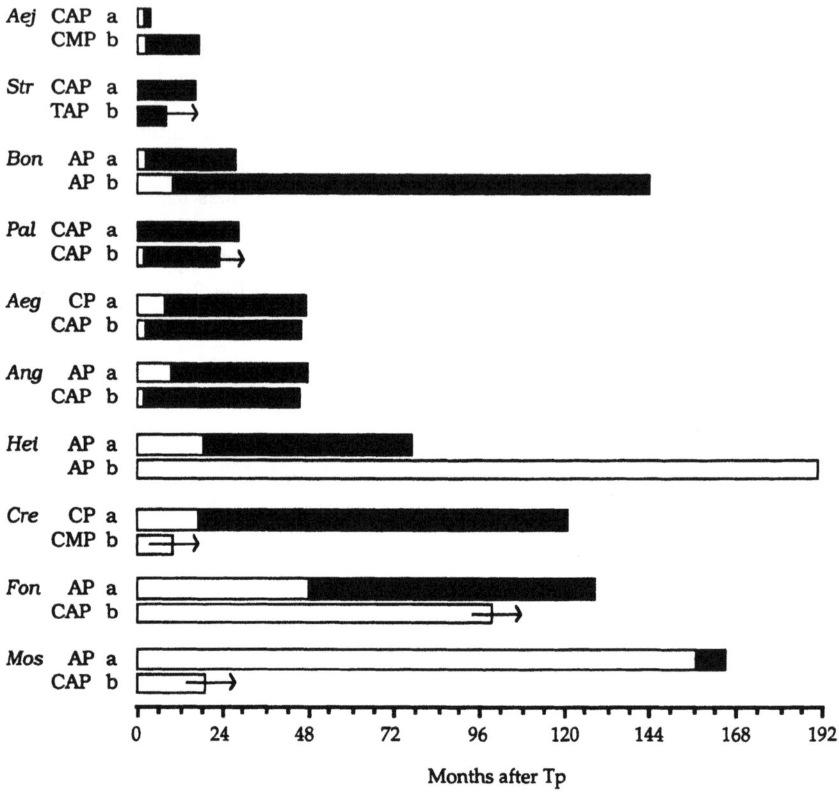

Fig. 2. Outcome of second graft in 10 patients with recurrence of MPG in the first graft. C: cyclosporine; A: azathioprine; P: prednisone; T: tacrolimus; M: mycophenolate. □ no recurrence; ■ recurrence; closed rectangles: graft lost; rectangles with arrow: functioning graft.

Table 1. Characteristics associated with recurrence of MPG in two successive renal grafts ($n = 10$)

	Recurrence in 2nd graft ($n = 6$)	No recurrence in 2nd graft ($n = 4$)
Early recurrence in 1st graft (within 12 months)	6/6	0/4
Glomerular crescents in 1st graft	5/6	1/4
Hypocomplementaemia (C3 < 50% of nl value)	2/4	1/4
HBV and/or HCV infection	1/6	2/4

Membranous nephropathy (Table 2)

Two men with documented MN in native kidneys received a first cadaver Tp at ages 42 and 58. HBs antigen was present in one of them and absent in the other; anti-HCV antibodies were absent in both of them. None had

Table 2. Recurrent membranous nephropathy in successive transplants

			First transplant					Second transplant			
Ref.	Age at first Tp Sex	Duration of MN in native kidney (months)	Source	IS therapy	Onset proteinuria	Proven recurrence (months)	Duration 1st Tp (months)	Interval end 1st Tp –2nd Tp (months)	Source	IS therapy	Outcome
Innes, 1994 [25]	51 M	?	CD	CyA-Pred	33	33	57	7	CD	Pred-Aza-CyA	Recurrence at 6 months. Renal failure
Josephson, 1994 [26]	47	62	CD	ALG-Pred-Aza-CyA	12	12	33	0	CD	OKT3-Pred-Aza-CyA	Recurrence at 12 months. Graft fct at 54 months
Lyon, 1997 (Ach)	42 M	216	CD	Aza-Pred	40	93	141	28	CD	ATG-Pred-Aza-CyA	No recurrence at 38 months. Graft fct at 38 months
Lyon, 1997 (Vil)	58 M	45	CD	ATG-Pred-Aza—CyA	3	38	45	25	CD	ATG-Pred-Aza-CyA	Recurrenct at 7 months. Graft fct at 29 months

CD: cadaver donor; IS: immunosuppressive; CyA: cyclosporine; Pred: prednisone; Aza: azathioprine; ALG: antilymphocyte globulins; ATG: antithymocyte globulins. Duration of MN in native kidneys: from diagnosis to end-stage renal failure.

binephrectomy. Immunosuppressive regimen included cyclosporine in one of them. In patient Ach, proteinuria appeared 40 months after Tp and recurrence was documented 53 months later; graft was lost at 141 months from associated recurrence and chronic rejection. In patient Vil, proteinuria appeared 3 months after Tp and recurrence was diagnosed 35 months later, leading to graft loss 45 months after Tp.

These two patients received a second cadaver Tp 28 and 25 months after first Tp failure. Both were given cyclosporine-based quadruple therapy. Patient Ach has currently a well functioning graft without proteinuria, 38 months after 2nd Tp; graft biopsy performed at 27 months did not reveal MN. Patient Vil developed proteinuria 7 months after Tp; biopsy performed at that time showed grade I MN; 29 months after Tp this graft is currently functioning with persistent proteinuria (2 g/24 h).

IgA nephropathy

A man with documented IgAN in native kidneys received a first cadaver Tp at age 23. He was given antilymphocyte globulins, prednisone and azathioprine post-operatively and cyclosporine at day 20. Sixteen months after Tp, graft biopsy (performed for a rise in serum creatinine) disclosed cellular rejection associated with recurrence of IgAN. Over the next 3 years, the patient was treated for 3 further rejection episodes. Progressive deterioration of graft function led to resumption of dialysis 49 months after Tp.

Twenty-three months after first Tp failure, this patient received a second cadaver Tp under quadruple immunosuppression. Fifty-two months after 2nd Tp, graft biopsy was performed for microscopic haematuria and proteinuria (5 g/24 h): crescentic IgAN together with mild cellular rejection was found. Currently, 59 months after 2nd Tp, graft function is impaired with persistent nephrotic syndrome.

Discussion

As FSG is the most common PG that is known to recur after Tp, one may be surprised by the small number of patients with this disease we collect in our study. This is likely to result from the strict criteria for the diagnosis of recurrent FSG we adopted: many cases of probable recurrent FSG had indeed to be excluded because of the lack of definite FSG diagnosis either in native kidney or in the graft. Together with previously published series [5–7], our data nevertheless provide a valuable assessment of the fate of a second Tp in patients with FSG who lost their first Tp from recurrence.

FSG reportedly recurs in 20–30% of first Tp, with subsequent graft loss in half of cases [1–4]. Recognized risk factors for recurrence are a rapid progression of the original disease and mesangial proliferation in the native kidney biopsy [1–3]. Contrary to previous beliefs, neither the use of living donors

[1, 8, 9] nor the persistence of native kidneys [8] makes recurrence more likely. Though cyclosporine does not prevent recurrence [1–5, 10] its early use was found to be associated with a decrease both in rate and severity of recurrence [11].

We observed recurrence in the second graft of every patient who had experienced recurrence in the first. This is in keeping with the literature, since the recurrence rate in this setting was reported to be 60–100% [5–7]. The outcome of second Tp most often reproduces that of the first one, a rapid recurrence in the first Tp nearly invariably predicting a similar course after the second, whether or not immunosuppressive regimen includes cyclosporine [6, 7].

Attempts at treatment of FSG recurrence are frequently unsuccessful. High-dose intravenous cyclosporine given early after recurrence was able to reverse nephrotic syndrome in a few children [12, 13]. Though tacrolimus was anecdotally reported to induce remission of FSG [14], this drug failed to prevent or cure recurrence in our experience. Our only patient entered remission after second Tp was treated early with a combination of plasmapheresis and cyclophosphamide, a strategy which has been proved to be successful in previous cases [15]. Immunoadsorption of plasma onto protein A has also been reported to reduce proteinuria, but most often transiently [7]. Anyway, the effect of plasma treatments demonstrated the presence of a circulating factor responsible for recurrence. Using an *in vitro* assay of glomerular permeability to albumin, Savin et al. recently showed an association between an increased permeability activity and post-Tp recurrence of FSG [16]. If both sensitivity and specificity of this test are confirmed, it could be used before embarking (re)Tp in FSG.

MPG type I reportedly recurs in 20–30% of patients [2, 3]. Risk factors for recurrence in a first Tp have not been clearly specified. A rapid progression of the disease in native kidneys may be associated with a similar course in the 1st Tp [17]. Whether persistent hypocomplementaemia predisposes to recurrence remains disputed. The diagnosis of recurrence may not be easy to establish since the main light microscopic changes (interposition of mesangial matrix and cells; reduplication of the glomerular basement membrane) are very similar to transplant glomerulopathy; glomerular crescents and early subendothelial C3 deposits without significant Ig deposits strongly suggest MPG recurrence, whereas associated obliterative vascular changes are more compatible with transplant glomerulopathy [18]. Using these criteria, we identified 10 patients with recurrent MPG type I in the first Tp and who were retransplanted.

We observed recurrence in the second Tp in 6 of 10 patients. This is the first available assessment of the rate of recurrence of MPG in a 2nd Tp following recurrence in the first one. Remarkably, all 6 patients who had experienced recurrence within 12 months following 1st Tp had again recurrence within the same time interval after second Tp, whatever the changes in immunosuppressive regimen. By contrast, recurrence did not occur so far in the second Tp of the 4 patients who had experienced late recurrence in the first Tp; as a note of caution, the short follow-up in two of them (Cre, Mos) does not exclude further development of a late recurrence.

Three cases of repeated recurrence of MPG type I in successive transplants were reviewed by Glicklich [19]. Interestingly, these three cases were characterized by a rapid and severe recurrence of the disease in the first Tp, as witnessed by the short time interval for both onset of recurrence (1–4 months after Tp) and graft loss (2–14 months after Tp).

Taken together, these observations strongly suggest that early recurrence of MPG type I in a first graft predicts a similar course in the second. We wondered whether some additional histological or serological markers were associated with repeated recurrence: though the small number of cases does not allow to draw any firm conclusion, the presence of glomerular crescents in 83% of first grafts with early recurrence versus 25% of those with late recurrence is noteworthy; neither hypocomplementaemia nor HBV/HCV infection emerge as a risk factor (Table 1).

None of the newer immunosuppressive agents (tacrolimus, mycophenolate) we used for the second Tp was able to prevent repeated recurrence. In a previously reported case of recurrent MPG type I in a first Tp, plasmapheresis and cyclophosphamide was suggested to control recurrence [20].

MN reportedly recurs in about 25% of patients [21–23]. No pretransplant clinical or serological characteristics were found to be associated with recurrence [22, 23]. As *de novo* MN develops in 1–2% of all transplants, it can be difficult to ascribe to recurrence MN lesions found in the graft of any patient with MN in native kidneys [24]. The time course of proteinuria may help distinguish the two processes: the mean time after Tp to the development of nephrotic syndrome is 10 months (range 1 week to 25 months) in recurrent MN vs 21 months (3–72 months) in *de novo* MN [21]. In this regard, a *de novo* variety remains a possibility in one of our patients (Ach) but seems reasonably excluded in the other (Vil). There is no data in the literature on the rate of repeated recurrence of MN in successive grafts. Only two isolated cases of repeated recurrence have been reported; no risk factors have been identified [25, 26]. Also in MN, the use of cyclosporin did not prevent recurrence, either in 1st or 2nd Tp (Table 2). Treatment of recurrence with increased immunosuppression seems unhelpful [25].

Many studies have documented the frequent recurrence of IgAN after Tp. Though IgA deposits are found in as many as 50% of patients, it has been thought for long that the clinical course was largely unaffected by histological recurrence [2]. This view is challenged by recent reports showing that with increasing time post-Tp recurrence of IgAN leads to progressive graft dysfunction and failure [27–29].

Surprisingly, our case is the first one demonstrating recurrence of IgAN in two successive grafts. The usual long time interval to clinical recurrence maybe explains the lack of previous reports. Interestingly, crescents were present in the second Tp but not in the first Tp nor in native kidneys. This occurred despite tritherapy including cyclosporin. Recurrent IgAN as crescentic glomerulonephritis in a first Tp has been previously reported in two patients [30, 31]; treatment with plasma exchange and cyclophosphamide was unsuccessful in one of them [30] and of possible some help in the other one [31].

Conclusions

Our study provides interesting information on the fate of a second kidney Tp in patients who experienced recurrence of FSG and MPG type I in their first Tp. The rate of repeated recurrence is 100% for FSG and at least 60% for MPG type I. The risk of repeated recurrence is the highest in patients who had an early recurrence in the first graft. The prognosis is the worst in case of FSG: it seems wise to discourage this subset of patients from retransplantation. The availability of a serological predictive test should be of great help.

Unfortunately, none of the newer immunosuppressive agents is able to prevent repeated recurrence. In patients with established FSG recurrence, treatment with plasmapheresis and cyclophosphamide may be attempted.

The actual risk of repeated recurrence of other PGs is currently unknown. Establishing a European registry could help answer this issue as well as design and test management strategies.

References

1. Cameron JS. Recurrent disease in renal allografts. Kidney Int. 1993; 44 (Suppl. 43): 91–94.
2. Ramos EL, Tisher CC. Recurrent disease in the kidney transplant. Am. J. Kidney Dis. 1994; 24: 142–154.
3. Davison AM. Renal transplantation: recurrence of original disease with particular reference to primary glomerulonephritis. Nephrol. Dial. Transplant. 1995; 10 (Suppl. 1): 81–84.
4. Michielsen M. Recurrence of the original disease. Does this influence renal graft failure? Kidney Int. 1995: 48 (Suppl. 52): 79–84.
5. Artero M., Biava C, Amend W, Tomlanovich S, Vincenti F. Recurrent focal glomerulosclerosis; natural history and response to therapy. Am. J. Med. 1992; 92: 375–383.
6. Stephanian E, Matas AJ, Mauer SM, Chavers B, Nevins T, Kashtan C, Sutherland DER, Gores P, Najarian JS. Recurrence of disease in patients retransplanted for focal segmental glomerulosclerosis. Transplantation 1992; 53: 755–757.
7. Dantal J, Soulillou JP. Récidive des hyalinoses segmentaires et focales après transplantation rénale. In: Funck-Brentano JL, Bach JF, Kreis L, Grünfeld JP (ed.). Act. Néphrol Hôp. Necker.: Flammarion Médecine-Sciences, Paris, 1995: 91–106.
8. Odorico JS, Knechtle SJ, Rayhill SC, Pirsch JD, D'Alessandro AM, Belzer FO, Sollinger HW. The influence of native nephrectomy on the incidence of recurrent disease following renal transplantation for primary glomerulonephritis. Transplantation 1996; 61: 228–234.
9. Tejani A, Stablein DH. Recurrence of focal segmental glomerulosclerosis posttransplantation: a special report of the North American Pediatric Renal Transplant Cooperative Study. J. Am. Soc. Nephrol. 1992; 2 (Suppl. 3): 258–263.
10. Banfi G, Colturi C, Montagnino G, Ponticelli C. The recurrence of focal segmental glomerulosclerosis in kidney transplant patients treated with cyclosporine. Transplantation 1990; 50: 594–596.

11. Pouteil-Noble C, Colon S, Donia-Maged A, Cochat P, Lacavalerie B, Touraine JL. Influence of cyclosporine A on the recurrence of focal segmental glomerulosclerosis after renal transplantation. XIIIth International Congress of Nephrology, Jerusalem, June 13–18, 1993, p. 31.
12. Ingulli E, Tejani A, Butt KMH, Rajpoot D, Gonzalez R, Pomrantz A, Ettenger R. High-dose cyclosporine therapy in recurrent nephrotic syndrome following renal transplantation. Transplantation 1990; 49: 219–221.
13. Ranchin B, Gagnadoux MF, Broyer M et al. Intérêt de la ciclosporine dans le traitement des récidives de néphrose après transplantation rénale. Néphrologie 1996; 17: 441–445.
14. McCauley J, Tzakis AG, Fung JJ, Todo S, Starzl TE. FK506 in steroid-resistant focal sclerosing glomerulonephritis of childhood. Lancet 1990; 335: 674.
15. Cochat P, Schell M, Ranchin B, Boueva A, Saïd MH. Management of recurrent nephrotic syndrome after kidney transplantation in children. Clin. Nephrol. 1996; 46: 17–20.
16. Savin VJ, Sharma R, Sharma M et al. Circulating factor associated with increased glomerular permeability to albumin in recurrent focal segmental glomerulosclerosis. N. Engl. J. Med. 1996; 334: 878–883.
17. McCoy R, Clapp J, Seigler HF. Membranoproliferative glomerulonephritis. Am. J. Med. 1975; 59: 288–292.
18. Habib R, Broyer M. Clinical significance of allograft glomerulopathy. Kidney Int. 1993; 44 (Suppl. 43): 95–98.
19. Glicklich D, Matas AJ, Sablay LB et al. Recurrrent membranoproliferative glomerulonephritis type 1 in successive renal transplants. Am. J. Nephrol. 1987; 7: 143–149.
20. Muczynski KA. Plasmapheresis maintained renal function in an allograft with recurrent membranoproliferative glomerulonephritis type I. Am. J. Nephrol. 1995; 15: 446–449.
21. Davison AM, Johnston PA. Allograft membranous nephropathy. Nephrol. Dial. Transplant. 1992; (Suppl. 1): 114–118.
22. Couchoud C, Pouteil-Noble C, Colon S, Touraine JL. Recurrence of membranous nephropathy after renal transplantation. Transplantation 1995; 59: 1275–1279.
23. Cosyns JP, Pirson Y, Squifflet JP, van Ypersele de Strihou C. Post-transplant recurrence of membranous nephropathy: prevalence and outcome. XIIIth International Congress of Nephrology, Jerusalem, June 13–18, 1993, p. 142.
24. Cosyns JP, Pirson Y, Squifflet JP et al. De novo membranous nephropathy in human renal allografts: report of nine patients. Kidney Int. 1982; 59: 177–183.
25. Innes A, Woodrow G, Boyd SM, Beckingham IJ, Morgan AG. Recurrent membranous nephropathy in successive renal transplants. Nephrol. Dial. Transplant. 1994; 9: 323–325.
26. Josephson MA, Spargo B, Hollandsworth D, Thistlethwaite JR. The recurrence of recurrent membranous glomerulopathy in a renal transplant recipient: case report and literature review. Am. J. Kidney Dis. 1994; 24: 873–878.
27. Odum J, Peh CA, Clarkson AR et al. Recurrent mesangial IgA nephritis following renal transplantation. Nephrol. Dial. Transplant. 1994; 9: 309–312.
28. Kessler M, Hiesse C, Hestin D, Mayeux D, Boubenider K, Charpentier B. Recurrence of immunoglobulin A nephropathy after renal transplantation in the cyclosporine era. Am. J. Kidney Dis. 1996; 28: 99–104.
29. Frohnert PP, Donadio JV, Velosa JA, Holley KE, Sterioff S. The fate of renal transplants in patients with IgA nephropathy. Clin. Transplantation 1997; 11: 127–133.
30. Diaz-Tejeiro R, Maduell F, Diez J et al. Loss of renal graft due to recurrent IgA nephropathy with rapidly progressive course: an unusual clinical evolution. Nephron 1990; 54: 341–343.
31. Streather CP, Scoble JE. Recurrent IgA nephropathy in a renal allograft presenting as crescentic glomerulonephritis. Nephron 1994; 66: 113–114.

6. Risk of liver retransplantation for viral hepatitis

DIDIER SAMUEL, BRUNO ROCHE, CYRILLE FERAY & HENRI BISMUTH

Introduction

The risk of viral recurrence after liver transplantation for viral related liver disease is high. Viral reinfection is characterized by a viral reactivation, high amount of virus, difficulty to control viral replication in these immunosuppressed patients, occurrence of graft disease, and sometimes graft failure. For these reasons, retransplantation for viral recurrence is controversial due to the high risk of recurrence on the second graft and to the overall poor results in a context of organ shortage.

Retransplantation for HBV recurrence

The risk of HBV reinfection is 80% in the absence of prophylactic measures [1]. In patients who receive long-term administration of high doses of anti-HBs immunoglobulins, the risk of HBV reinfection is almost nil in fulminant hepatitis B, 15% in patients with viral B-delta cirrhosis, 25–30% in patients with HBV DNA negative viral B cirrhosis, and 80–90% in those with HBV DNA positive HBV cirrhosis [2, 3]. Patients with HBV recurrence developed graft disease, which lead in some cases to acute liver failure and in the majority of cases to chronic hepatitis then liver cirrhosis. The course of the disease is obviously accelerated in comparison to immunocompetent patients, the reason being a very high amount of viral particles. This very high viral load is favored by the immunosuppressive treatment and probably mainly but not exclusively by the steroids since there is a steroid receptor on HBV. Interferon is not very efficient in this setting and there is a risk of rejection [4], ARA AMP has only a transient antiviral effect and due to high neurological toxicity, it cannot be administered for more than 6 weeks [5, 6]. Ganciclovir, which has a potent antiviral effect against HBV, is well tolerated [6]. However, it should be administered for a period of at least several months and should be given intravenously which is not convenient; in addition it is not licensed for the treatment of HBV infection. Famciclovir and Lamivudine, 2 nucleoside analogues are 2 promising antiviral drugs, they have a high antiviral potency, both

J.L. Touraine et al. (eds.), Retransplantation, 39–43.

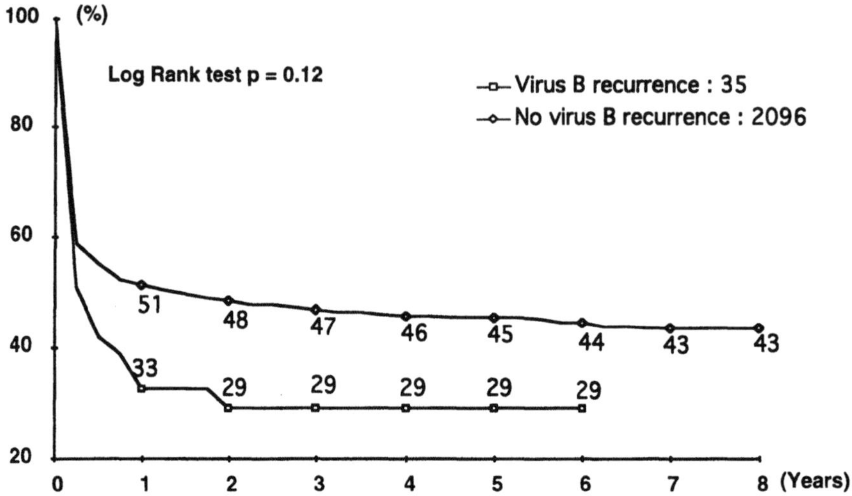

Fig. 1. Survival after retransplantation for HBV recurrence in 35 patients in comparison to 2096 patients retransplanted for other causes in Europe (from the European Liver Transplant Registry).

are well tolerated, and should be given for several months or years since there is a risk of viral rebound at discontinuation of the drug [7, 8]. Lamivudine is the more potent: its antiviral action is rapid, however, 20–25% of patients will develop an escape mutant virus due to a point mutation in the polymerase gene. In case of failure of these treatments, liver retransplantation may be considered. However, liver retransplantation for HBV recurrence is highly controversial and is usually considered as a contraindication. Indeed, results from a multicenter report and from the European Liver Transplant Registry are poor [9]. The one year survival in the ELTR report is 30% at 1 year and 29% at 5 years, which is significantly lower than retransplantation for other indications (Figure 1). Most of the patients have died from sepsis in the early postoperative period or from HBV recurrence on the second graft. In addition, this recurrence is accelerated after each retransplantation. For all these reasons, liver retransplantation for HBV recurrence is usually not performed. In our own center, 10 patients have been retransplanted for HBV recurrence; 5 before 1992 (group 1), 5 after 1992 (group 2); patients of group 1 were retransplanted at a median of 4 months after the first transplantation, all were HBsAg positive and HBV DNA positive at time of retransplantation. All had massive hepatic necrosis on liver graft histology, they received anti-HBs Ig after the second transplantation according to our classical protocol in order to maintain anti-HBs titer above 100 IU/l. All died, 3 in the postoperative period (they remained HBsAg positive), 2 from recurrence of HBV in the second graft. In group 2, the median delay for retransplantation was significantly longer: 43 months (1–110), all were HBsAg positive but 4 became HBV DNA negative at time of retransplantation after antiviral treatment. In addition, after the retransplantation they received anti-HBs Ig in order to maintain the titer of anti-HBs above 500 IU/l and prophylactic IV Ganciclovir for a minimum of 1 year. One patient developed recurrence and died 50 months after the retransplantation from liver graft failure, the 4 other patients are still HBsAg negative and are alive at a median of 27 months after the retransplantation.

Retransplantation for HCV recurrence

HCV recurrence is almost constant after liver transplantation, indeed HCV RNA is present in 90% of cases after transplantation in serum [10–12]. There are no prophylactic measures to protect the graft from HCV recurrence. Survival after liver transplantation for HCV cirrhosis is 78% at one year in our center. However, at 5 years, 60% of the patients have lesions of chronic hepatitis, and 10% have lesions of cirrhosis [11]. This accelerated course on the graft is probably facilitated by the high viral load which may be a consequence of the immunosuppressive treatment. The treatment of chronic hepatitis on the graft is difficult, because of the high amount of virus on one hand and because of the risk of rejection due to the antiviral treatment on the other hand. Interferon, the most potent antiviral agent against HCV in immunocompetent patients, has a poor antiviral effect. Indeed during Interferon treatment, most of the liver transplanted patients remain HCV RNA positive in serum, and in the few responder patients, HCV RNA became again HCV positive after the discontinuation of the treatment [13]. In addition, some groups including our group have described the occurrence of rejection phenomenon on the graft during Interferon treatment [14, 15]. We have shown the occurrence of vanishing bile duct syndrome (disappearance of interlobular bile ducts), in 5 out of 14 patients treated with Interferon, 3 of them being retransplanted [15]. Ribavirin alone is a therapeutic option [16]. The first results showed a diminution of the transaminases and GGT level in most patients, however, HCV RNA remained positive in all and liver histology did not seem to improve. Promising results of a combination treatment of Interferon and Ribavirin have been reported by the group of Lyon in a pilot study including patients with acute or non severe chronic hepatitis on the graft [17]. These results need to be confirmed in a randomized controlled study. Retransplantation for HCV infection on the graft is the consequence of a failure of these treatments. In most cases, the graft is affected with cirrhosis, and in few cases the histology showed a severe acute hepatitis. Few reports on retransplantation for HCV infection have been published. In one report from the group of Mount Sinai in New York, 14 patients have been retransplanted for HCV infection on the graft. 6 of these patients died: 4 in the postoperative period from sepsis, one at 45 days from HCV recurrence on the second graft and one from CMV infection after 3 months [18]. The 4 patients who died in the postoperative period were all at the end stage of the disease with ascites,

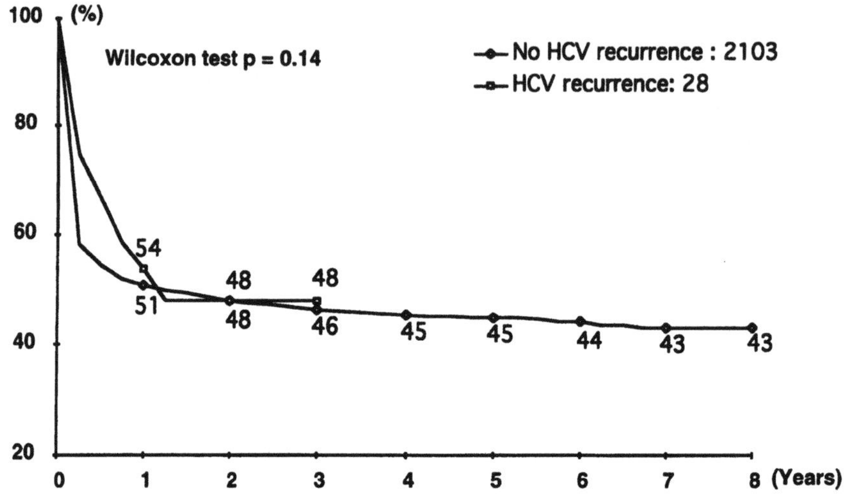

Fig. 2. Survival after retransplantation for HCV recurrence in 28 patients in comparison to 2103 patients retransplanted for other causes in Europe (from the European Liver Transplant Registry).

low albumin level and renal failure in comparison to those who survived. This important point suggests that survival after retransplantation for HCV recurrence is related to the general status of the patient and that retransplantation should not be performed too late. In addition, except in one case, there was no accelerated course of HCV infection on the 2nd graft as seen in patients retransplanted for HBV recurrence. In the European Liver Transplant Registry, there were 28 cases of retransplantation recorded on a total of 2103 retransplantations (Figure 2). Survival after retransplantation for HCV recurrence was not different from that observed after retransplantation for other indications: 51% at 1 year and 45% at 5 years.

Conclusion

Patients who are candidates for retransplantation for HBV infection on the graft are usually not considered for retransplantation because of the poor results and of the risk of accelerated course of HBV reinfection on the second graft. However, our recent experience shows that an aggressive approach including antiviral treatment pretransplantation with negativation of HBV DNA, combined administration after transplantation of very high doses of anti-HBs Ig and antiviral treatment may dramatically improve the results of retransplantation. Patients who are candidates for retransplantation for HCV recurrence on the graft have a similar outcome to other indications of retransplantation. An accelerated course of HCV reinfection on the second graft seems not to be the rule. Results are dependent on the clinical status of the patient at the time of retransplantation, this means that retransplantation should be performed before the end-stage of the graft disease.

References

1. Todo S, Demetris AJ, Van Thiel D, Teperman L, Fung J, Starzl TE. Orthotopic liver transplantation for patients with hepatitis B virus related liver disease. Hepatology 1991; 13: 619–626.
2. Samuel D, Bismuth A, Mathieu D et al. Passive immunoprophylaxis after liver transplantation in HBsAg-positive patients. Lancet 1991; 337: 813–815.
3. Samuel D, Muller R, Alexander G, Fassati L, Ducot B, Benhamou JP, Bismuth H. and the investigators of the European concerted action on viral hepatitis study. Liver transplantation in European patients with the hepatitis B surface antigen. N. Engl. J. Med. 1993; 329: 1842–1847.
4. Terrault NA, Combs Holland C, Ferrel L, Hahn JA, Lake JR, Roberts JP, Asher NL, Wright TL. Interferon alfa for recurrent hepatitis B infection after liver transplantation. Liver Transplant. Surg. 1996; 2: 132–138.
5. Marcellin P, Samuel D, Loriot MA, Areias J, Bismuth H, Benhamou JP. Anti-viral effect of adenine arabinoside monophosphate (ARA-AMP) in patients with recurrence of hepatitis B virus (HBV) infection after liver transplantation (abstract) Hepatology 1990; 12: 966.
6. Gish RG, Lau JYN, Brooks L, Fang JWS, Steady SL, Imperial JC, Garcia-Kennedy R, Esquivel CO, Keefe EB. Ganciclovir treatment of hepatitis B virus (HBV) infection in liver transplant patients. Hepatology 1996; 23: 1–7.
7. Kruger M, Tillmann HL, Trautwein C, Bode U, Oldhafer K, Maschek H, Böker KHW, Broelsch CF, Pichlmayr R, Manns MP. Famciclovir treatment of hepatitis B virus recurrence after liver transplantation: a pilot study. Liver Transplant. Surg. 1996; 2: 253–262.
8. Perillo R, Rakela J, Martin P, Levy G, Schiff E, Wright T, Dienstag J, Gish R, Villeneuve J et al. Lamivudine for Hepatitis B after liver transplantation. Hepatology 1996; 24: 182A.
9. Report of the European Transplant Registry, Hopital Paul-Brousse, Villejuif, France, 1994.
10. Wright TL, Donegan E, Hsu H, Ferrell L, Lake J, Kim M, Combs C, Fennessy S, Roberts J, Asher N. Recurrent and acquired hepatitis C viral infection in liver transplant recipients. Gastroenterology 1992; 103: 317–322.
11. Feray C, Gigou M, Samuel D et al. The course of hepatitis C virus infection after liver transplantation. Hepatology 1994; 20: 1137–1143.
12. Gane E, Portmann BC, Naoumov NV, Smith HM, Underhill JA, Donaldson PT, Maertens G, Williams R. Long-term outcome of hepatitis C virus infection after liver transplantation. N. Engl. J. Med. 1996; 334: 815–820.
13. Wright TL, Combs C, Kim M, Ferrell L, Bacchetti P, Ascher N, Roberts J, Wilber J, Sheridan P, Urdea M. Interferon-alpha therapy for hepatitis C virus infection after liver transplantation. Hepatology 1994; 20: 773–779.
14. Dousset B, Conti F, Houssin D, Calmus Y. Acute vanishing bile duct syndrome after interferon therapy for recurrent HCV infection in liver transplant recipients. N. Engl. J. Med. 1995; 330: 1160–1161 (letter).
15. Feray C, Samuel D, Gigou M, Reynes M, Bismuth H. An open trial of interferon alpha recombinant for hepatitis C after liver transplantation: antiviral effects and risk of rejection. Hepatology 1995, 22: 1084–1089.
16. Gane E, Tibbs CJ, Ramage JK, Portmann BC, Williams R. Ribavirin therapy for hepatitis C infection following liver transplantation. Transplant. Int. 1995; 8: 61–64.
17. Bizollon T, Ducerf C, Trepo C. New approaches to the treatment of hepatitis C virus infection after liver transplantation using ribavirin. J. Hepatol. 1995; 23 (Suppl. 2): 22–25.
18. Sheiner PA, Schluger LK, Emre S, Thung SN, Lau JYN, Guy SR, Schwartz ME, Miller CM. Retransplantation for recurrent hepatitis C. Liver Transplant. Surg. 1997; 2: 130–136.

7. Risks of recurrence of posttransplant lymphoproliferative disease, Hodgkin's disease or Kaposi's sarcoma after retransplantation

ISRAEL PENN

Lymphomas and lymphoproliferations comprise 24% of posttransplant malignancies and Kaposi's sarcoma (KS) 6%, if non-melanoma skin cancers and *in situ* carcinomas of the uterine cervix are excluded, as they are from most studies of patterns of malignancy [1]. A gratifying feature is that following treatment 41% of lymphomas and 36% of KS undergo complete remission. In some patients a complication of such therapy is loss of the allograft, which may necessitate retransplantation. A question that arises is whether retransplantation, with reinstitution of full dose immunosuppressive therapy will precipitate recurrence of the neoplasm. The current study examined the data accumulated by the Cincinnati Transplant Tumor Registry (CTTR) from the fall of 1968 till May 1997 to address this question.

Results

Lymphomas and lymphoproliferations

There were 1593 patients with 49 posttransplant lymphomas and lymphoproliferations (PTLD), 63 with plasmacytomas and multiple myeloma, and 49 with Hodgkin's disease (HD). Of 1133 patients with PTLD on whom detailed information was available 879 (78%) underwent treatment, 196 (17%) had no treatment and for 58 patients (5%) no treatment data are available. Of the treated patients 335 (38%) had complete remissions. Thirty recipients with PTLD who had complete remissions and three with HD who had complete remissions underwent retransplantation. These 33 treated patients underwent 35 transplants prior to development of their lymphomas and 37 retransplants after development of the PTLD/HD. Eighteen were male and 15 female. Their ages at the time of their first transplants ranged from 6 months to 59 years (average 24) years. Seventeen recipients (52%) were aged 18 years or less at the initial transplantation. The initial transplants were liver (18), kidney (8), heart (3), bone marrow (2), combined heart-lung (1), and lung (1). With the exception of 3 living related donors all donors were cadaveric. Incomplete information were available regarding immunosuppressive therapy in 2 recipients

J.L. Touraine et al. (eds.), Retransplantation, 45–53.

Table 1. Treatments causing regression of PTLD/HD

Treatment	No. of patients
Reduction or cessation of immunosuppressive therapy	24(6)*
Excision†	16†
Antiviral therapy	7
Local radiation therapy	7(2)*
Cancer chemotherapy	6(1)*
Alpha-interferon	4
Monoclonal anti-B cell antibodies	1
Autologous bone marrow transplantation	1

*The figures in parentheses represent the number of patients in whom this was the only treatment used.
†Includes removal and immediate retransplantation of 5 liver allografts and removal of 5 kidney allografts.

(bone marrow 1, liver 1). Another bone marrow recipient received total body irradiation, cyclosporine, prednisone and multiple cancer chemotherapeutic agents. Of the other 30 recipients 22 received triple therapy (cyclosporine, azathioprine, prednisone), 4 received cyclosporine and prednisone and 4 received azathioprine and prednisone. Additional immunosuppressive agents used in these 30 recipients included ALG (16), OKT3 (6), Tacrolimus (4), mofetil mycophenolate (3), splenectomy (1), local radiation therapy to a kidney allograft (1) and actinomycin (1).

The PTLD/HD appeared from 0.33 to 68 (average 16) months after the initial transplantation. The disease was widespread in 18 patients (including the 3 patients with HD who had widespread nodal involvement), and localized to a single organ or site in 15 recipients, including 8 patients in whom the disease was localized to the allograft (4 hepatic; 4 renal). The treatments given for PTLD/HD are listed in Table 1. Retransplantation was performed from 0 to 146 (average 31) months after diagnosis of the PTLD/HD. The 37 retransplantations consisted of 29 single retransplants while 4 patients each had two retransplants, of whom two were liver and 1 heart transplant recipients, while 1 heart transplant recipient subsequently required 2 liver transplants because of non-A non-B viral hepatitis (Tables 2 and 3; patients 5, 12, 29, 30). The indications for the 37 retransplantations were rejection or probable rejection (23), treatment of a lymphomatous allograft (9), non-A non-B hepatitis (2), coronary artery disease in a cardiac allograft (1), recurrent HD (1), and unstated (1).

Three patients (9%) had recurrence or persistence of PTLD after retransplantation. The first patient (Patient 2, Table 2) developed widespread PTLD, including the liver allograft, one month after initial transplantation. The immunosuppression was reduced and the hepatic allograft was removed and replaced with a healthy liver, but the patient died one week later of persistent PTLD and sepsis. The second patient was a kidney allograft recipient

Table 2. Outcome of retransplantation: group 1

Patient	Initial organ tx	Time of appearance of PTLD/HD (mos)	Indication for ReTx	Time from diagnosis of PTLD/HD to ReTx (mos)	Follow-up after first ReTx (mos)	Outcome
1	Liver	5	PTLD in allograft	0	8.5	A
2	Liver	1	PTLD in allograft	0	0.25	D(PTLD)
3	Liver	10	PTLD in allograft	2	7	A
4	Liver	9	PTLD in allograft	0	2	DO
5	Liver	0.33	PTLD in allograft	0.5	14.5	
			? Rejection	9.5	19.5	A
6	Kidney	8	PTLD in allograft	13.5	40.5	A
7	Kidney	1.5	PTLD in allograft	17.5	5.5	A
8	Kidney	20	PTLD in allograft	0	0.75	D(PTLD)
9	Kidney	1.5	PTLD in allograft	27.5	27.5	A
10	Bone marrow	40	Recurrent HD	24.5	47.5	A

Mos = Months; ReTx = Retransplantation; D(PTLD = Dead (PTLD); DO = Dead (other causes); A = Alive and free of PTLD/HD.

Table 3. Outcome of retransplantation: Group 2

No.	Initial organ tx	Time of appearance of PTLD/HD (mos)	Indication for ReTx	Time from diagnosis of PTLD/HD to ReTx (mos)	Follow-up after first ReTx (mos)	Outcome
11	Liver	68	Rejection	3.5	0.5	D(PTLD)
12	Liver	6	Rejection	31.5	102.5	
			? Rejection	134	103.25	A
13	Liver‡	6	Rejection	?	?	A*
14	Liver	23	Rejection	6	56.5	DO
15	Liver	6	Rejection	6.5	67.5	A
16	Liver	2	Rejection	8	19	DO
17	Liver	0.75	Rejection	0.75	6	DO
18	Liver	6.5	? Rejection	5	25	A
19	Liver	40.5	? Rejection	13.5	13	A
20	Liver	6.5	? Rejection	4	16.5	A
21	Liver	31	Rejection	6.5	20.5	A
22	Liver	12	Rejection	2.5	0	DO
23	Liver	0.5	Rejection	?	?	A†
24	Kidney	4	Rejection	41.5	52	A
25	Kidney‡	67	Rejection	45	110	A
26	Kidney	22	Rejection	92.5	1	A
27	Kidney	10.5	Rejection	60	11.5	A
28	Heart	4.5	Atherosclerosis of coronary arteries	182	51	A
29	Heart	20.5	NANB hepatitis	117§	20	DO
			NANB hepatitis	146§	21.5	
30	Heart	48.5	? Rejection	?	?	
			? Rejection	24	0	DO
31	Bone marrow	32.5	Not stated	10	1	DO
32	Lung	5	? Rejection	18.5	1.5	DO
33	Heart-lung	2	? Rejection	16.5	0	DO

*Alive 32 months after diagnosis.
†Alive 8.5 months after diagnosis.
‡Patient had HD.
§Liver transplants in a cardiac allograft recipient.
Mos = Months; ReTx = Retransplantation; D(PTLD) = Dead (PTLD); DO = Dead (other causes); A = Alive and free of PTLD/HD; NANB = Non-A non-B hepatitis.

(Patient 8, Table 2) who developed PTLD involving the allograft and the spleen 20 months after initial transplantation. The renal allograft was removed and replaced with a healthy one, but the patient died of acute lymphocytic leukemia (presumably a leukemic phase of the lymphomatous process) 3 weeks after retransplantation. The third patient was a liver allograft recipient (Patient 11, Table 3) who developed widespread PTLD 68 months after initial transplantation. Immunosuppressive therapy was reduced and the graft gradually failed. Retransplantation was performed 3.5 months after diagnosis of PTLD. The patient died 2 weeks later. Autopsy examination showed microscopic evidence of residual PTLD.

The outcomes of the patients after retransplantation can be divided into two broad groups (Tables 2 and 3). In group 1 (patients 1–10), patients 1–9 were retransplanted after a allograft, involved by PTLD, was removed (5 liver, 4 kidney), and patient 10 was retransplanted for recurrent HD. This patient had undergone bone marrow transplantation from a sibling for treatment of severe aplastic anemia and developed HD posttransplantation. It regressed after surgical excision, combined with radiotherapy and chemotherapy, but relapsed, necessitating autologous bone marrow transplantation, which caused regression of the disease (Table 1). These 10 patients were characterized by a short time interval between diagnosis of the PTLD/HD and retransplantation (range 0–27.5, average 9) months and a relatively short follow-up after the first retransplantation (range 0.25–47.5, average 16 months). Two of three recurrences were in this group (patients 2 and 8).

In contrast group 2 (patients 11–33), who were mostly retransplanted for rejection, had a much longer time interval between diagnosis of the PTLD/HD and retransplantation (range 0.75–182, average 42 months) and a longer follow-up after the first retransplantation (range 0–110, average 30 months). The one recurrence in this group (patient 11) resembled the patients in group 1 in that there was a short time interval between diagnosis of PTLD and retransplantation.

The 3 patients with recurrent PTLD following retransplantation died of this disease. Ten other patients died of other causes. The remaining 20 patients are alive and free of neoplasia including all three patients with HD. Of the 31 patients, whose length of follow-up after retransplantation is known (Tables 2 and 3), 15 (48%) were followed for less than 12 months. Three of them (patients 22, 30, 33) died within hours or a day or two following retransplantation. The remaining 16 patients were followed from 13 to 110 (average 43) months after the first retransplantation.

Kaposi's sarcoma

Of 416 patients with posttransplant KS 127 of 240 patients (53%) with non-visceral disease had complete remissions following various treatments, as did 49 of 173 patients (28%) with visceral disease. In both groups 74 of 176 (42%)

Table 4. Recurrence of Kaposi's sarcoma after retransplantation

No.	Type of KS	Time of appearance of KS post-tx (mos)	Time from diagnosis of KS to ReTx (mos)	Recurrence	Follow-up after ReTx	Outcome
1	NV	26.5	47	–	121	*
2	NV	12	43.5	+	> 72	†
3	NV	9	28	+	107	‡
4	V	6	56	+	19	§

mos = months; NV = non-visceral; V = visceral.
*Alive and well.
†Discontinuation of immunosuppression → rejection of allograft. Complete remission of KS.
‡ReTx lost to rejection after 3 weeks. KS regressed. Well on dialysis.
§Allograft lost to rejection 3.5 months after ReTx. KS regressed completely.

of complete remissions occurred in patients when the only treatment was reduction or cessation of immunosuppressive therapy. In 22 of 34 (65%) of these patients in whom allograft function was reported, loss or impairment of allograft function occurred. Four patients with complete regression of KS underwent retransplantation from 28 to 56 (average 44) months after the KS was diagnosed. Regression of KS was accomplished following reduction of immunosuppression in 3 patients, surgical excision of lesions in 2 patients, and local radiation therapy in one. All required retransplantation because of loss of their allografts to rejection. Three of the 4 patients developed recurrent KS after retransplantation (Table 4). All 3 allografts were subsequently lost because of rejection and the KS again underwent complete regression.

Discussion

There are several reasons why retransplantation may be necessary in some patients after treatment of PTLD/HD and KS. Sometimes, as occurred in 9 patients in this series, it is necessary to remove an allograft affected by PTLD. In renal allograft recipients it would be wise to wait for at least 12 months before attempting retransplantation, until all evidence of PTLD has regressed, and the patient has recovered from the effects of immunosuppressive therapy. However, in liver transplant recipients immediate replacement of the lymphomatous allograft is necessary. The need to give full doses of immunosuppressive agents to such patients, who may have microscopic foci of PTLD elsewhere, is likely to be associated with recurrence as occurred in 2 patients in this series. This experience is reinforced by the finding that 11 transplant patients at the University of Pittsburgh, who had complete clinical remissions of PTLD following reduction or cessation of immunosuppressive therapy (among other treatments), later had second episodes of Epstein–Barr virus (EBV) related lesions (10 PTLD, 1 smooth muscle tumor) [3] presumably when immunosuppressive therapy was either reinstituted or the dosage increased.

The major indication for retransplantation after treatment of PTLD/HD or KS is acute or chronic rejection, as occurred in the majority of patients in this series. Most cases followed reduction or cessation of immunosuppressive therapy. Thus, this treatment caused impaired function or allograft loss from rejection in 22 of 34 recipients treated for KS [4]. Similarly, in a series of 14 renal recipients whose PTLD was treated (among other methods) by reduction or cessation of immunosuppression, 8 of 12 survivors lost their allografts [5].

Some agents used to treat PTLD and KS may unintentionally stimulate the immune response. Alpha-interferon (IFN) is a potent immune modulator that increases membrane expression of class I antigens of the major histocompatibility complex, T-cell mediated cytotoxicity, and natural killer cell function [6]. Thus, it may stimulate rejection. However, conflicting findings have been reported in renal allograft recipients. Two studies showed an increased number of acute rejection episodes leading to graft failure, when either high-dose or low-dose IFN was used immediately after transplantation, whereas two other studies showed no difference in the incidence of rejection or graft dysfunction using low-dose regimens [7]. Although IFN may also induce rejection of liver allografts, neither this possibility nor the factors that predispose to it have been clearly defined [7].

Questions arise as to whether it is safe to resume immunosuppressive therapy, without neoplastic recurrence, in patients whose tumors had regressed after reduction or cessation of immunosuppression. If possible, retransplantation should be delayed until the PTLD/HD or KS has been in remission for several months. All recurrences in the present series occurred in patients in whom there was only a brief interval between diagnosis of lymphoma and retransplantation. In the present series only 9% of patients, who underwent retransplantation after treatment of PTLD/HD, developed recurrences. This figure may be unduly optimistic as 48% of the patients were followed for less than a year after retransplantation and some may still develop a recurrence. Furthermore, not all the patients, who died of various causes during this period, had autopsy examinations and some recurrent lymphomas may have been missed.

One would make several recommendations to try to prevent recurrent PTLD after retransplantation. First, retransplantation should be delayed for at least a year, if at all possible. Second, whenever feasible, one should ensure optimal HLA matching in order to minimize the risk of rejection, and hence increased immunosuppression that could favor recurrence of PTLD. Third, immunosuppressive therapy should be kept at as low a level as is compatible with allograft survival. In particular, one should try to avoid using antilymphocyte preparations, such as ALG and OKT3, in addition to standard immunosuppressive agents, as overimmunosuppression is a risk factor for development of PTLD [8]. Fourth, as most cases of PTLD are related to EBV infection antiviral prophylaxis is desirable. Although only sketchy data are available regarding their use after retransplantation it may be wise to treat patients for 3–6 months with agents such as acyclovir or ganciclovir.

Experience with retransplantation after treatment of KS is very limited [9–11]. It is disturbing that recurrences occurred in 3 of 4 patients despite an interval averaging 44 months between the diagnosis of KS and retransplantation. This concern is reinforced by a study of 4 renal allograft recipients, whose posttransplant KS regressed after reduction of immunosuppressive therapy, only to recur when immunosuppressive therapy was reinstituted or steroid pulses were given [9]. Subsequent reduction of immunosuppression caused regression of KS in all 4 patients, but two recipients lost their allografts. In addition, there is a case of a patient who was successfully treated for KS 234 months prior to renal transplantation, who developed recurrence of the disease 9 months after transplantation and treatment with prednisone, azathioprine and cyclosporine [9, 12]. If human herpes virus type 8 proves to be a major cause of posttransplant KS, as EBV has done with PTLD, it is possible that antiviral prophylaxis may be of value in patients with KS who require retransplantation. In the meantime, because of the risk of KS recurrence with immunosuppressive therapy, some physicians may prefer not to offer transplantation to patients with a history of KS, while others will undertake the procedure only after informing patients of the risk involved. If retransplantation is undertaken most of the recommendations made regarding prevention of recurrent PTLD are applicable in this situation.

Acknowledgment

The author wishes to thank his many colleagues throughout the world who have generously contributed data concerning their patients to the CTTR.

References

1. Penn I. Epidemiology of cancer in transplant patients. In: Touraine JL, Traeger J, Betuel H, Dubernard JM, Revillard JP, Dupuy C (eds.), Cancer in Transplantation, Prevention and Treatment. Dordrecht: Kluwer Academic Publishers, 1996: 3–15.
2. Penn I. Malignancy. Surg. Clin. N. Am. 1994; 74: 1247–1257.
3. Wu T-T, Swerdlow S, Locker J et al. Pathologic analysis of recurrent posttransplant lymphoproliferative disorders. Transplant. Proc. 1995; 27: 1193–1194.
4. Penn I. Sarcomas in organ allograft recipients. Transplantation 1995; 60: 1485–1491.
5. Hickey DP, Nalesnik MA, Vivas CA et al. Renal retransplantation in patients who lost their allografts during management of previous post-transplant lymphoproliferative disease. Clin. Transplant. 1990; 4: 187–190.
6. Peters M. Mechanisms of action of interferons (Review). Semin Liver Dis. 1989; 9: 235–239.
7. Min AD. Does interferon precipitate rejection of liver allografts? (Editorial). Hepatology 1995; 22: 1333–1335.
8. Penn I. Immunosuppression – a contributory factor in lymphoma formation. Clin. Transplant. 1992; 6: 214–219.

9. Doutrelepont JM, De Pauw L, Gruber SA et al. Renal transplantation exposes patients with previous Kaposi's sarcoma to a high risk of recurrence. Transplantation 1996; 62: 463–466.
10. Poch E, Oppenheimer F, Del Rio R et al. Reinstitution of immunosuppression in a renal transplant recipient after remission of Kaposi's sarcoma. Transplantation 1992; 54: 162–163.
11. Al-Sulaiman MH, Mousa DH, Dhar JM, Al-Khader AA. Does regressed posttransplantation Kaposi's sarcoma recur following reintroduction of immunosuppression? Am. J. Nephrol. 1992; 12: 384–386.
12. Penn I. Effects of immunosuppression on preexisting cancers. Transplantation 1993; 55: 742–747.

8. How should we retransplant patients after graft loss due to noncompliance?

EDUARDO A. SANTIAGO-DELPIN

Introduction

Noncompliant behavior – considered for a long time as an important risk factor in cardiovascular and cancer treatments – is now being recognized as an important element in organ transplantation outcome. Its existence is most vexing to the members of the transplant team and to the patient's family since it is universally recognized that a large amount of effort and sacrifice goes into organ donation and transplantation. Careful analysis of this problem is necessary in order to identify its exact prevalence, the magnitude of the problem, the importance of noncompliance in patient death and graft loss, as well as in other post transplant complications.

Organ transplantation is the only currently available 'cure' for endstage organ disease [1].

Also, quality of life demonstrably improves [2], as do the employability of recipients [3] and rehabilitation after transplantation [4, 5]. Further arguments to give the best care possible to the transplanted organ stem from its cost [6] and the cost-effectiveness of a complication-free post transplant course [7]. Furthermore, the waiting lists for organ transplantation continue to grow rapidly [8], especially importantly in regions with low donation rates such as Latin America [9] because of cultural factors [10, 11] although this has recently improved [12].

In this chapter, I will review several aspects of noncompliant behavior, its magnitude, its scope, causes associated and predictive factors, its prevention and management, all in the context of whether or not to retransplant a patient who has lost his first kidney due to noncompliance, or even whether or not to transplant a patient with noncompliance at all.

Noncompliance as a risk factor for organ transplantation

Even before the term 'outcomes analysis' became popular, surgeons in general and transplanters in particular have recognized the importance of results as part of their autocritical philosophy. In transplantation, the main emphasis has been on medical, surgical and immunological factors [13, 14]. This has been especially important in reviews of second kidney transplants in adults [15]

J.L. Touraine et al. (eds.), Retransplantation, 55–63.

Table 1. General concepts and factors in the successful evolution of organ transplantation

Prevention, awareness and early detection of infection and rejection
Improvement in monitoring of organ specific function
Advancement in non-invasive and invasive diagnosis of infections and rejections
Improved immunosuppression
Improvements in fundamental knowledge of the immune response and the continuing study of this phenomenon
Outcomes analysis
Clinical and basic research and their public discussion in regional and world forums.
The development of transplant 'programs' with dedicated, committed, well-trained personnel
Efficient, specialized hospital infrastructure
Enhanced communication between transplant programs around the world
The interdisciplinary team approach to organ transplantation
Transplantation in the context of a total quality management program
National, regional and international transplant registries and organizations

Table 2. Specific factors associated with outcome in organ transplantation

Histocompatibility	Preservation time
Sensitization	Warm ischemia time
Lessons from living unrelated donors	Good initial function
Multiple transplants	Initial non-function
Race	Early rejection
Original disease	Technical complications, early and late
Recipient weight	Infection
Blood transfusions	The different immunosuppressive regimes
Age	The 'center effect'
Marginal cadaver donors	Noncompliance
Marginal cadaver organs	

and children [16] where the main focus is immunological, such as sensitization, immunosuppression, etc. More recently, both immunological [17] and non-immunological [18] factors have been described in late graft failure.

Nonetheless, there is also a number of other non-medical factors which have an effect on the overall quality of care and infrastructure, which in turn, affects the success of organ transplantation. Table 1 lists general factors which have affected transplantation outcomes in developed countries, while Table 2 enumerates specific factors which either historically or currently have been considered as important in the success or failure of organ transplantation.

It is only recently that noncompliance has been recognized as contributing to the risk of organ transplantation. Indeed, none of the available text books on transplantation in the English language, whether European, Middle Eastern or North American, or whether on kidney, liver or pancreas transplantation discuss noncompliance in this context. It is only in the last ten years in which attention has been focused on this factor as important in patient and graft loss. The initial papers called attention to this problem in specific groups such as

Table 3. Protean manifestations of noncompliance

Discontinuation of immunosuppressive medications or unauthorized dose modifications
Intentional or irresponsible manipulation of anti-hypertensive and other medications
Ingestion of over-the-counter or natural non-prescribed medications and substances and foods
Missing clinic appointments
Missing laboratory appointments
Denying or minimizing symptoms including fever, malaise and respiratory and urinary symptoms, and not seeking medical attention promptly
Obesity
Excessive salt ingestion
Poor control of diabetes
Poor control of blood pressure
Smoking
Alcohol abuse

African-Americans and Hispanics [19–23]. Promptly however, children and adolescents where found to have a particularly high prevalence [24–26]. The exact incidence however defies quantification, since identification depends on awareness and there are different definitions, criteria and approaches to the study of noncompliance. Importantly, noncompliance is being recognized as everpresent and highly prevalent as a determinant of graft survival [27]. Similarly, in children the real prevalence is difficult to estimate but it is felt to be underestimated and overlooked by health care providers [26].

Noncompliance: causes, determinants and consequences

Noncompliance is an ill-defined vague term which is loosely applied to a patient's lack of adherence to a particular treatment. However, definitions have varied in the literature and with the definition, the magnitude of the problem, the effects on the results and the prevalence. Prospective searching for noncompliance can take the form of a monthly pill count [28] but this measure only focuses on medications rather than on the overall management strategy. Others have defined noncompliance retrospectively as acceptance by the patient of not adherance to immunosuppression, resulting in graft loss [29]. We have included several factors in defining noncompliance in a previous study [23]. The noncompliant patient was defined as a patient with poor attendance to clinics or to laboratory appointments, who delayed in the notification of problems, showed poor adherence to diets and/or consistently gained weight, and showed poor adherence to the drugs schedule, including minor deviations. We feel that noncompliance takes many forms and that eventhough the most dangerous manifestation is stopping or modifying the immunosuppressive drug regime, other factors too can result in an increased risk for morbidity, mortality or graft lost. Table 3 enumerates some manifestations of noncompliance which can have a deleterious effect on the overall results. Certainly obesity is a risk

Table 4. 'Causes' of noncompliant behavior

Ignorance or poor education	Misplaced priorities
Poor insight	Peer pressure
Social or marital problems	External locus of control
Denial	Depression
False sense of security and a feeling of omnipotence	Mistrust of physician, service or treatment regime
Equivocal interpretation of the Bible or religion	Pessimism; skepticism; fatalism
Youth and adolescence	Concern on side effects
'Revenge' against spouse or parents	The cost of treatment

factor after kidney and kidney–pancreas transplantation [30]; alcoholism is also an important factor for all organ transplants because of the attendant increase in liver toxicity, and certainly in liver transplantation [31] (where it is a true recurrence of the original disease). Refractory hypertension can also signify nonadherance to treatment [32]. The factors enumerated in Table 3 are seldom considered in studies of noncompliant patients. It should be noted that minor deviations from the prescribed regime can be additive to other conditions such as coincidental viral infection or uncontrolled blood pressure. Indeed, suboptimal immunosuppression may contribute to the development of chronic rejection [33], and subclinical noncompliance with immunosuppressive therapy results in more acute late rejections, even when violations are minimal [34]. Again, because of problems with the definition as well as lack of awareness, noncompliance seems to be underestimated [26].

Virtually all publications on the topic report a uniform deleterious effect on graft and even patient survival [19–24]. It is one important cause of late mortality in pediatric liver transplant recipients [35] and a major cause of graft failure in other countries as well [23, 36].

What are the causes of noncompliant behavior? Why would a patient who has regained health and has improved his or her quality of life engage on behavior which increases the risk of losing all that has been gained? The answers to these questions come mostly from studies on treatment adherance in hypertension and cancer although more recent on organ transplantation too. Although there are a number of factors associated with this type of behavior, the actual 'cause' is not known. It is not unusual to hear patients say "after many years with no problems I was sure the kidney belong to me; I could stop my medications and nothing would happen": a sence of false security. "I had so much work and my hours were so erratic that I started missing my medications and before I knew, I wasn't sure of what I was taking anymore": a case of misplaced priorities. And, "I had facial hair, I became obese, I had fear that I would lose my husband": a case of external locus of control and/or manipulation from the family. Table 4 lists some 'etiological' factors in non-compliant behavior. Many studies have indicated that individuals do physically

Table 5. Measureable factors associated with noncompliance

Scholarity
Socio-economic problems
Marital status
Distance from the transplant center and transportation
Capacity for self care
Problems with family
Noncompliant problematic behavior during dialysis, including fluid and electrolyte control, dialysis visits, appointments, etc.
Obesity and associated complications
Edema and associated complications
Drug toxicity
Refractory hypertension

and emotionally better when they have a sense of self-control [37]. But these are only factors related to patients and patient beliefs. However, others have stressed organizational factors influencing adherence such as infrastructure, continuity of care, personalized care, scheduling, relationship with the medical personnel, patient participation, etc. [38].

Of more importance however is identifying measurable factors associated with noncompliance which may predict this behavior or at least allow for an early detection. Table 5 identifies some of these factors as reported in the literature, including studies by our group [23, 26, 34, 38–40].

Of very important predictive value both for the new patient as well as for the patient who has lost the kidney due to noncompliance, is the adherance to treatment during the dialysis phase. Noncompliance on dialysis takes many forms of which important is noncompliance to fluid restriction. This has been found mostly in young males with an external health locus of control [41], although seasonal factors are apparently operant also [42]. In a previous study, noncompliance during dialysis was highly predictive of noncompliance after transplantation ($P = 0.0004$) [23]. Psychosocial parameters as well as economic problems cannot be underestimated in this context.

Prevention and management of noncompliance

A cursory glance at the previous tables identifies problem of such magnitude that cast doubt on the prognosis of some patients. The problems are of two types, external problems, and problems related to image, locus of control, or emotional-personality problems. Perhaps a more important practical question to formulate is how to initially identify noncompliant behavior, especially in the context of a graft loss? Also of importance is the continuous awareness of the different manifestations of noncompliance in the medical history and in the medical interview as well as the interview by the psychologist, dietitian and medical social worker. The possibility of the problem should also be considered if some of the factors determinant of this type of behavior are identified. The

Table 6. Prevention and management of noncompliance

Awareness and identification of risk causal factors
Identification of predictive factors
Monitoring for manifestations of non-compliant behavior
(Computerized) tracking of clinic and laboratory appointments
Persons of Hispanics or African-American extraction, the young and males, will need special attention
Pre-transplant counseling of patients and family
Discussions in the transplant committees
The Medical Social Worker as an essential team member
Empathy and identification with the patient's problems, and assistance in their solution.
Communication, direct counseling, group discussions, participation of other patients
Behavior modification techniques

possibility should be everpresent during deliberations of the transplant committee, in decision making meetings and in case discussions and interdisciplinary planning meetings. It is only through awareness that noncompliant or 'subcompliant' behavior can be consistently detected [23, 36]. The importance of the medical social worker, of outcome analysis, of total quality management approach, of the dietitian, of the ward nursing staff, and the transplant secretary cannot be underestimated since non-medical personnel frequently develops good rapport and better personal communication than the surgical and medical staff. Calls from relatives alerting staff to undesirable behavior on the part of the transplanted patient should not go unheeded. Table 6 enumerates some important factors in the approach to this problem.

Attention to the particular factor of the case, especially in the context of previous serious complications such as infections, rejections, graft loss, may correspondingly result in a very gratifying change of attitude and behavior. Specifically, most investigators recommend education and reinforcement as key elements in adherance to treatment [43]. Once a noncompliant recipient is identified the team approach shoud be initiated. The transplant nurse, medical social worker [44], and the psychologist should make direct interventions in order to further identify internal as well as external factors, and work towards their correction together with the patient. Communication is critical [37], and group discussions will be of great value as they are in other aspects of organ donation and transplantation [45].

Patients who have lost their kidneys or who have been severely ill may share their experiences in these group sessions, and their advice is frequently taken up by other patients quite easily because of identification. Relationship between the patient and the health care provider most be optimized and enhanced, since ultimately it is trust in the system which will allow for effective communication. In the case of children and adolescents who may not understand the consequences of their behavior and who generally are encumbered by poor insight, participation of the family is critical. Even formal behavior modification approaches may be started, including self regulatory skills and other interventions [38]. Empathy and understanding about the specific concerns of the patient is important in achieving behavior modification. In all techniques, education is foremost [46].

How should we retransplant patients after graft loss due to noncompliance?

First of all should we even transplant noncompliant patients? Indeed, there is a sense of betrayal when a patient loses a kidney in an irresponsible manner. Physicians and transplant personnel verbalize hostility because of a perceived affront to the medical personnel, to the institution, but above all, to the donor or his family who have altruistically given a gift of life. Almost 50% of US centers polled in a recent study will not transplant noncompliant patients from a living donor [47]. However, we have seen that not all noncompliant behavior is irresponsible or a manifestation of an erratic mind.

Noncompliance takes many forms, has many manifestations and has many multiple causes. It is by prospective attention to these causes that we can control non-medical factors, which are as determinant of success as surgical, medical and immunological factors. It is my contention that awareness of noncompliance should be everpresent and not only in patients already identified as noncompliant because of a previous graft loss. The experience of our group and others [29, 36, 48] indicate that appropriate identification and management of these factors may result in behavior modification which is beneficial to the outcome of that kidney.

Therefore, the answer to the question on retransplantation of noncompliant patients rests on the efforts that the particular program may invest in attending all appropriate details. Retransplantation of the noncompliant patients should only be carried out after careful analysis of the pertinent risk, etiological and determinant factors, and after addressing and correcting the specific factors in question of the recipient: careful evaluation and selection. Pretransplant counseling of the patient and the family as well as the participation of the medical social worker and other members of the transplant team should apply to all candidates for primary and retransplantation as part of the routine management.

References

1. Najarian JS. The making of the Transplantation Society. Transplant. Proc. 1997; 29: 7–11.
2. Adang EMM, Engel GL, Van Hoof JP, Koostra G. Comparison before and after transplantation of pancreas-kidney and pancreas-kidney with loss of pancreas – prospective controlled quality of life study. Transplantation 1996; 62: 754–758.
3. Matas AJ, Lawson W, McHugh L et al. Employment patterns after successful kidney transplantation. Transplantation 1996; 61: 729–733.
4. Matos-Alvarado D, Rodríguez-Palmer N, Santiago RI et al. La rehabilitación del paciente transplantado. Bol. Asoc. Med. P. Rico 1980; 72: 91–94.

5. Santiago-Delpín E, Amadeo JH, Ramírez-González R. Results of living related kidney transplantation in Puerto Rico. Transplantation 1986; 41: 606–610.
6. Rettig RA. The social contract and the treatment of permanent kidney failure. JAMA 1996; 275: 1123–1126.
7. Lewis RL, Canafax DM, Pettit KG et al. Use of Markov modelling for evaluating the cost-effectiveness of immunosuppressive therapies in renal transplant recipients. Transplant. Proc. 1996; 28: 2214–2217.
8. UNOS Update, United Network for Organ Sharing, Richmond, VA (USA). Jan 1997.
9. Santiago-Delpín EA. Organ donation and transplantation in Latin America. Transplant. Proc. 1991; 23: 2516–2518.
10. Fernández M, Zayas E, González ZA et al. Factors in a meager donation pattern of a Hispanic population. Transplant. Proc. 1991; 23: 1799–1801.
11. René PP, Viera E, Jiles R, Daniels DE. Organ donation awareness: Knowledge, attitudes and beliefs in a Puerto Rican Population. Transplant. Proc. 1995; 27: 1893–1896.
12. Santiago-Delpín EA, Duro-García V, Chameh O. Forty thousand organ transplants in Latin America. Transplant. Proc. 1997; 29: 1586–1589.
13. Terasaki PI (ed.). Clinical kidney transplants – 1985, UCLA Tissue Typing Lab. Los Angeles, CA (USA) 1985.
14. Terasaki PI, Cecka JM (eds.). Clinical transplants – 1995, UCLA Tissue Typing Lab, Los Angeles, CA (USA), 1995.
15. Mahoney RJ, Norman DJ, Colombe BW et al. Identification of high- and low-risk second kidney grafts. Transplantation 1996; 61: 1349–1355.
16. Tejani A, Sullivan EK. Factors that impact on the outcome of second transplants in children. Transplantation 1996; 62: 606–611.
17. Hiesse C, Riev P, Larve JR et al. Late graft failure and death in renal transplant recipients: Analysis in a single-center population of 1500 patients. Transplant. Proc. 1997; 29: 240–242.
18. Häyry P, Yilmaz S. Chronic allograft rejection: An update. Transplant. Proc. 1994; 26: 3159–3160.
19. Didlake RH, Dreyfus KRH, Van Buren CT, Kahan BD. Patient non-compliance: A major cause of late graft failure in cyclosporine-treated renal transplants. Transplant. Proc. 1988; 10: 63–66.
20. Rovelli M, Palmieri D, Vossler E et al. Non-compliance in organ transplant recipients. Transplant. Proc. 1989; 21: 833–834.
21. Schweitzer RT, Rovelli M, Palmieri P et al. Non-compliance in organ transplant recipients. Transplantation 1990; 49: 374–376.
22. Dunn J, Golden D, Van Buren C et al. Causes of graft loss beyond two years in the cyclosporine era. Transplantation 1990; 49: 349–352.
23. Rodríguez A, Díaz M, Colón A, Santiago-Delpín EA. Psychosocial profile of non-compliant transplant patients. Transplant. Proc. 1991; 23: 1807–1809.
24. Meyers KEC, Weiland H, Thomson PD. Pediatric renal transplantation non-compliance. Pediatr. Nephrol. 1995; 9: 189.
25. Korsch BM, Fine RN, Negrete VF. Non-compliance in children with renal transplants. Pediatrics 1978; 61: 872.
26. Meyers KEC, Thomson PD, Weiland H. Non-compliance in children and adolescents after renal transplantation. Transplantation 1996; 26: 186–189.
27. Pirsch JD, Ploeg RJ, Gange S et al. Determinants of graft survival after kidney transplantation. Transplantation 1996; 61: 1581–1586.
28. Hilbrands LB, Hoitsma AJ, Koene RAP. Medication compliance after renal transplantation. Transplantation 1995; 60: 914–920.
29. Troppmann C, Benedetti E, Gruessner RWG, Najarian JS, Matas AJ. Should patients with renal allograft loss due to non compliance be retransplanted? Transplant. Proc. 1995; 27: 1093.
30. Bumgardner GL, Henry ML, Elkhammas E et al. Obesity as a risk factor after combined pancreas/kidney transplantation. Transplantation 1995; 60: 1426–1430.

31. Fabrega F, Foster PF, Sankary HN et al. Liver transplantation for patients with alcoholic cirrhosis. Transplant. Proc. 1997; 29: 465–466.
32. Setaro JF, Black HR. Refractory Hypertension. N. Engl. J. Med. 1992; 327: 543–547.
33. Simic S, Djukanovic L, Stojkovic D et al. Does suboptimal immunosuppression contribute to chronic rejection? Transplant. Proc. 1995; 27: 909–910.
34. De Geest S, Borgemans L, Genoets H et al. Incidence, determinants, and consequences of subclinical non compliance with immunosuppressive therapy in renal transplant recipients. Transplantation 1995; 59: 340–347.
35. Sudan DL, Shaw BW, Langnas AN. Causes of late mortality in pediatric liver transplant recipients. Transplant. Proc. 1997; 29: 430–431.
36. García V, Bittar A, Keltel E et al. Patient non-compliance as a major cause of kidney graft failure. Transplant. Proc. 1997; 29: 252–254.
37. Jacobs C. The word we call 'Compliance'. Transplant. Chronicles 1996; 3: 17–18.
38. Meichenbaum D, Turk DC. Facilitating treatment adherence. Plenum Press, New York, 1987.
39. Rovelli M, Palmieri D, Vossler E et al. Non compliance in renal transplant recipients: Evaluation by socioeconomic groups. Transplant. Proc. 1989; 21: 3979–3980.
40. Kalil RSN, Hein-Duthoy KL, Kasiske BL. Patients with a low income have reduced renal allograft survival. Am. J. Kidney Dis. 1992; 10: 63.
41. Everett KD, Sletten C, Carmack C et al. Predicting non-compliance to fluid restrictions in hemodialysis patients. Dialysis Transplant. 1993; 22: 614–618.
42. Desmond FE, Tucker CM. Seasonal variation of fluid intake adherence in hemodialysis patients. Cont. Dial. Nephrol. March 1993: 15–16.
43. Perkins KA. Applicability of health promotion strategies to increasing organ donation. In: Shanteau J, Harris RJ (eds.), Organ Donation and Transplantation: Psychological and Behavioral Factors. American Psychological Association, Washington, DC; 1990: 179–188.
44. Souchet MM. La evaluación social y el grave problema de no-cumplimiento. Bol. Asoc. Med. P. Rico 1995; 87: 114–115.
45. Townsend ME, Rovelli MA, Schweitzer RT. Value of discussion groups in educating blacks about organ donation and transplantation. Transplant. Proc. 1990; 22: 324–325.
46. Beck DE, Fennell RS, Yost RL et al. Evaluation of an educational program on compliance with medication regimens in pediatric patients with renal transplants. J. Pediatr. 1980; 96: 1094.
47. Ramos EL, Kasiske BL, Alexander SR et al. The evaluation of candidates for renal transplantation. Transplantation 1994; 57: 490–497.
48. Matas AJ, Gillighan KJ, Payne WD et al. A third kidney transplant: Cost-effective treatment for end-stage renal disease? Clin. Transplant. 1996; 10: 516–520.

9. Influence of rejection of the first transplant on the outcome of subsequent transplants

YONG W. CHO & PAUL I. TERASAKI

Introduction

Patients who receive second cadaver transplants continued to pose unique challenges as they are considered to be immunized by their previous grafts. However, the success rates for renal retransplantation have significantly improved in recent years as a result of improved pretransplant screening and posttransplant management, including sensitive crossmatching, better HLA matching, and more potent immunosuppressive agents [1–3]. The present study is an updated report on second cadaver donor transplants in the United States.

Materials and methods

The subjects of this study were second cadaver donor transplant recipients reported to the UCLA Kidney Transplant Registry between January 1981 and December 1987, and the United Network for Organ Sharing (UNOS) Kidney Transplant Registry between January 1988 and December 1995. We excluded transplant cases without follow-up. To study previous graft survival time (PGST) and the waiting time (WTIME) between the previous graft failure and retransplantation, we linked patients who received second grafts to their first transplant results in the UCLA and UNOS databases, and in some cases a first transplant reported to the UCLA Registry was linked to the patient's second graft reported to UNOS (see Figures 3 and 7). Graft survival rates were estimated by the product-limit method and patient deaths were considered graft loss regardless of the functional status of the graft. The χ^2 and t-tests were used for group comparisons. The log-rank test was utilized to compare entire survival curves. All reported p-values were two-tailed. Potential risk factors for second cadaver transplants were identified using univariate analyses. To confirm the influence of risk factors on graft outcome in the univariate analyses, the Cox proportional hazard models were applied, which considered donor age, PGST, WTIME, peak panel reactive antibody, cause of primary graft failure, and the number of HLA-A,B,DR antigens mismatched (ABDR mismatch). Split HLA-DR antigens were converted to their broad specificities. Missing observations were discarded from the multivariate analysis.

J.L. Touraine et al. (eds.), Retransplantation, 65–78.

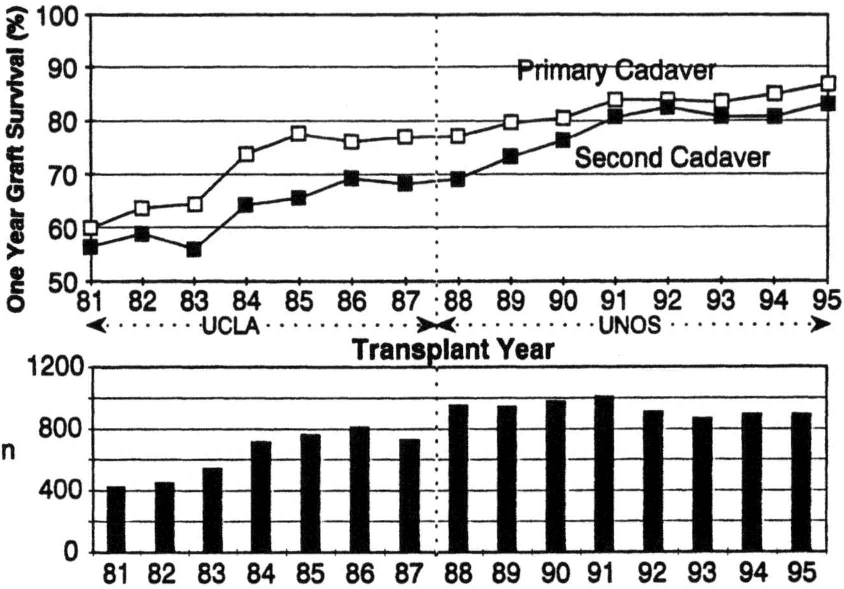

Fig. 1. One year graft survival and the number of second cadaver donor transplants performed per year.

Results

Figure 1 shows the annual number of second cadaver transplants. A steady increase in the number of second cadaver transplants was observed until 1991 after which time the number stabilized at about 900 after 1992. In the influence of rejection of the first transplant on the outcome of UCLA data, one-year graft survival rates for second cadaver donor transplants improved steadily from 56% in 1981 to 69% in 1987. One-year survival rates for second cadaver grafts continued to increase steadily during the UNOS era and reached 83% by 1995.

A significant stepwise increase in second cadaver graft survival curves was noticed from 1988 to 1991 (Figure 2). After 1991, there was no significant improvement in graft survival. The major difference between survival curves from 1988 to 1991 occurred within 3 months posttransplant. One possible cause has been the improvement in crossmatching techniques during this period. With respect to longer term graft survival, no significant improvement was noted.

There was a gradual increase in the proportion of patients whose previous graft survived more than 2 years from 23% in 1981 to 57% in 1995 (Figure 3). There was a corresponding decrease in the proportion of patients whose previous graft failed between one and 6 months posttransplant, from 30% in 1981 to 12% in 1995. This suggests that clinicians may have consciously selected

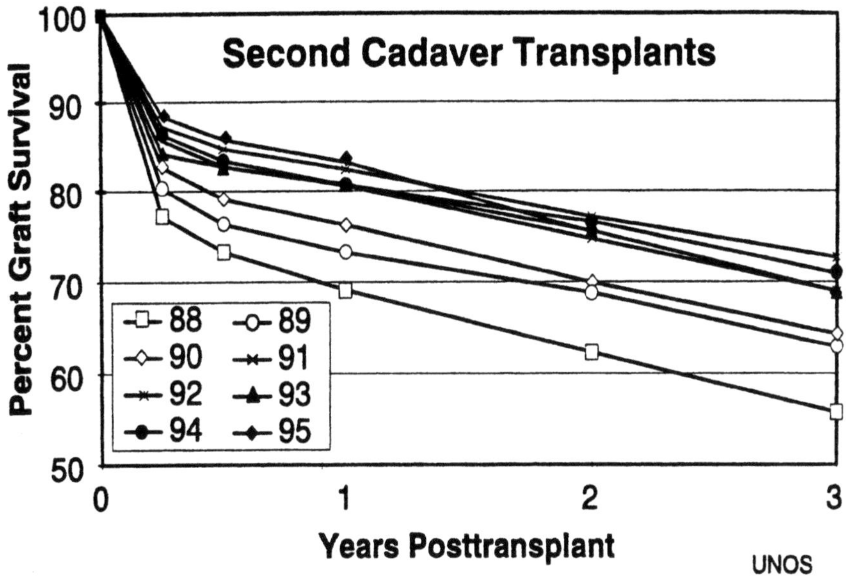

Fig. 2. Yearly graft survival for second cadaver donor transplants in the UNOS database.

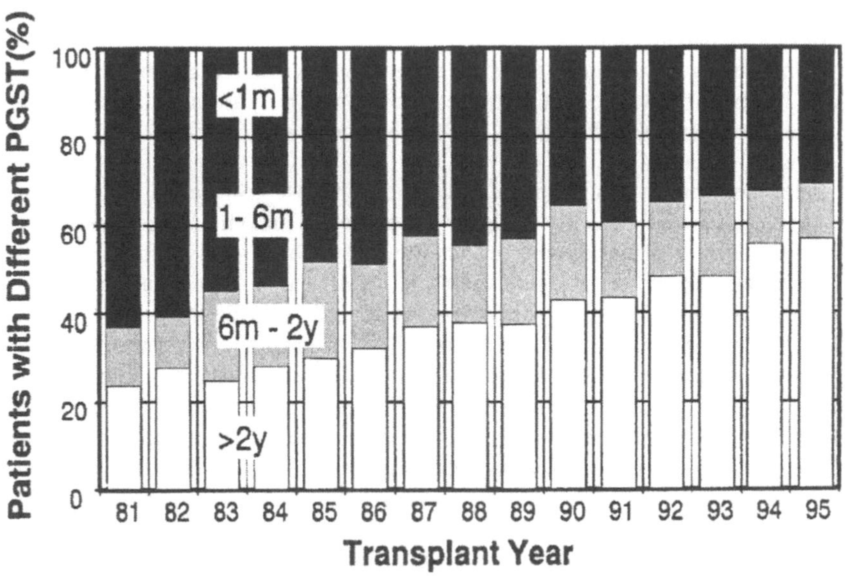

Fig. 3. Proportion of patients with different levels of PGST.

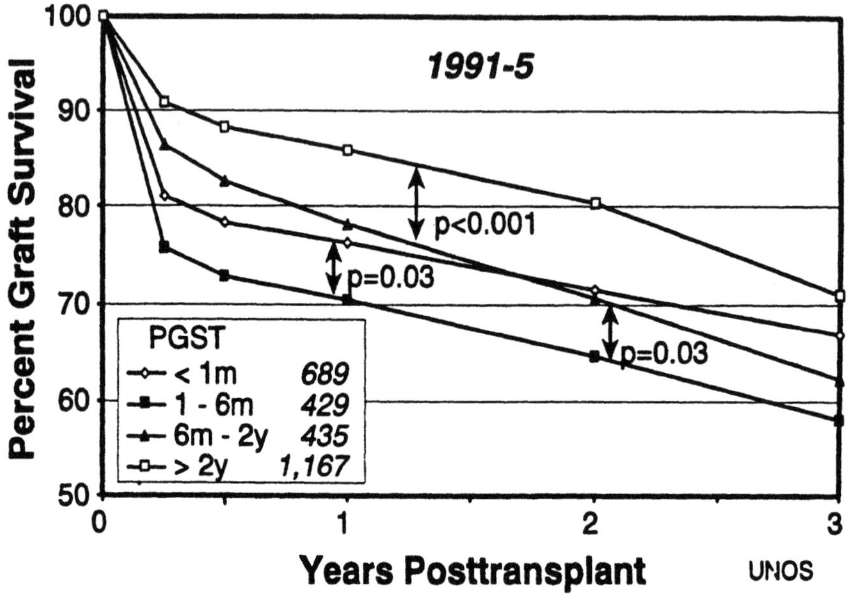

Fig. 4. Second graft survival performed from 1991 to 1995 according to PGST.

patients with longer first graft survival times ahead of those with shorter first graft survival. Higher rates of sensitization among patients who rejected their first transplant early also may have affected the composition of the waiting pool of retransplant candidates.

Graft survival was the highest in patients whose first graft survived more than 2 years, and was lowest in those whose primary graft failed between one and 6 months posttransplant. The difference for all periods was highly significant (Figure 4).

The one-year graft survival rate of patients whose graft failed as the result of chronic rejection was 15% higher than that of patients who experienced acute rejection of their primary grafts (Figure 5). Graft survival for those who experienced chronic rejection of their first graft was almost identical to that for patients whose first graft survived more than 2 years, as shown in Figure 4.

A plot was constructed of the actual one-year graft survival rates for high- and low-risk groups (PGST 1–6 months and >2 years, respectively) each year from 1981–1995. The difference between the actual graft survival rate and that of patients whose primary graft survived longer than 2 years decreased gradually from 17% in 1981 to 4% in 1995 (Figure 6). We conclude that much of this decrease can be attributed to the increasing selection of patients with longer first graft survival times.

The waiting time for patients whose primary graft failed increased every year (Figure 7). In 1981, 52% of patients received second cadaver graft within 1 year compared to 30% in 1995.

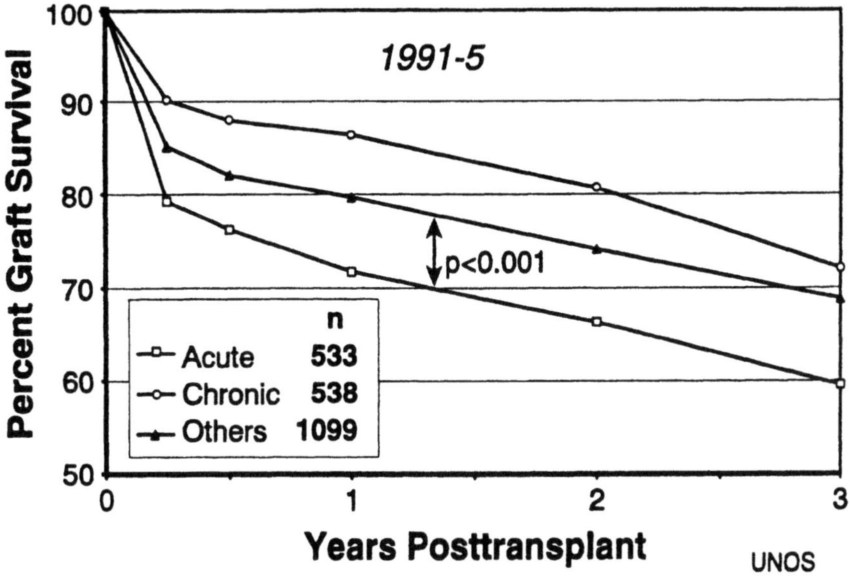

Fig. 5. Cause of previous graft failure and second graft survival.

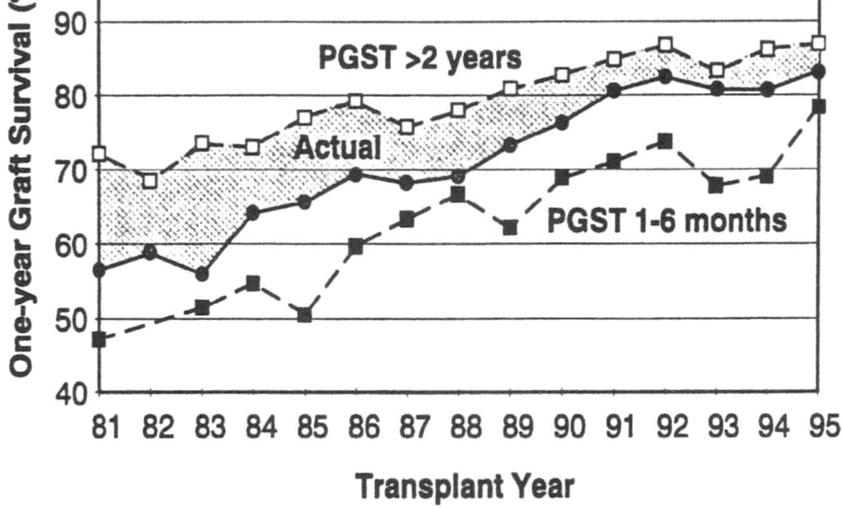

Fig. 6. Impact of PGST on second graft survival from 1981 to 1995.

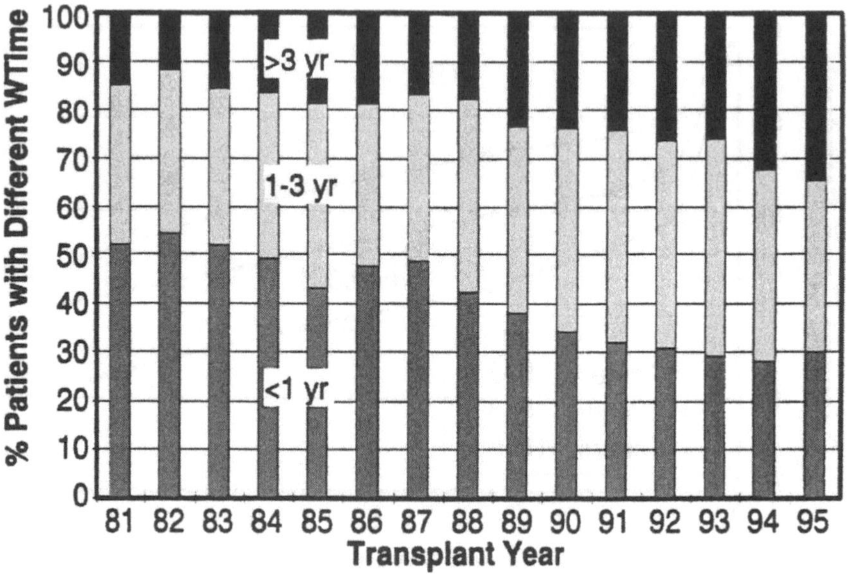

Fig. 7. Proportion of patients with short and long waiting times for second transplants.

Patients who waited less than 1 year had a better graft survival than those who waited for longer periods (Figure 8). There was a 13% difference in one-year graft survival rate between patients who had waited longer than 3 years and those who waited less than 1 year.

The proportion of zero HLA-A,B,DR antigen mismatched patients increased from 5% in 1988 to 22% in 1995 (Figure 9). The 6 antigen match program of UNOS has had a marked impact in the proportion of second grafts with zero HLA-A,B,DR antigen mismatched.

A significant matching effect has already been seen within 3 months post-transplant (Figure 10). Five or 6 HLA-A,B,DR antigen mismatched transplants had an 11% lower 3-month graft survival rate compared with the zero mismatched group

HLA matching had the greatest effect on patients who had acute rejections or other causes of failure of the first graft (Figure 11). HLA matching had a relatively small effect on those who rejected their first graft chronically. Thus, despite the level of HLA mismatch, patients with chronic first graft rejections had a higher graft survival than patients with acute rejections.

The proportion of nonsensitized patients (0–20% PPRA) increased from 41% in 1988 to 52% in 1995, suggesting second grafts into sensitized patients have been increasingly avoided (Figure 12). The broadly sensitized patients are probably more often excluded by more sensitive crossmatch tests. Patients with high levels of anti-HLA antibodies (>80%) had a significantly lower graft

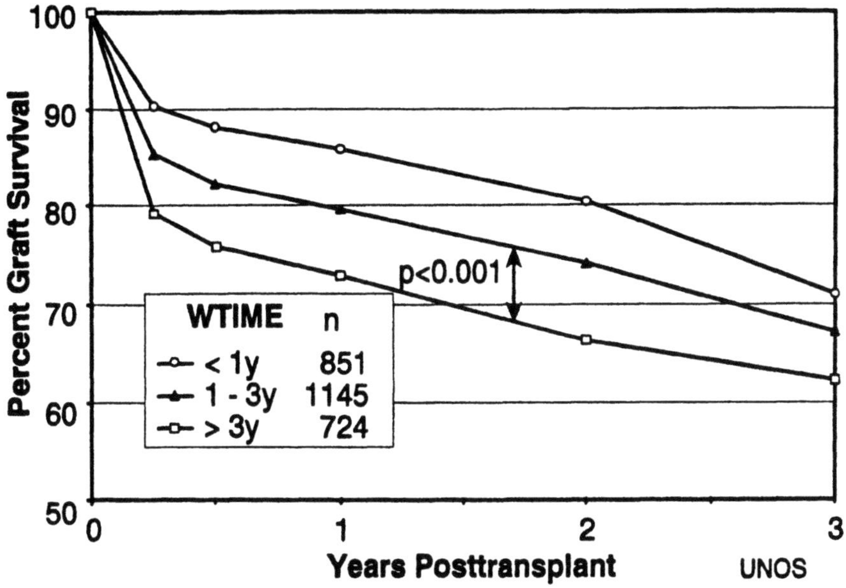

Fig. 8. Second graft survival and waiting time.

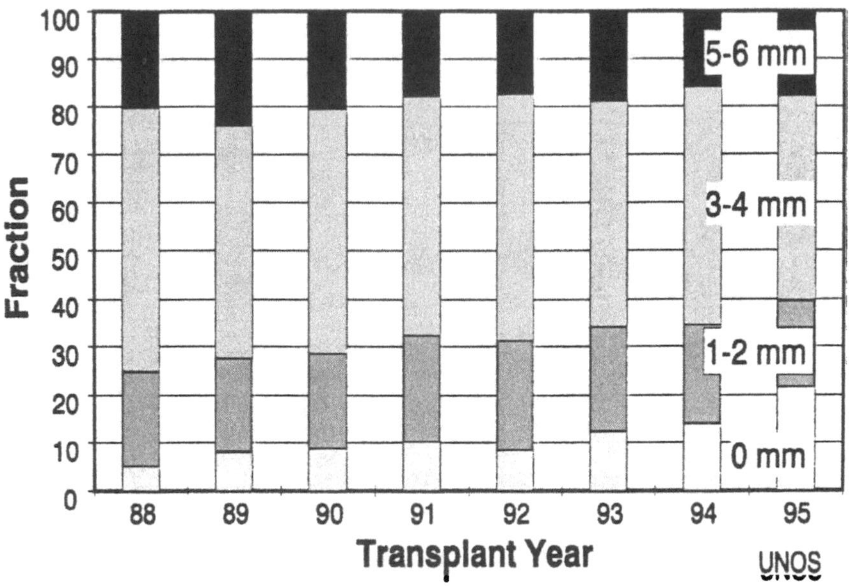

Fig. 9. HLA matching and second cadaver donor transplants.

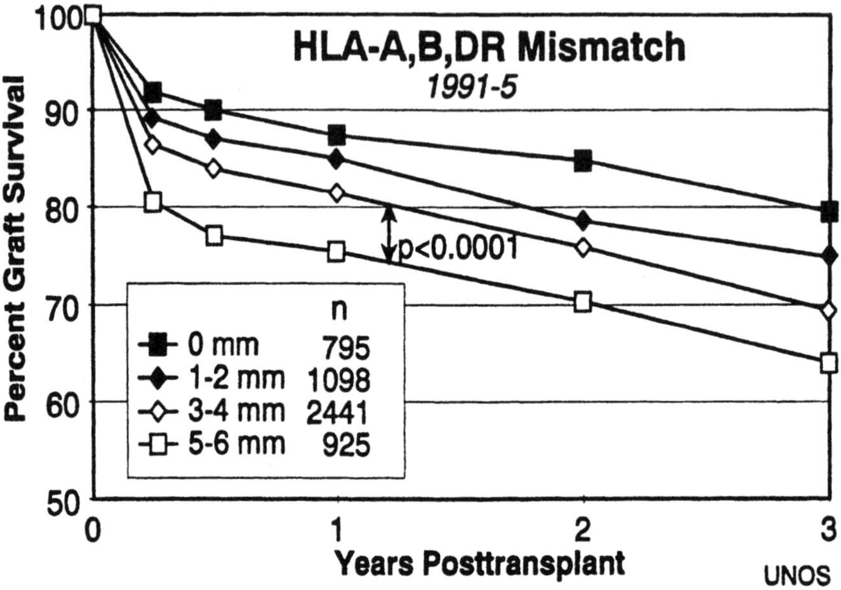

Fig. 10. Matching for HLA-A,B,DR antigens resulted in improved graft survival for second cadaver donor transplants.

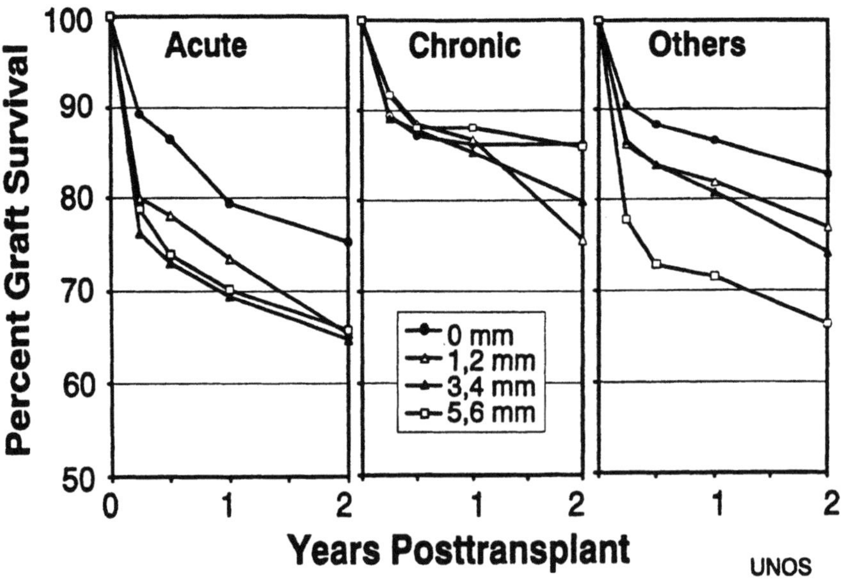

Fig. 11. Effect of HLA matching on second grafts in patients with acute and chronic rejection of the first graft.

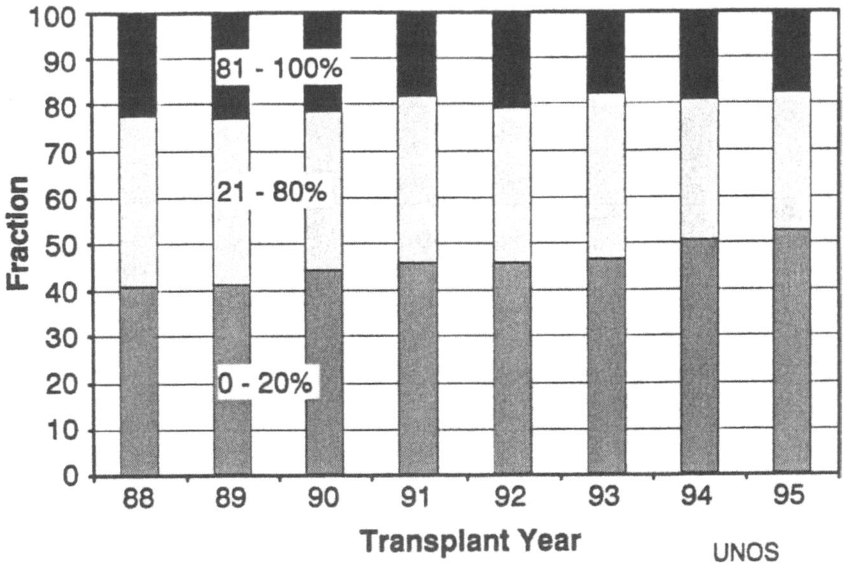

Fig. 12. Proportion of presensitized patients retransplanted.

survival rate compared with those with intermediate (21–80%) or low (0–20%) levels of antibody (Figure 13).

The number of kidneys transplanted from donors older than 50 years of age nearly doubled between 1988 and 1995 (Figure 14). The graft survival for donors aged 16–40 was 17% higher at one year than that for donors more over age 60 (Figure 15). This difference increased to 22% by 3 years. Note that the graft survival of kidneys from donors aged 16–40 was similar to the high graft survival seen for patients with first graft survival times more than 2 years.

The fraction of patients treated for rejection during the initial hospitalization period decreased significantly from 39% in 1988 to 17% in 1995, suggesting considerable improvement of early posttransplant management (Figure 16). Better crossmatching methods also may have selected for donors against whom presensitization had not occurred. During the same period, there was a significant 8% reduction in patients who required dialysis in the first week. Reductions in the percentage of patients with no urine output in the first day and primary nonfunctioning kidneys (PNF) were marginal during this period.

Forty-two percent of patients whose second graft failed as a result of acute rejection had also lost their first graft due to acute rejection (Figure 17). Similarly, 40% of patients whose second graft failed because of chronic rejection had already experienced chronic rejection of their primary graft.

The donor's age, the number of HLA-A,B,DR antigens mismatched, the primary graft survival time, broad sensitization, and acute rejection as a cause of the primary graft failure were significant risk factors in second cadaver

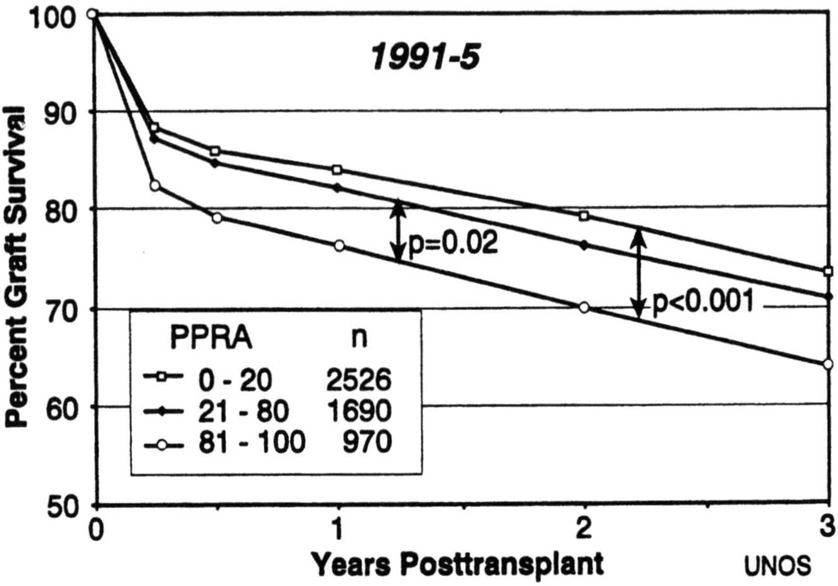

Fig. 13. Second graft survival in patients with different levels of sensitization.

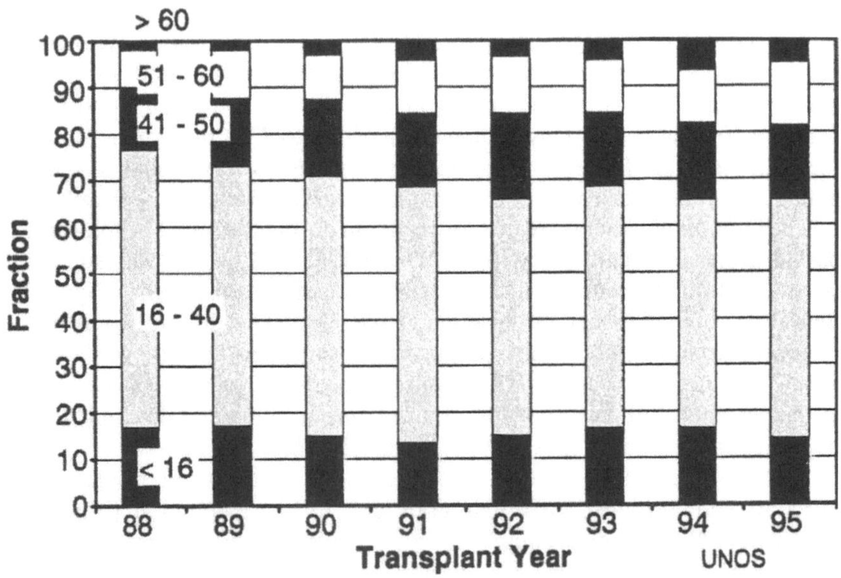

Fig. 14. Proportion of patients who received grafts from donors of various ages.

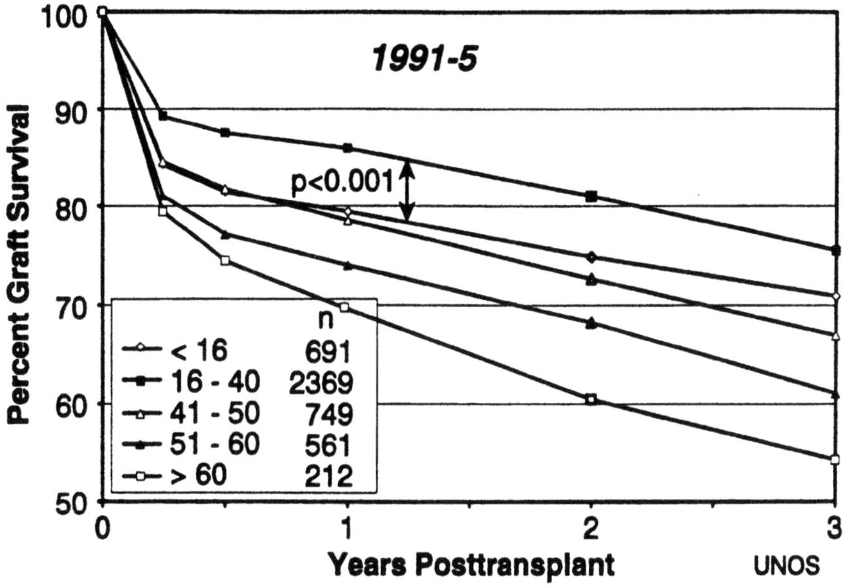

Fig. 15. Second graft survival according to donor age.

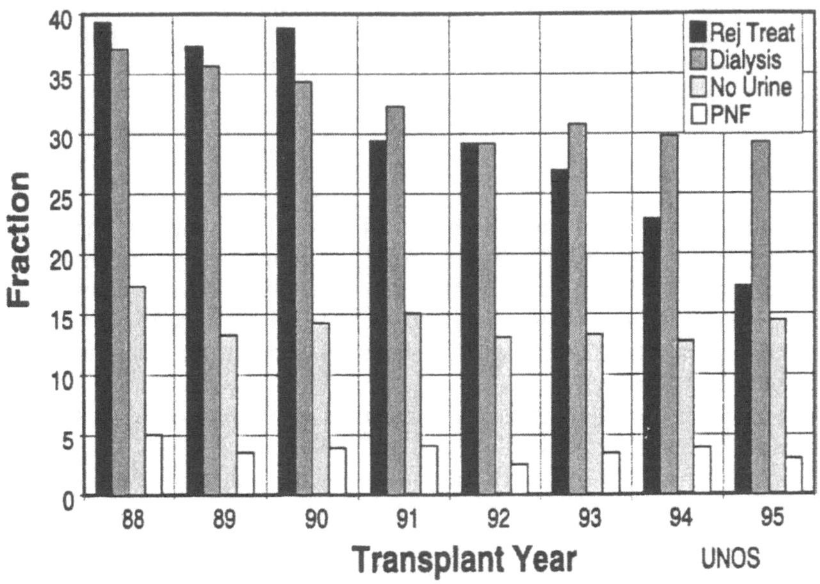

Fig. 16. Early graft function of second cadaver grafts.

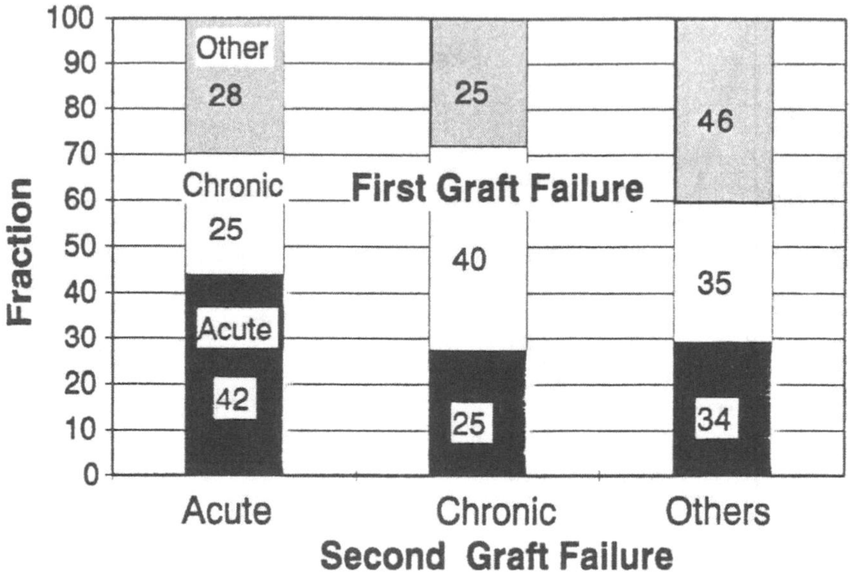

Fig. 17. Association between causes of first and second graft failures.

donor transplants after adjusting for all other factors (Table 1). The effect of longer waiting times following previous graft failure did not reach statistically significant levels after adjusting for other factors, and may have been confounded by sensitization.

Discussion

The major factors that influence second graft survival are similar to those that affect first grafts. Donor age is a very strong factor, as recently emphasized for cadaver grafts [4]. Transplants from donors older than 50 have almost twice the relative risk of those from younger donors. As in first grafts, HLA matching has a graded effect from best to worst mismatches. Presensitization as measured by PRA is also a factor.

The unique factors that influence second grafts are the previous graft survival time [1, 2, 3, 5] and the cause of the first graft failure. Transplants which failed after more than 2 years usually failed as a result of chronic rejection, thus linking these two influential factors. Interestingly, these patients with long previous graft survival times were apparently unaffected by the level of HLA mismatches in their second graft (Figure 11). These patients' immune systems may have become anergized by long exposure to the mismatched alloantigens of their first grafts, as mismatched regrafts survived at the same rate as matched regrafts.

Table 1. Cox proportional hazard analysis

Factors	Relative risk	*p* value
Donor age (year)		
<16	1.37	0.007
16–40	1.0	
41–50	1.46	<0.001
>50	1.93	<0.001
No. of HLA-A, B, DR antigen mismatched		
0	1.0	
1,2	1.23	0.164
3,4	1.42	0.010
5,6	1.70	<0.001
Previous graft survival time		
>2 years	1.0	
6 months–2 years	1.56	<0.001
1 month–6 months	1.62	<0.001
<1 month	1.34	0.012
Peak panel reactive antibody		
0–80%	1.0	
>80%	1.30	0.001
Cause of first graft failure		
Acute rejection	1.26	0.010
Other causes	1.0	
Waiting time for regraft		
>3 years	1.0	
1–3 years	1.17	0.092
<1 year	1.19	0.133

From the evidence provided here, it appears that much of the improvement in second graft survival seen in recent years is the result of selecting patients whose first graft had longer graft survival times. This selection is likely to be deliberate on the part of transplant physicians. In order to obtain the best survival of the valuable cadaver donor resource, this policy can probably be justified.

Summary

Second cadaver donor grafts had exhibited an improvement in one-year graft survival from 56% in 1981 to 83% in 1995. One of the strongest factors influencing second graft survival was the previous graft survival time. The one-year graft survival was 87% for second grafts in patients with a first graft survival of more than 2 years. An important reason for increased regraft survival with time has been the increased selection of patients with long surviving first grafts. More than half of the patients who received a second graft in 1995 had first grafts that survived more than 2 years. Patients who lost their first graft as a result of chronic rejection had a 87% one-year graft survival rate compared with 72% for those who lost their first grafts to acute rejection.

In univariate analyses, patients who received zero ABDR antigen mismatched transplants had the highest survival of 88% at one year and 79% at 3 years. The corresponding value for 5 or 6 ABDR mismatched grafts was 75% and 64%. Patients who lost their first grafts as a result of chronic rejection had high second graft survival despite the level of ABDR mismatches. Among patients who lost their first grafts as a result of acute rejection, only those with zero ABDR mismatches had higher survival. Patients who had 0–20% PPRA had a one-year graft survival rate of 84% compared with 76% for those with 81–100% PRA. The lowest graft survival was noted in second grafts from donors aged 60 or more. Their one-year graft survival rate was 70% and their 3-year survival was 54%. This contrasted the 86% one-year graft survival rate and 75% 3-year graft survival for donors aged 16–40. Waiting time for a second graft following a first graft loss was significant in the univariate analysis, but not statistically significant in the multivariate Cox regression analysis. All the other previously mentioned factors important in the univariate analyses were also significant in the multivariate analysis.

References

1. Cho YW, Terasaki PI. Cadaver-donor renal retransplants. In: Terasaki PI, Cecka JM (eds.), Clinical Transplants 1993, Los Angeles, UCLA Tissue Typing Laboratory 1994; 469–484.
2. Hirata M, Terasaki PI. Renal retransplantation. In: Terasaki PI, Cecka JM (eds.), Clinical Transplants 1994, Los Angeles, UCLA Tissue Typing Laboratory 1995; 419–433.
3. Imagawa DK, Cecka JM. Renal regrafts. In: Terasaki PI and Cecka JM (eds), Clinical Transplants 1988, Los Angeles, UCLA Tissue Typing Laboratory 1989; 387–398.
4. Terasaki PI, Gjertson DW, Cecka JM et al. Significance of the donor age effect on kidney transplants. Clin. Transplant. (in press).
5. Heise ER, Thacker LR, MacQueen JM, Peters TG. Repeated HLA mismatches and second renal graft survival in centers of the South-Eastern Organ Procurement Foundation. Clin. Transplant. 1996; 10: 579–585.

10. Retransplantation in aged patients

F. OPPENHEIMER

An increase in the risk factors influencing renal transplant survival has been observed over the last few years. Among them, one must consider the age of recipients and retransplanted patients.

Objective

To determine the influence of age on patient and graft survival in kidney retransplanted patients.

Subjects

1133 patients receiving a cadaver kidney transplant between 1978 and 1996 (973 first transplants and 160 retransplants). Third transplants, living related donors and combined kidney-pancreas transplants were excluded.

Methods

Patients were grouped according to number of transplants (1st or 2nd) and age range (<20, 20–39, 40–59, >60). Kaplan–Meier analysis and the Mantel–Henzel test were used to estimate and compare patient and graft survival. Infection rates were analysed with chi-square and Fisher's exact test.

Results

One and five year survival was the same in first (93.3% and 86.6%) and second (90.2% and 83.4%) transplants. Similarly, there were no significant differences in graft survival (78.4% and 62.7% versus 83.2% and 64.5% respectively). However, patient age was a significant negative factor: in 54 recipients between the ages of 40 to 59 years, one and five year patient (77.3% and 65.5%) and graft (65.4% and 50.7%) survival was significantly worse than between the ages of 20 and 39 years (96.1% and 89.9% patient, and 96.4% and 67.7% graft one and five year survival).

Infection (50%) was the most common cause of early death (in the first year), whereas liver failure (58%) was responsible for most long term fatalities. In first time transplants, early infection (36%) and cardiovascular complications (40%) were the main causes of death. The incidence of death secondary to

J.L. Touraine et al. (eds.), Retransplantation, 79–80.

infection was significantly higher in retransplanted patients over the age of 40 (41% versus 22% for younger patients).

Conclusion

The combination of age over 40 and retransplantation represents a high risk, with significant negative implications in terms of patients and graft survival. A difficult situation develops in balancing the need for aggressive immunosuppression in retransplanted patients (to counteract their increased immune response), and the increased susceptibility to infection in older patients.

11. Organ retransplantation in inherited inborn of metabolism

PIERRE COCHAT, NEVILLE V. JAMIESON, LAURENCE DUBOURG, JANUSZ FEBER & PAULO C. KOCH NOGUEIRA

Introduction

From the clinical point of view, the conditions associated with recurrence in the transplanted kidney can be classified into 3 groups: (i) inherited inborn errors of metabolism (IEM), (ii) systemic diseases with multiple organ involvement and (iii) glomerulonephritis [1]. Organ transplantation has been introduced during the last 15 years as a possible therapy of IEM. Such a management requires an accurate diagnosis, an early intervention in most cases and a precise knowledge of the biochemical defect. Because of the possible consequences and risks of transplantation, the place of organ replacement is the following issue of conventional therapy of IEM, i.e. treatment at the clinical phenotype level, at the metabolic level and at the dysfunctional protein level [2]. In most cases, transplantation provides the normal protein in its physiological cellular and subcellular locations with respect to its substrates and cosubstrates. Four main conditions can be considered (Tables 1 and 2): (1) transplantation as a

Table 1. Rationale for liver transplantation (LTx) in some examples of inborn errors of metabolism [1]

Primary disease	LTx as a protein source	LTx for hepatic failure	Associated risk of malignancy
α1-anti-trypsin deficiency	+	+	+
Criggler–Najjar I	+		
Cystic fibrosis		+	
Hypercholesterolemia	+		
Galactosemia	+	+	+
Glycogen storage disease I–IV	+	+	+
Hemochromatosis		+	+
L-cholesterol-acyl-transferase deficiency	+		
Ornithine transcarbamylase deficiency	+		
Primary hyperoxaluria I	+		
Protein C deficiency	+		
Protoporphyria	+	+	
Tyrosinemia I	+	+	+
Wilson disease	+	+	+

J.L. Touraine et al. (eds.), Retransplantation, 81–88.

Table 2. Examples of combined organ transplantation (Tx) in inherited inborn errors of metabolism [1]

Primary disease	Organ Tx as a protein source	Associated Tx as replacement of damaged organs					
Primary hyperoxaluria I	Liver	Kidney					
Glycogen storage disease	Liver	Kidney	Heart				
α1-antitrypsine deficiency	Liver		Heart	Lung			
Hypercholesterolemia	Liver	Kidney	Heart				
L-CAT deficiency	Liver	Kidney					Cornea
Tyrosinemia I	Liver	Kidney	(Heart)				
Hemochromatosis	(Liver)		Heart			Pancreas	
Diabetes mellitus	Pancreas	Kidney	Heart				
Cystinosis		Kidney				Pancreas	Cornea
Cystic fibrosis			Heart	Lung	Liver		

replacement of an isolated damaged target organ, such as kidney in nephropathic cystinosis or heart in familial hypercholesterolemia; (2) transplantation as a source for a deficient protein such as displacement marrow transplantation in lysosomal storage diseases or orthotopic liver transplantation in primary hyperoxaluria type 1 (PH1); (3) transplantation as a concommittent protein source and replacement of damaged organ, such as liver transplantation in α1-antitrypsin deficiency or tyrosinemia type 1; (4) in cases of combined transplantation, another organ has to be grafted as a replacement of the damaged native one, such as liver + heart in familial hypercholesterolemia or liver + kidney in PH1 [2]. According to the mechanism of IEM, such a treatment may be palliative (kidney in cystinosis or PH1, lung in cystic fibrosis) or curative (liver in ornithine transcarbamylase deficiency, tyrosinemia type 1 or PH1). Theoretically, isolated organ transplantation is capable to bring the deficient activity; however the intrinsic risk of transplantation has allowed to wait for multiorgan failure before transplanting both the damaged organ and the source of deficient protein. In the whole cases, it has been shown that the isolated replacement of a damaged organ cannot be successful if the protein source is not restored at the same time or by a previous transplantation. The choice for an optimal timing remains an acute problem since the source of enzyme – mainly the liver – is always normally functioning except the specific deficiency [1]. The timing will be given by the degree of deterioration of the most damaged target-organ. In such condition, the organ replacement will be either early when recovery is possible, or late after end-stage organ involvement has occurred.

Kidney transplantation is not considered as a protein source but as the replacement of a damaged organ. In most cases, the native kidneys are the main target organs of the disease, but isolated renal transplantation may be involved by the recurrence of a multisystemic disease if enzyme replacement has not previously been performed; a good example is provided by primary hyperoxaluria type 1 [2]. In some other situations, kidney replacement is a part of the treatment of systemic involvement without localized enzyme deficiency, like cystinosis.

Heart and lung transplantation may be required in IEM, since they represent target organs in some diseases (familial hypercholesterolemia, cystic fibrosis, α1 anti-trypsin deficiency).

The problem of retransplantation

Retransplantation must be considered in IEM when rejection has lead to graft loss or when the recurrent metabolic defect has damaged the transplant. In cases of late onset recurrence of the primary IEM (Fabry's disease, lecithine cholesterol acyltransferase deficiency, sickle cell disease), the same organ – usually the kidney – may be retransplanted; this condition is often related to a systemic metabolic defect. In case of early onset recurrent IEM (PH1, familial hypercholesterolemia), both the damaged organ and the protein source, usually the liver, must be transplanted. Some IEM (such as cystinosis) are not associated with the risk of recurrence.

Primary hyperoxaluria type 1

PH1 is the most common condition where retransplantation is required on the basis of the consequences of a protein deficiency (alanine: glyoxylate aminotransferase, AGT). There has been recent advances in the understanding and management of the disease [2]. Because of the rarity of the disease, no controlled information on large series of patients is available upon which therapeutic decisions could be based. Nevertheless, some rational strategies have emerged from recent insights into the pathogenesis.

Prognosis of the disease

Prognosis is generally poor and 30–50% of patients reach end-stage renal failure by 15 years of age. The median age at the beginning of renal replacement therapy is 25 years. Past experience with isolated renal transplantation has mostly, but not universally, been negative. The availability of liver transplantation has provided a novel form of enzyme substitution therapy. Although combined renal and hepatic transplantation is indicated in most cases, no clear consensus regarding transplant strategy has emerged, some authors advocating isolated kidney transplantation, others combined liver-kidney transplantation and others even isolated liver transplantation [3–9]. Selection of the correct procedure requires some insight into the underlying principles, and we speculate that there is not one treatment for one disease but adapted treatments for individual patients.

Basis of transplantation strategy

Before considering organ transplantation, it is essential to prove the diagnosis enzymologically and to test pyridoxine responsiveness. A second step is the assessment of oxalate storage [10]. Third, one must have a clear target for therapy: kidney transplantation will correct end-stage renal failure, liver transplantation will correct the metabolic defect (even before significant renal damage has occurred) and combined liver-kidney transplantation will correct both the enzyme defect and the renal failure. Whatever the procedure, early transplantation should be planned while the patient still has some residual renal function and is not seriously and irreversibly incapacitated by systemic oxalosis.

Experience with kidney transplantation

More than 100 isolated kidney transplantations have been performed worldwide. This procedure does not reliably prevent recurrent nephrocalcinosis: massive elimination of oxalate from a pool of accumulated oxalate adds to unabated endogenous production [6]. Some recipients develop oxalate stones or nephrocalcinosis in the graft, others do not and the amount of oxalate accumulated in the graft is variable [3, 10]. In Europe, allograft survival at 3 years was 23% for recipients of grafts from living related donors (15 patients) and 17% for recipients of grafts from cadaver donors (79 patients); 3 year patient survival was no more than 26% [11]. Similar poor data were reported by the North American Pediatric Registry Transplant Cooperative Study [12]. Our French experience includes 15 recipients of cadaveric donor grafts with more than 1 year follow-up: only 1 patients has a functioning graft, 6 have died, 5 had subsequently received combined liver-kidney transplantation and the others are on regular haemodialysis [2].

Role of liver transplantation

The liver is the only organ in which glyoxylate is transformed to alanine by AGT, so that interconversion of glyoxylate to oxalate is prevented. It is therefore necessary not only to transplant the donor liver and to provide enzyme replacement therapy, but also to remove the host liver deficient in AGT [13, 14]. It follows from the above that partial or auxiliary liver transplantation will not be of significant benefit, quite apart from its technical difficulties. It is of interest that overall results of liver transplantation for IEM are better than those of liver transplantation performed to treat liver failure [1].

Results of combined liver and kidney transplantation

Between 1984 and 1996, 81 PH1 patients in Europe received 87 liver grafts [15]; the mean age at transplantation was 17.3 ± 11.7 years (range 1.0–50.7). The type of liver transplant performed was the following: orthotopic with simultaneous kidney 68, orthotopic reduced with simultaneous kidney 8, orthotopic alone 7, orthotopic reduced alone 2, orthotopic alone with delayed kidney 1, auxiliary partial orthotopic with simultaneous kidney 1. Actuarial graft and patient survival was 87% at 1 year and patient survival at 5 years was 79%. Fifty-nine patients received no prior renal transplant whereas 30 previous isolated kidney grafts (4 were from living donors) were performed in 22 patients (16 patients received 1 graft, 5 patients received 2 grafts and 1 patient received 4 grafts). There was definite recurrence of oxalosis in 20 cases; several kidneys never functioned, including most of the remaining 10, and oxalate was presumed to have been a major component. According to this European experience the indication for combined liver-kidney transplantation is in (i) infants with severe primary hyperoxaluria type 1, (ii) retransplantation due to failure of a previous isolated kidney graft, (iii) first-line treatment of patients on dialysis, and (iv) first-line treatment of patients with advanced renal failure.

In contrast to patients with isolated kidney transplantation, those with combined liver-kidney transplantation do not experience the slow and relentless deterioration of their renal grafts, with the exception of the occasional patients who have been on dialysis for a long time, have acquired a large oxalate burden and experience prolonged elimination of high amounts of oxalate.

The problem of retransplantation

In patients who were first elected for isolated renal transplantation, there is no rationale to consider retransplantation of the kidney alone after graft loss due to recurrence of the disease. In those patients, combined liver-kidney transplantation must be scheduled before end-stage renal failure has occurred because of the risk and the timing should consider the increased risks associated, i.e. when the GFR has dropped to 30–20 ml/min/1.73 m^2.

It seems that correct therapeutic decisions require great experience with this rare condition; this requirement is only met if such patients are treated in specialized centres.

Other inborn errors of metabolism

In other conditions of localized protein deficiency, the replacement of the damaged graft due to recurrence of the primary disease should be associated with enzyme replacement therapy. According to the clinical course of the disease, isolated heart (and/or kidney) transplantation may be proposed to patients with familial hypercholesterolemia as a first step. In case of early recurrence of the disease or in case of associated severe lesions, liver transplantation should be proposed together with heart (and/or kidney) retransplantation.

In most cases of systemic metabolic defect, retransplantation might be required after late onset recurrence of the disease.

Fabry's disease

Anderson–Fabry's disease is a rare, sex-linked recessive disorder of glycosphingolipid metabolism characterized by the accumulation of ceramide trihexoside in many tissues. It is caused by a deficiency of a specific enzyme α-galactosidase A and results in accelerated cardiovascular disease and progressive renal failure. The recurrence of the ceramide accumulation in the kidney graft may cause graft loss. Limited histological recurrences can be seen but their clinical relevance is limited [16–18].

Sickle cell disease

Sickle cell anemia results from a single amino acid substitution at position 6 of the hemoglobin locus for the sickle cell gene. It has been reported to be responsible for 0.32% of renal transplant recipients in one series [19]. There may be 2 pathways to graft failure related to sickle cell disease: one can result from an acute vaso-occlusive crisis leading to early failure or renal vascular thrombosis, the other can follow a more indolent course that recapitulates the primary injury, either in homozygous or in heterozygous patients. Because of the very late onset of the recurrence, one can speculate that kidney retransplantation is available. However, the prognosis of the disease will be given at this stage by extrarenal involvement, like stroke or cardiac failure.

Other IEM may lead to retransplantation

Retransplantation of the damaged target organ may be available for chronic renal failure in lecithin cholesterol acyltransferase deficiency syndrome [20], acute porphyria [21], mannosidosis [22], etc. In some cases, there is no risk of recurrent disease in the target damaged organ.

In nephropathic cystinosis, a disease which is caused by a local lysosomal storage disorder, patient and graft survival is equal or better than in non-cystinotic patients [23, 24]. Cystine crystals are present in graft-infiltrating cells, but do not seem to affect kidney allograft function [25]. In the long term, patient's survival and quality of life may be compromized by extrarenal involvement, i.e. hypothyroidism, diabetes mellitus, vision disturbances and brain atrophy [23, 25]. In the next future, we can speculate that the wide use of cystine-depleting agents will delay the need for renal replacement therapy and the consequences of extrarenal involvement.

Conclusion

Apart from graft loss due to allograft rejection, there are two main conditions leading to retransplantation in inborn errors of metabolism: (i) in case of late onset recurrence of the primary disease, retransplantation of the target organ is available whereas (ii) in case of early recurrence, retransplantation of the damaged organ should be avoided and concommittent replacement of both the protein source and the target organ is required. In the latter condition, a combined transplantation is therefore recommended as a first step treatment in order to avoid morbidity associated to retransplantation.

References

1. Cochat P, Guibaud P. Principles of organ transplantation in inborn errors of metabolism. In: Touraine JL et al. (eds.), Transplantation and Clinical Immunology XXII. Amsterdam: Elsevier Science, 1991: 73–81.
2. Cochat P, Mahmoud A. Transplantation in primary hyperoxaluria type 1. Nephrol Dial Transplant. 1995; 10: 1293–1296.
3. Katz A, Mauer SM. Transplantation in primary hyperoxaluria type 1. Am. J. Med. 1992; 92: 341–342.
4. Scheinman JI, Najarian JS, Mauer SM. Successful strategies for renal transplantation in primary oxalosis. Kidney Int. 1984; 25: 804–811.
5. Thervet E, Legendre C, Daudon M et al. Is there a place for isolated renal transplantation in the treatment of type 1 primary hyperoxaluria? Experience from Paris. Nephrol. Dial. Transplant. In press.
6. Watts RWE, Calne RY, Rolles K et al. Successful treatment of primary hyperoxaluria type 1 by combined hepatic and renal transplantation. Lancet 1987; 2: 474–475.
7. Cochat P, Schärer K. Should liver transplantation be performed before advanced renal insufficiency in primary hyperoxaluria type 1? Pediatr. Nephrol. 1993; 7: 212–218.
8. Haffner D, Cochat P, Otto G, Steffen H, Schärer K. When should isolated liver transplantation be performed in hyperoxaluria type 1? Follow-up report of two children. Nephrol. Dial. Transplant. 1995; 10: 47–52.
9. Cochat P, Faure JL, Divry P et al. Liver transplantation in primary hyperoxaluria type 1. Lancet 1989; 1: 1142–1143.
10. Watts RWE. Treatment of primary hyperoxaluria type 1. J. Nephrol. 1994; 7: 208–214.
11. Broyer M, Brunner FP, Brynger H et al. Kidney transplantation in primary oxalosis: data from the EDTA Registry. Nephrol. Dial. Transplant. 1990; 5: 332–336.
12. Scheinman JI, Alexander M, Campbell ED, Chan JC, Latta K, Cochat P. Transplantation for primary hyperoxaluria in the USA. Nephrol. Dial. Transplant. 1995; 10: 42–46.
13. Watts RWE, Mansell MA. Oxalate, livers, and kidneys. Combined renal and hepatic transplants transform the outlook in primary hyperoxaluria type 1. Br. J. Med. 1990; 301: 772–773.
14. Danpure CJ, Jennings PR. Peroxisomal alanine: glyoxylate aminotransferase deficiency in primary hyperoxaluria type 1. FEBS Lett. 1986; 201: 20–24.
15. Jamieson NV. PH1 Transplant Registry Report 1984–1997. Fourth Workshop on Primary Hyperoxaluria, Torino, 7–8 March 1997.
16. Michielsen P. Recurrence of the original disease. Does it influence graft failure? Kidney Int. 1995; 48 (Suppl. 52): S79–S84.
17. Friedlander MM, Kopolovic J, Rubinger D et al. Renal biopsy in Fabry's disease eight years after successful renal transplantation. Clin. Nephrol. 1987; 27: 206–211.
18. Mosnier JF, Degott C, Bedrossian J et al. Recurrence of Fabry's disease in a renal allograft eleven years after successful renal transplantation. Transplantation 1991; 51: 759–762.

19. Montgomery R, Zibari G, Hill GS, Ratner LE. Renal transplantation in sickle cell nephropathy. Transplantation 1994; 58: 618–620.
20. Horina JH, Wirnsberger G, Horn S et al. Long term follow-up of a patient with lecithin cholesterol acyltransferase deficiency syndrome after kidney transplantation. Transplantation 1993; 56: 233–236.
21. Nunez DJ, Williams PF, Herrick AL, Evans DB, MacColl KEL. Renal transplantation for chronic renal failure in acute porphyria. Nephrol. Dial. Transplant. 1987; 2: 271–274.
22. Segoloni GP, Colla L, Messina M, Stratta P. Renal transplantation in a case of mannosidosis. Transplantation 96; 61: 1654–1655.
23. Ehrich JHH, Brodehl J, Byrd DI et al. Renal transplantation in 22 children with nephropathic cystinosis. Pediatr. Nephrol. 1991; 5: 708–714.
24. Kashtan CE, McEnery PT, Tejani A, Stablein DM. Renal allograft survival according to primary diagnosis: a report of the North American Pediatric Renal Transplant Cooperative Study. Pediatr Nephrol 1995; 9: 679–684.
25. Almond PS, Matas A, Nakhleh RE et al. Renal transplantation for infantile cystinosis: long-term follow-up. J. Pediatr. Surg. 1993; 28: 232–238.

PART THREE

Immunology of retransplantation and immunosuppression

12. Immunological pathways of rejection in sensitized recipients

KATHRYN J. WOOD

Introduction

In allotransplantation the common causes of sensitization are blood transfusion, pregnancy and rejection of an allograft. An additional route of sensitization that should not be overlooked is the potential crossreactivity of T cells responding to enviromental antigens or pathogens that may be able to cross react with alloantigens expressed by the antigen presenting cells (APC) within an organ graft. In this situation the T cells of the host would be sensitized to the alloantigens of the organ donor even though the donor alloantigens themselves had not been encountered previously. The frequency of crossreactive T cells present in a recipient and their contribution to the rejection of allografts is extremely difficult to assess with the tools currently available.

Sensitization by whatever route will result in the activation of both the innate and adaptive arms of the immune response. The inevitable consequence of this activation process (see below) is that when the same antigen, or one that is cross reactive, is encountered for a second time a more rapid and augmented immune response involving both the innate and adaptive arms will occur.

The rejection of a graft by a presensitized host are a complex process. The dynamics of the rejection process can vary depending on the status of both the recipient and the graft. Thus the precise contribution of different components of the response will be different in different circumstances. For example, if preformed antibodies to major histocompatibility (MHC) antigens expressed by the graft or the graft endothelial cells are present in the recipient at the time of transplantion rejection of the graft can occur within minutes after reanastomosis [1, 2]. Whereas if transplantation is performed in an individual who has a current negative but previously positive crossmatch rejection may still occur in an accelerated time frame within the first few days after transplantation. The former process is known as hyperacute rejection and the latter is most frequently referred to as accelerated rejection.

Overview of the rejection response in naive recipients

As a framework for understanding the rejection response in hosts already sensitized to the alloantigens of the donor by whatever means the cellular and

J.L. Touraine et al. (eds.), Retransplantation, 91–96.

molecular events that ultimately result in graft destruction in naive recipients will be considered first.

The immunological nature of graft rejection was established more than 40 years ago when Medawar and his colleagues observed that skin grafts transplanted between genetically disparate rabbits underwent rapid necrotic changes and were eventually sloughed off (e.g. [3]). Our understanding of this immunological process is still developing as more information is obtained from analysing the individual events involved and as understanding of the events that occur during normal physiological immune responses to foreign antigens evolves [4]. The rejection process can be divided into two arms, afferent and efferent. The afferent response involves the activation of the immune system as a result of recognition of the foreign histocompatibility antigens (alloantigens) of the organ donor of the graft. The efferent arm occurs as a later event and results from the triggering of the humoral and cellular effector mechanisms of the immune system; it is these that are ultimately responsible for the destruction and elimination of the transplant.

In brief, donor alloantigens are presented directly to recipient T lymphocytes by immunostimulatory APC or passenger leukocytes present within transplanted tissues. The number and phenotype of these APCs present varies between organs [5]. After transplantation the passenger leukoctyes migrate from the graft to the host lymphoid tissue [6]. It is believed that primary sensitization of the host to the donor alloantigens occurs centrally in the host lymphoid tissue as a result of the migration and maturation of the passenger cells [7]. Thus direct presentation of donor alloantigens to recipient T cells is the primary route of antigen recognition in a naive host. As the response progresses APCs of donor and host origin will participate in the rejection process presenting alloantigens directly and indirectly to T cells respectively [8].

T cells are essential for the rejection of primary grafts [9–11]. APCs of both donor and recipient origin are thought to be involved in triggering the activation of allospecific helper T cells (T_H) [8, 12, 13]. The T_H population influences both qualitative and quantitative aspects of the response [14–16]. Following antigen recognition by a T cell receptor (TCR), an activation signal is delivered to the T cell via the CD3 complex (signal 1). In addition to signals through the TCR itself additional interactions and signals, referred to as costimulation or signal 2, have to be delivered to trigger full T cell activation [17]. The T cell then blast transforms and begins to produce a number of new cell surface and soluble molecules.

The cell surface molecules are referred to as activation antigens, as they are only expressed by T cells following activation and include molecules that both augment and down regulate the response. In the former category are adhesion molecules that will promote cellular interactions and expression of cytokine receptors, such as CD25, the α chain of the interleukin-2 receptor (IL-2R) that are required for the generation of effector cells. Other molecules, for example

CTLA4 are expressed after T cell activation and have been shown to limit the duration of the response after activation [18]. The soluble molecules belong to a family of mediators known as cytokines [19], and include interleukin-2 (IL-2) and gamma interferon (IFNγ). The microenvironment at the time of T cell activation will determine the precise nature of the T_H population that predominates in the response. T_H1 cytokine phenotype is characteristic of the rejection response in naive recipients [20].

As a result of both direct cell contact and cytokine mediated interactions the T_H cells trigger the effector arm of the response. The cellular events supported by activated T_H cells include (i) the triggering of the maturation of cytotoxic precursor cells into mature cytotoxic T cells (T_C) with cytotoxic or killing potential towards target cells expressing the appropriate alloantigen; (ii) the growth and differentiation of B cells that produce antibody reactive against the transplant; (iii) the activation of macrophages that can develop cytocidal activity; (iv) an increase in the lytic potential of natural killer cells; (v) the attraction of other leukocytes to the site of the immune activation resulting in amplification of the response and (vi) the increased expression and induction of MHC antigens and other molecules, such as adhesion molecules on the transplanted organ. The relative contribution of each of these effector mechanisms to graft destruction is still hotly debated and may vary depending on the status of the recipient's immune system before transplantation.

Rejection in sensitized recipients

Hyperacute rejection results in the rapid destruction of the graft as a result of preformed antibodes binding to antigens expressed by the transplanted tissue, in particular by the endothelial cells within the graft. As a result of antibody binding a number of changes occur including activation of complement. This will result in the release of inflammatory mediators, such as C5a, initiating the rapid infiltration of inflammatory cells including eosinophils and polymorphonuclear leukocytes into the graft. The release of inflammatory mediators by the infiltrating cells, will further activate the endothelial cells causing them to upregulate adhesion molecules very rapidly thereby augmenting infiltration of the graft by leukcoytes. In addition, the activation of complement will result in the activation of other pathways that contribute to innate immunity that are present in the plasma, including the coagulation and kinin systems [4]. All of these changes result in the highly characteristic pathology of grafts undergoing hyperacute rejection observed both in experimental studies and in clinical transplantation [21]. These include injury to the microvasculature with the formation of platelet thrombi, aggregates of red blood cells deposition of fibrin and the infiltration of polymorphonuclear leukocytes.

As histocompatiblity laboratories routinely screen and document the MHC antibody status of recipients on transplant waiting lists hyperacute rejection due to anti-HLA antibodies is now observed only very rarely after allotransplantation. However, most laboratories do not screen routinely for anti-endothelial cell antibodies thus is some cases rejection can still be initiated by preformed antibodies to endothelial cells. Renewed interest in xenotransplantation has also stimulated further analysis of the processes occuring during hyperacute rejection [22].

Inflammation always occurs after transplantation as a consequence of organ harvesting and storage as well as the surgical procedure itself. The death of cells in the transplanted organ due to ischaemic injury and the wound healing process that is triggered by the surgery will inevitably result in infiltration by mononuclear cells and activation of the endothelial cells of the graft. The magnitude of this response will vary considerably depending on the time between organ harvesting and transplantation and nature of the transplant procedure itself.

In naive recipients the influence of inflammatory response on the rejection process although still undesirable is less significant than in sensitized recipients as the leukocytes that participate in the adaptive arm of the response have yet to be activated to respond to the donor alloantigens. In sensitized recipients even in the absence of preformed antibodies the rapid infiltration of a wide variety of leukocytes into the graft can have potentially serious consequences. Polymorphonulear leukocytes will be triggered to release inflammotory meidators such as IL-1 and TNF and as a consequence the endothelial cells of the graft will themselves be activated.

The requirements for the initiation of secondary immune responses are thought to be much less stringent than those for primary responses. In a primary immune response only specialized populations of APCs most widely believed to be dendritic cells are thought to be capable of triggering T cell activation [23]. Indeed endothelial cells within the graft may switch naive T cells off rather than on [24]. In contrast, in sensitized recipients any cell expressing the appropriate MHC peptide complex can effectively present antigen and trigger T cells to respond. Thus in the latter situation the endothelial cells of the graft will be capable of presenting alloantigens directly to host T cells in addition to the passenger leukocytes. The indirect pathway of allorecognition will also be relatively more important in sensitized recipients as B cells and macrophages of host origin will all be capable of presenting processed alloantigenic peptides to host T cells. For example, in a sensitized recipient B cells may express cell surface immunoglobulin receptors specific for alloantigens expressed by the transplanted tissue thereby facilitating processing and presentation of allopeptides. Thus the overall frequency of T cells responding to the donor alloantigens will be much higher than in naive hosts. Moreover, the threshold for T cell activation is lower in sensitized recipients where the T cells are already primed [25]. Sensitized T cells express cell surface molecules such as CD40L that can participate in T cell costimulation.

As a result of antigen presentation by endothelial cells T cell activation will take place within the graft rather than centrally in the lymphoid tissue. This will potentially provide a source of cytokines and of effector cells and molecules in situ. As one of the most important features of the activity of cytokines is that they act over short distances within local microenvironments, production of effector cytokines within the organ graft itself may have a dramatic effect on graft function. The kinetics of cytokine production in grafts transplanted into sensitized recipients has been documented in a cardiac allograft model in rats [26]. Both the kinetics and repertoire of cytokines produced is distinct from that found within grafts transplanted into unsensitized recipients.

Endothelial cell activation may be triggered by the binding of anti-endothelial cell antibodies or as a result of the infiltration by mononuclear cells and release of chemokines [27]. Activation of endothelial cells in the graft will also trigger the upregulation of adhesion molecules thereby augmenting leukocyte infiltration and transmigration into the tissue.

The precise effector mechanism or mechanisms responsible for graft destruction in sensitized recipients is a source of major debate. A number of immune effector mechanisms have been shown to be capable of destroying an organ graft in experimental systems, including the T_C, DTH reactions, NK cells, antibody dependent cell mediated cytotoxicity (ADCC) and complement dependent antibody mediated cytotoxicity. The relative contribution of the different effector mechanism is certainly different when rejection in naive and sensitized recipients is compared. For example in a mouse model $CD4^+$ T cells were shown to be dominant in the rejection of cardiac allografts transplanted into naive recipients [28], whereas $CD8^+$ T cells were more important in sensitized recipients [29]. The relative roles of each of these mechanisms may be different in each individual situation in sensitized recipients.

References

1. Kissmeyer-Nielsen F, Olsen S, Petersen V, Fjeldborg O. Hyperacute rejection of kidney allografts, associated with pre-existing humoral antibodies against donor cells. Lancet 1966; 2: 662–665.
2. Jordan S, Yap H, Sakai R, Alfonso P, Fitchman M. Hyperacute rejection mediated by anti-vascular endothelial cell antodies with a negative myocyte cross match. Transplantation 1988; 46: 585–587.
3. Medawar P. A second study of the behaviour and fate of skin homografts in rabbits. J. Anat. 1945; 79: 157–176.
4. Austyn J, Wood K. Principles of cellular and molecular immunology. Oxford University Press, 1993.
5. Wood K, Sachs D. Chimersim and transplantation tolerance: cause and effect. Immunol. Today 1996; 12: 584–587.
6. Larsen C, Morris P, Austyn J. Migration of dendritic leukocytes form cardiac allografts into host spleens: a novel pathway for initiation of rejection. J. Exp. Med. 1990; 171: 307–314.
7. Larsen C, Steinman R, Witmer-Pack M, Morris P, Austyn J. Migration and maturation of Langerhans cells in skin transplants and explants. J. Exp. Med. 1990; 172: 1483–1493.

8. Shoskes D, Wood K. Indirect presentation of MHC antigens in transplantation. Immunol. Today 1994; 15: 1–7.
9. Rolstad B, Ford WL. Immune responses of rats deficient in thymus-derived lymphocytes to strong transplantation antigens (Ag-B). Graft versus host activity, allograft rejection and the factor of immunisation. Transplantation 1974; 17: 405–415.
10. Rygaard J. Skin grafts in nude mice. Ann. Intern. Med. 1974; 82: 93–104.
11. Hall BM, Dorsch S, Roser B. The cellular basis of allograft rejection *in vivo*. I. The cellular requirements for first-set rejection of heart grafts. J. Exp. Med. 1978; 148: 878–889.
12. Lechler RI, Batchelor JR. Restoration of immunogenicity to passenger cell-depleted kidney allografts by the addition of donor strain dendritic cells. J. Exp. Med. 1982; 155: 31–41.
13. Austyn JM, Steinman RM. The passenger leukocyte – a fresh look. Transplant. Rev. 1988; 2: 139–176.
14. Loveland BE, Hogarth PM, Ceredig R, McKenzie IFC. Cells mediating graft rejection in the mouse. I. Lyt-1 cells mediate skin graft rejection. J. Exp. Med. 1981; 153: 1044–1057.
15. Dallman MJ, Mason DW, Webb M. The roles of host and donor cells in the rejection of skin allografts by T cell deprived rats injected with syngeneic T cells. Eur. J. Immunol. 1982; 12: 511–518.
16. Mosmann TR, Schumacher JH, Street NF et al. Diversity of cytokine synthesis and function of mouse CD4+ T cells. Immunol. Rev. 1991; 123: 209–229.
17. Schwartz RH. Costimulation of T lymphocytes: the role of CD28, CTLA-4, and B7/BB1 in interleukin-2 production and immunotherapy. Cell 1992; 71: 1065–1068.
18. Krummel M, Allison J. CD28 and CTLA-4 have opposing effects on the response of T cells to stimulation. J. Exp. Med. 1995; 182: 459–465.
19. Dallman MJ, Wood KJ, Hamano K et al. Cytokines in transplantation tolerance. Immunol. Rev. 1993; 133: 5–18.
20. Dallman MJ, Larsen CP, Morris PJ. Cytokine gene transcription in vascularised organ grafts: analysis using semiquantitative polymerase chain reaction. J. Exp. Med. 1991; 174: 493–496.
21. Hisatake G, Hammond E, Ives M, Griffith J, Shelby J, Eichwald EJ. Hyperacute rejection of the transplanted mouse heart. Transplantation 1989; 47: 996–1000.
22. Parker W, Saadi S, Lin S, Holzenecht Z, Bustos M, Platt J. Transplantation of discordant xenografts: a challenge revisited. Immunol. Today 1996; 17: 373–384.
23. Inaba K, Steinman RM. Resting and sensitized T lymphocytes exihibit distinct stimulatory requirements for growth and lymphokine release. J. Exp. Med. 1984; 160: 1711–1735.
24. Marelli-Berg F, Hargreaves R, Carmichael P, Dorling A, Lombardi G, Lechler R. Major histocompatibility complex class II-expressing endothelial cells induce allospecific nonresponsiveness in naive T cells. J. Exp. Med. 1996; 183: 1603–1612.
25. Kundig T, Shahinian A, Kawai K et al. Duration of TCR stimulation determines costimulatory requirement of T cells. Immunity 1996; 5: 41–52.
26. Hancock WW, Distefano R, Braun P, Schweizer RT, Tilney NL, Kupiec-Weglinski JW. Cyclosporine and anti-interleukin 2 receptor monoclonal antibody therapy supress accelerated rejection of rat cardiac allografts through different effector mechanisms. Transplantation 1990; 49: 416–421.
27. Mantovani A, Bussolino F, Introna M. Cytokine regulation of endothelial cell function: from molecular level to the bedside. Immunol. Today 1997; 18: 231–240.
28. Madsen JC, Peugh WN, Wood KJ, Morris PJ. The effect of anti-L3T4 monoclonal antibody on first-set rejection of murine cardiac allografts. Transplantation 1987; 44: 849–852.
29. Madsen JC, Wood KJ, Morris PJ. Effects of anti-L3T4 and anti-Lyt2 monoclonal antibody therapy on cardiac allograft survival in presensitised recipients. Transplant. Proc. 1989; 21: 1022.

13. Tolerance and cytokine profiles in sensitized transplant recipients

JOCHEN BINDER & JERZY W. KUPIEC-WEGLINSKI

Introduction

The immediate and fulminant rejection of human renal allografts in sensitized recipients was first described more than 30 years ago [1]. The process of hyperacute rejection, occurring within minutes or hours after revascularization, is thought to be primarily mediated by pre-existing anti-donor antibodies (Abs) [2]. That it has become rare in recent years is primarily ascribed to improved crossmatching techniques [3]. However, at present, over 20% of patients with end-stage renal disease on waiting transplant lists are considered highly sensitized. Apart from prior failed allografts, this may result from blood transfusions or pregnancies. These highly sensitized patients experience an increased rate of graft rejection, compared to unsensitized individuals, which is often irreversible and unresponsive to currently used immunosuppressive therapy.

The initial concept was that allograft rejection in sensitized hosts is driven primarily by the humoral component of the alloresponse. Current knowledge, however, emphasizes the interdependency of the humoral and the cellular responses, and recognizes a key role for T cells, primarily of the CD4-positive phenotype, as well as macrophages in initiating and controlling B cell differentiation and Ig production through elaboration of a number of cytokine mediators.

The terminology of transplant rejection in sensitized patients and in experimental settings is not uniform. Some clinicians define hyperacute rejection as an irreversible deterioration and cessation of allograft function within the first days after transplantation; others have described its occurrence within minutes after revascularization of the organ. Some investigators have arbitrarily established transplant rejection within 24 h as 'hyperacute', whereas those lost during the first few days are said to have been rejected in an 'accelerated' manner [4]. However, as both pathologic and immunologic patterns are largely similar in these two processes, local factors and variations in balance between a multitude of mechanisms seem to determine the speed of rejection. In any case, as the cascade of immune events leading to graft destruction in sensitized recipients differs from the acute process in unsensitized hosts not only in its rapid time course, but in its unique interaction of humoral and cellular alloresponses, the strategies for tolerance induction in this setting are thought to be equally distinct.

J.L. Touraine et al. (eds.), Retransplantation, 97–105.

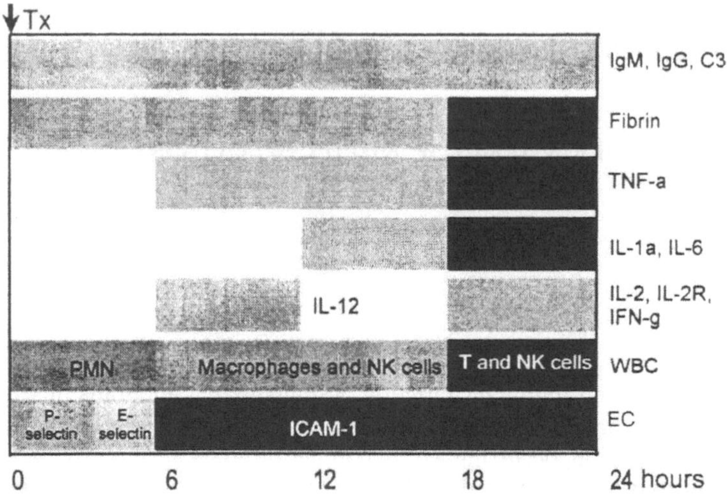

Fig. 1. Time course of events resulting in accelerated (< 24 h) rejection of cardiac allografts in sensitized rat recipients. Increasing densities of indicator bars provide a qualitative assessment of the intensity and/or extent of labeling for a given cell, cytokine, or humoral factor. Adapted from [8].

Allograft rejection in sensitized graft recipients

Preformed cytotoxic Abs, binding to Ags on donor endothelium, as well as the complement, coagulation, and kinin cascades are instrumental for the rejection response in sensitized recipients. In addition, host cellular immune mechanisms appear to play an equally important role.

Macroscopic and histologic changes in grafts undergoing rejection in sensitized recipients are characteristic, regardless of the organ studied. For instance, hearts rejected within 24 h by presensitized rats and mice become distended and cyanotic. The histology reveals widespread edema and massive vascular engorgement [5–7]. Interstitial hemorrhage and formation of platelet microthrombi in small vessels only are the hallmark lesion. In renal grafts, aggregates of fibrin, erythrocytes and platelet microthrombi are found, along with accumulating polymorphonuclear neutrophils (PMN) within glomeruli, juxtaglomerular arterioles, and intertubular capillaries. Prominent features are platelet aggregation and increase in leukocytes in glomerular and peritubular capillaries.

The events during development of accelerated (<24 h) rejection of (LEW × BN)F1 rat cardiac in sensitized LEW recipients are summarized in Figure 1 [8]. Morphologically, sections of cardiac transplants collected at 6 hr show a considerable mixed leukocyte infiltrate within capillaries, in addition to mild edema and small numbers of extravasated leukocytes, which were observed in direct contact with myocardial cells. By 18 h, heart grafts showed a dense cellular infiltrate of mononuclear cells (MNC) with considerable edema and focal myocyte necrosis. Allografts harvested at the time of complete rejection (24 h) showed marked edema and hypercellularity with lymphoblasts in direct contact with myocardial fibers, widespread myocyte degeneration and necrosis, diffuse interstitial hemorrhages and intravascular and perivascular thromboses.

Immunolabeling for humoral factors revealed dense deposits of IgM, IgG and C3 on graft endothelium by 3 h, whereas only trace amounts of fibrin deposition were seen. Thus, dense deposition of Ig and C were not sufficient to activate coagulation or cause rejection in this model. However, fibrin deposition on capillary and small vessel endothelium increased progressively during the time after transplantation, and by 18–24 h, just prior to rejection, deposition of IgM and IgG (mainly IgG2b) was coupled with occlusion of essentially all capillaries and venules by dense fibrin deposits. Interestingly, intragraft fibrin was significantly increased from 6 h, when cross-linked fibrin was demonstrated around infiltrating tissue factor (TF)-positive cells. Microvascular endothelial cells also showed induction of TF expression and downregulation of thrombomodulin by 18–24 h, when dilated small vessels were packed with MNC and fibrin thrombi.

The intragraft accumulation of leukocytes, mainly PMN, began during the first hr after engraftment. A dramatic (> 20-fold) increase in heart graft cellularity, due to an influx of equal numbers of PMN and MNC (> 75% macrophages, 10–20% T/NK cells, < 1% B cells) was apparent from 6 h and thereafter. This correlated with induction of E-selectin expression on arterioles at 3–6 h, followed at 6–12 h by ICAM-1 on all cardiac endothelial cells. Prior to this time, ICAM-1 expression was confined to large vessels, as in normal hearts. The 24 h rejection of heart grafts was associated with an early increase in the intermyocyte and endothelial deposition of laminin and fibronectin, the major extracellular matrix proteins, which preceded cellular infiltration localizing in fibronectin-rich cardiac interstitial and perivascular areas [9].

Cytokine labeling revealed small numbers of TNF-α+ and IL-12+ MNC at 6 h after engraftment. By 18 h, dense TNF-α expression by MNC, microvascular endothelial cells, and focal myocytes was present. IL-1β and IL-6 expression by mononuclear and endothelial cells was also observed, and increased particularly from 18 h after engraftment. Labeling for IL-2 and IFN-γ was first noted at 18 h. IL-2 labeling was restricted to 10–15% of MNC, whereas IFN-γ showed dense staining of 20–50% of leukocytes and most adjacent microvascular endothelium. Thus, monokine expression, particularly TNF-α was present from 6 h but additional monokines, endothelial cell activation, and the expression of IL-2 and IFN-γ correlated with an influx of IL-2R+ cells from 18 h after grafting. This influx of IL-2R+ cells correlated with progressive deterioration in myocardial contractility, leading to ultimate, irreversible rejection.

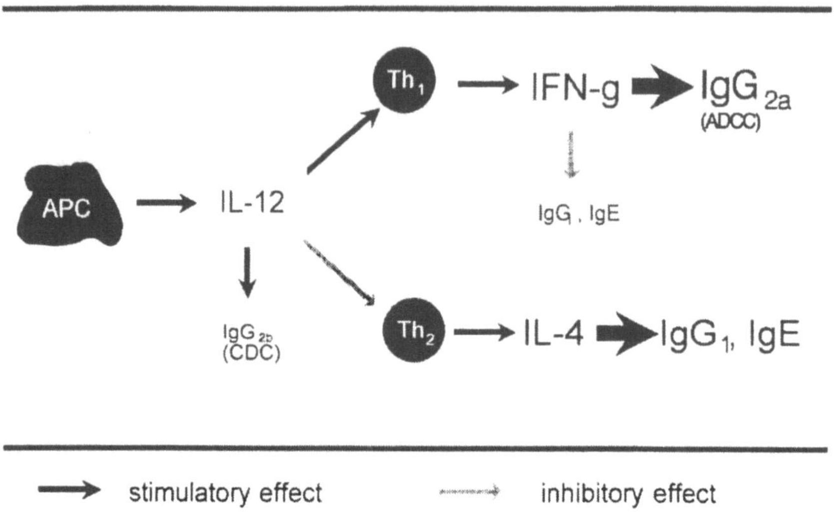

Fig. 2. Regulation of antibody production and Ig isotype selection by cytokines. Both stimulatory and inhibitory effects of APC-derived IL-12 and Thl/Th2-type cytokines upon stimulation and proliferation of B cells, and their subsequent differentiation into Ig-secreting cells are shown. These interactions are critical for host sensitization.

Cytokine pattern and allo-Ab networks in sensitized graft recipients

Allo-Ab responses and Ig isotype switching involve complex interactions of T cells and B cells, which are thought to be regulated by host cytokine networks. CD4 T cells may be divided into at least two mutually exclusive and functionally distinct subsets based on their heterogeneous cytokine elaboration profiles [10]. Thus, Th1 cells produce IL-2, IFN-γ, and TNF-α; these promote delayed-type hypersensitivity reactions. In contrast, Th2 cells secrete IL-4, IL-5, IL-6, and IL-10 and provide helper activity for Ig synthesis by B cells. The generation of Thl and Th2 cells is regulated by the equilibrium between these different cytokine groups, with dominant effects of IL-12 and IL-4. Thl and Th2 responses, on the other hand, are maintained by both positive and negative feedbacks, with the effect of IL-4 being dominant over that of IL-12.

After the initial Ag presentation, both Th subsets are activated to elaborate lymphokines, which stimulate B cells to proliferate and secrete Ig production. Figure 2 depicts a simplified scheme of a complex network of suppressive and enhancing interactions between both Th subsets, and B cells through T-cell and macrophage derived cytokine mediators. These interactions are believed to be critical for host sensitization. Although Thl–derived IL-2 and IFN-γ affect primarily cell-mediated responses, IFN-γ by itself may also stimulate B cells for Ab production. Moreover, IFN-γ can also suppress the Th2 subset and thus, the production of other lymphokines, such as IL-4, IL-5, IL-6, and

IL-10, which are responsible for direct stimulation and proliferation of B cells, and their subsequent differentiation into Ig-secreting cells. IL-12, the macrophage product, affects primarily Th1 cells and their cytotoxic effects. However, IL-12 is also the major stimulator of IFN-γ, and it may also act directly at B cells, and influence their allo-Ab production.

In the rat, IgG1 and IgG2a are mostly elicited by T cell-dependent Ags, whereas the generation of IgM, IgG2b and IgG2c allo-Ab is relatively T cell-independent [11]. The generation of IgG responses appears to be under the control of CD4+ T cells, with the Th2-derived IL-4 pivotal for the isotype switch to IgG1 and IgE; the Th1-type IFN-γ seems critical for the induction of IgG2a, which in the rat system is the most effective subclass in triggering antibody-dependent cell cytotoxicity (ADCC) *in vitro* [12, 13]. IFN-γ has also been shown to play a role in human IgG subclass induction by suppressing IgG1 and enhancing IgG2 production [14]. The generation of IgG2b subclass, stimulated by APC-derived IL-12, may be critical for the immune response triggered by a secondary allo-Ag challenge in sensitized recipients. Indeed, IgG2b has been shown to be highly effective in lysing $CD4^+$ T cells *in vitro* (as measured in complement-dependent cytotoxicity [CDC] assay) and depleting $CD4^+$ cells *in vivo* [15]. Low levels of circulating allospecific IgG2b at 24 h (around the time of graft rejection) in sensitized hosts undergoing ACCR were accompanied by a strong labeling for intragraft endothelial IgG2b, suggesting rapid and preferential absorption of Ab to the graft itself [16].

Treatment strategies to combat accelerated rejection have been shown to shift the immune response away from early production of IgG2b following secondary allo-Ag challenge. Inoculation of allogeneic spleen cells into the thymus of sensitized rat recipients of cardiac allografts resulted in elevated systemic production of donor reactive IgG1 and IgG2a subclasses and reduced production of IgG2b. Accordingly, the IgG deposits in well functioning grafts consisted predominantly of IgG1 and IgG2a [16]. Long term survival of allografts following Rapamycin treatment of sensitized hosts was associated with persistent expression of IL-4 and IL-10 mRNAs and strong expression of IL-12(p40) mRNA (Figure 3). The detection of IL-12 in long term surviving transplants (>20 days) may reflect the presence of activated macrophages. Coupled with the late appearance of anti-donor IgG2b in the circulation, this may ultimately contribute to the form of early transplant arteriosclerosis noted in this model [17].

Tolerance in sensitized graft recipients

A decrease of Th1-type cytokines in parallel with a sustained or enhanced expression of Th2-type cytokines is manifested in the majority of transplant acceptance models in unsensitized rodents, including neonatal tolerance [18], therapy with CTLA4Ig [19], colchicine [20], and donor-specific blood transfusion [21]. A similar pattern of cytokine modulation has been observed after

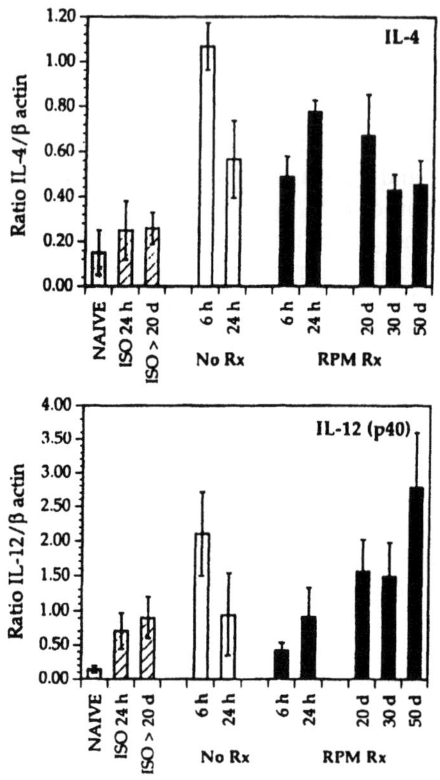

Fig. 3. Gene transcript expression of IL-4 and IL-12 (p40) in cardiac grafts in sensitized hosts treated with rapamycin, as analyzed by competitive template RT-PCR. Each column represents the average ratio ($\pm$SE) of wild-type cDNA per competitive template DNA for the cytokine, normalized against β-actin. IL-4 and IL-12 (p40) mRNAs were readily detectable during accelerated rejection and were inhibited after RPM treatment. In long term surviving grafts (>20 days), however, IL-4 and IL-12 (p40) transcripts reached levels comparable to those occurring during rejection. This was associated with considerable labeling for IL-4 and IL-12 in immunohistochemistry. No Rx, no treatment; RPM Rx, treatment with RPM (0.25 mg/kg/day from day -7 to day -1); ISO, isograft. Adapted from [17].

treatment strategies abrogating accelerated graft rejection in sensitized recipients [22–25]; however, a model of transplantation tolerance in sensitized recipients has become available only recently.

We have found that the induction of tolerance to MHC-incompatible cardiac allografts in sensitized rat recipients could be achieved by monotherapy with RIB-5/2, an anti-rat nondepleting CD4 mAb [26]. The prolonged graft survival of >200 days was associated with characteristic features of an infectious tolerance [27]. The tolerant cells in mAb-treated hosts could disable naive or alloimmune cells, so that they failed to trigger graft rejection. Moreover, a

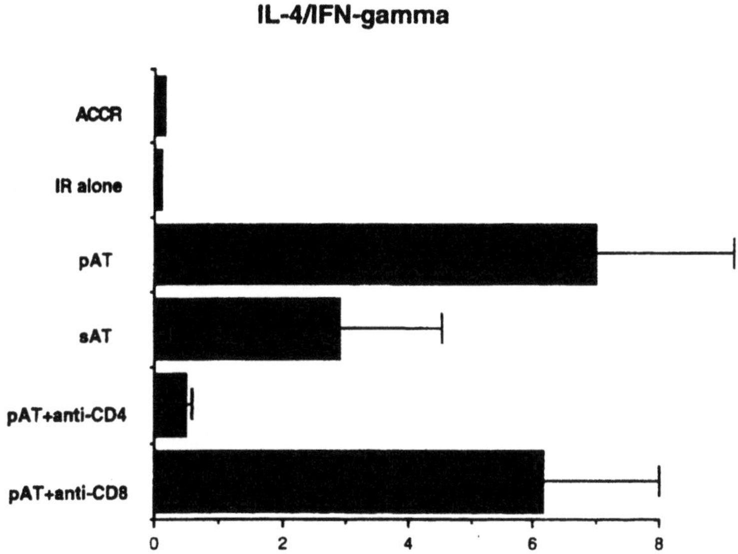

Fig. 4. Intragraft IL-4 to IFN-γ mRNA ratio based on the competitive template PT-PCR analysis of cardiac grafts from sensitized recipients. ACCR, no treatment; IR alone, γ-irradiated hosts undergoing acute graft rejection; pAT, primary test recipients after transfer of infectious tolerance by spleen cells from RIB-5/2mAb-treated hosts (day 70); sAT, secondary test recipients after transfer of infectious tolerance by spleen cells from primary test recipients (day 70); pAT+anti-CD4, primary test recipients undergoing rejection of cardiac allografts after infusion of OX-36mAb (day 6); pAT+anti-CD8, primary test recipients bearing functioning grafts after infusion of OX-8mAb (day 10). Adapted from [28].

donor-specific but organ non-specific tolerant state could be transferred by spleen cells into new generations of primary or secondary test recipients. Long term cardiac graft survival was accompanied by profound depression of both Th1 and Th2 cytokines (IL-2, IFN-γ; IL-4, IL-10) [28]. Contrarily, the expression of IL-4 and IL-10 was selectively up-regulated after transfer of infectious tolerance by spleen cells into new sets of primary and secondary test recipients. Therapy with cytolytic anti-CD4, but not anti-CD8, mAb recreated rejection of test cardiac allografts with simultaneous down-regulation of IL-4 mRNA expression and, in parallel, the IL-4/IFN-γ ratio, as depicted in Figure 4. These results show an important role of putative Th2–like regulatory IL-4 producing cells in the development of infectious tolerance in this model of graft rejection in sensitized recipients.

We share the self-critical judgment that we have probably only scraped the surface in identifying immunosuppressive cytokines [29]. In the case of tolerance induction in the sensitized graft recipient, this statement is even more appropriate.

References

1. Kissmeyer-Nielsen F, Olsen S, Petersen VP, Fjeldborg O. Hyperacute rejection of kidney allografts associated with preexisting humoral antibodies against donor cells. Lancet 1966; 2: 662–665.
2. Jordan SC, Yap HK, Sakai RS, Alfonso P, Fichtman M. Hyperacute allograft rejection mediated by anti-vascular endothelial cell antibodies with a negative monocyte crossmatch. Transplantation 1988; 46: 585–587.
3. Sanfilippo FP, Vaughn WK, Peters TG et al. Factors affecting the waiting time of cadaveric kidney transplant candidates in the United States. JAMA 1992; 267: 247–252.
4. Guttmann RD. A genetic survey of rat cardiac allograft rejection in presensitized recipients. Transplantation 1976; 22: 583–588.
5. Hisatake G, Hammond E, Ives M, Griffith J, Shelby J, Eichwald EJ. Hyperacute rejection of the transplanted mouse heart. Transplantation 1989; 47: 996–1000.
6. Hancock W, DiStefano R, Braun P, Schweizer RT, Tilney NL, Kupiec-Weglinski JW. Cyclosporine and anti-interleukin 2 receptor monoclonal antibody therapy suppress accelerated rejection of rat cardiac allografts through different effector mechanisms. Transplantation 1990; 49: 416–421.
7. Shelby J, Wakely E, Jorgensen C, Eichwald JE. Cell-mediated hyperacute rejection. VI. Prolonged survival of heterotopic mouse heart transplants. J. Surg. Res. 1986; 40: 133–137.
8. Hancock WW, Bach FH. The immunopathology of discordant xenograft rejection. Xeno 1994; 2: 68–74.
9. Coito AJ, Binder J, de Sousa M, Kupiec-Weglinski JW. The expression of extracellular matrix proteins during accelerated rejection of cardiac allografts in sensitized rats. Transplantation 1994; 57: 599–605.
10. Nickerson P, Steurer W, Steiger J, Zheng XX, Steele AW, Strom TB. Cytokines and the Th1/Th2 paradigm in transplantation. Curr. Opin. Immunol. 1994; 6: 757–764.
11. Der Balian GP, Slack J, Clevinger BL, Bazin H, Davie JM. Subclass restriction of murine antibodies. J. Exp. Med. 1980; 152: 209–218.
12. Snapper CM, Peschel C, Paul WE. IFN-γ stimulates IgG2a secretion by murine B cells stimulated with bacterial lipopolysaccharide. J. Immunol. 1988; 140: 2121–2127.
13. Finkelman FD, Holmes J, Katona IM, Urban JF Jr, Beckmann MP, Park LS et al. Lymphokine control of *in vivo* immunoglobulin isotype selection. Annu. Rev. Immunol. 1990; 88: 303–333.
14. Kitani A, Strober W. Regulation of Cg subclass germ-line transcripts in human peripheral blood B cells. J. Immunol. 1993; 151: 3478–3488.
15. Rashid A, Auchincloss H Jr, Sharon J. Comparison of GK1.5 and chimeric rat/mouse GK1.5 anti-CD4 antibodies for prolongation of skin allograft survival and suppression of alloantibody production in mice. J. Immunol. 1992; 148: 1382–1388.
16. Binder J, Hancock WW, Watschinger B, Wasowska B, Sayegh MH, Kupiec-Weglinski JW. The alloantibody network following intrathymic immunomodulation of sensitized rat recipients of cardiac allografts. Transplantation 1995; 59: 590–597.
17. Wasowska B, Wieder KJ, Hancock WW et al. Cytokine and alloantibody networks in long-term cardiac allografts in rat recipients treated with rapamycin. J. Immunol. 1996; 156: 395–404.
18. Donckier V, Wissing M, Bruyns C et al. Critical role of interleukin 4 in the induction of neonatal transplantation tolerance. Transplantation 1995; 59: 1571–1576.
19. Sayegh MH, Akalin E, Hancock WW et al. CD28-B7 blockade after alloantigenic challenge *in vivo* inhibits Th1 cytokines but spares Th2. J. Exp. Med. 1995; 181: 1869–1874.
20. Akalin E, Hancock WW, Perico N et al. Blocking cell microtubule assembly inhibits the alloimmune response *in vitro* and prolongs renal allograft survival by selective inhibition of Th1 and sparing of Th2 cell function *in vivo*. J. Am. Soc. Nephrol. 1995; 5: 1418–1425.
21. Takeuchi T, Lowry RP, Konieczny B. Heart allografts in murine systems. Transplantation 1992; 53: 1281–1294.

22. Papp I, Wieder KJ, Sablinski T et al. Evidence for functional heterogeneity of rat CD4+ T cells *in vivo*: differential expression of IL-2 and IL-4 in recipients of cardiac allografts. J. Immunol. 1992; 148: 1308–1314.
23. Hancock WW, Sayegh MH, Kwok CA, Weiner HL, Carpenter CB. Oral, but not intravenous, alloantigen prevents accelerated allograft rejection by selective intragraft Th2 cell activation. Transplantation 1993; 55: 1112–1118.
24. Binder J, Graser E, Hancock WW et al. Downregulation of intragraft IFN- expression correlates with increased IgG1 alloantibody response following intrathymic immunomodulation of sensitized rat recipients. Transplantation 1995; 60: 1516–1524.
25. Binder J, Lehmann M, Graser E et al. The effects of nondepleting CD4 targeted therapy in presensitized rat recipients of cardiac allografts. Transplantation 1996; 61: 804–811.
26. Onodera K, Lehmann M, Akalin E, Volk HD, Sayegh MH, Kupiec-Weglinski JW. Induction of 'infectious' tolerance to MHC-incompatible cardiac allografts in CD4 mAb-treated sensitized rat recipients. J. Immunol. 1996; 157: 1944–1950.
27. Qin S, Cobbold SP, Pope J et al. 'Infectious' transplantation tolerance. Science 1993; 259: 974.
28. Onodera K, Hancock WW, Graser E et al. Type 2 helper T cell-type cytokines and the development of 'infectious' tolerance in rat cardiac allograft recipients. J. Immunol. 1997; 158: 1572–1581.
29. Nickerson P, Steiger J, Zheng XX et al. Manipulation of cytokine networks in transplantation. Transplantation 1997; 63: 489–494.

14. T cell sensitization and graft rejection

F. CLAAS, D. ROELEN, L. VAESSEN and W. WEIMAR

In order to study the association between donor-specific alloimmune T cell responses *in vitro* and graft rejection, non-radioactive limiting ditlution assays have been developed to quantify the number of T cells involved.

Cytotoxic T cell precursor frequencies were determined both in highly sensitized patients and in patients rejecting an allograft.

These studies revealed that sensitization and rejection is not reflected by a significant increase of the number of donor reactive T cells.

In a further series of experiments we tested whether immunization was associated with qualitative differences in the alloreactive T cell involved. Inhibition studies with anti-CD8 and anti-CD4 antibodies showed that rejection was associated with the presence of high avidity cytotoxic T cells, which cannot be inhibited by these antibodies. Furthermore, these cytotoxic T cells were found to be more resistant to cyclosporin A (*in vitro*).

High avidity CTLs were found after different immunizing events, such as pregnancy, blood transfusion and graft rejection.

A clinical relevance for these CTLs is suggested by a pilot study in patients transplanted despite a positive historical crossmatch due to IgG antibodies directed against donor HLA mismatches.

In patients with high avidity CTLs these transplants failed in an early phase, while in patients with low avidity CTLs at the day of transplantation a good graft survival was obtained. These studies suggest that monitoring the T cell allorepertoire may be helpful for the selection of donors in sensitized recipients.

J.L. Touraine et al. (eds.), Retransplantation, 107.

15. Do re-grafts require more aggressive immunosuppression?

AMANDA J. ROBERTSON and PETER J. MORRIS

Introduction

This study was performed to investigate whether recipients of second or subsequent renal cadaveric allografts require more intensive immunosuppression than recipients of first grafts. Oxford data demonstrates that the outcome of patients with regrafts is overall identical to those with first cadaveric grafts [1] although Registry data has shown that regrafts do not do so well [2, 3], with regraft survival up to 10% lower than first grafts [4]. In most transplant centres this difference in survival between first and second grafts has decreased in the last 15 years and this has no doubt been influenced by the use of cyclosporine [5, 6]. Hirata et al. [7] describe a difference of as little as 1% between first and second graft survival in their patients, compatible with our own data. Kidney regraft candidates now comprise about 27% of all patients awaiting renal transplantation, but only receive 13–14% of the annual cadaveric transplants [8]. The reasons for this are multifactorial, but include high sensitization and associated positive crossmatches, and a presumption of worse outcome for regrafts [9]. Patients awaiting regrafting share the common experience of having lost a previous transplant and having been exposed to foreign HLA antigens. Only some of these graft losses will be the result of rejection, others having been lost to technical problems such as renal vein or artery thrombosis or to primary non-function. It is the sub-group who have mounted an immunological response sufficient to reject the primary graft that are likely to be the more difficult group in which to achieve success with a regraft, and in whom more aggressive immunosuppression might be indicated.

Clinical material and results

Graft survival of cadaveric transplants receiving triple therapy at the Oxford Transplant Centre is 82.5% for first grafts and 83.6% for second grafts at one year. Five year graft survival is 67.9% vs 68.1% and 10 year graft survival is 48.7% vs 53.1% for first vs second grafts (Figure 1). In view of the similar outcome of regrafts to first grafts in Oxford, we have looked at recipients of second cadaveric renal allografts, all of whom were immunosuppressed with triple therapy (cyclosporine, azathioprine and prednisolone) to assess graft survival, cause of early graft loss, the use of more aggressive

J.L. Touraine et al. (eds.), Retransplantation, 109–119.

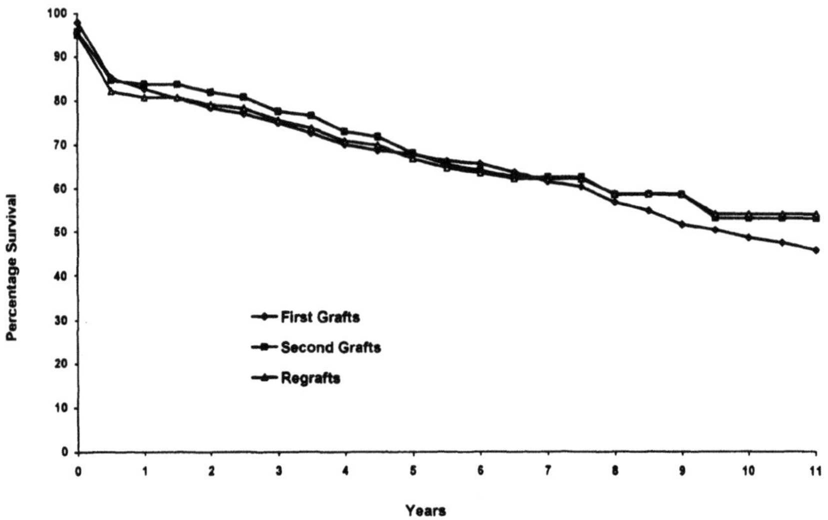

Fig. 1. Cadaveric graft survival for first grafts ($n = 624$), second grafts ($n = 123$) and all regrafts ($n = 155$) in Oxford.

Table 1. Number of primary grafts and regrafts by donor type

	Graft no.					
Donor type	1	2	3	4	5	Total
Cadaveric	624	123	25	5	2	779
Living donor	71	5	2	–	–	78
Total	695	128	27	5	2	857

immunosuppression, and graft function. From May 1985 (start of triple therapy) to the end of 1995, 862 renal transplants were performed at the Oxford Transplant Centre, and 857 received triple therapy. Of the triple therapy group, 695 were first grafts and of these 624 were cadaveric transplants. During this period, 162 retransplants were performed, of which 128 were second grafts including five living related transplants (Table 1).

Induction therapy

A large percentage of our retransplanted patients were given additional immunosuppression as induction therapy. Of the 155 cadaveric regrafts at our centre, 70 (45.1%) received induction therapy, in addition to standard triple therapy. This compares with only 9.9% of patients receiving a first cadaveric graft (Figure 2 and Table 2). Induction therapy comprised methylprednisolone

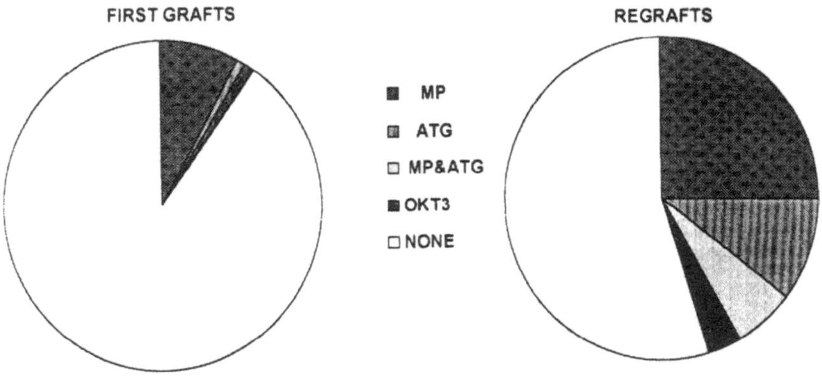

Fig. 2. Use of induction therapy in addition to triple therapy in cadaveric grafts, both first grafts and regrafts in Oxford (1985–1995). MP = methyl prednisolone 0.5 G/day IV × 3 days; ATG = antithymocyte globulin; MP + ATG = methyl prednisolone and antithymocyte globulin; OKT = anti T cell (CD3) monoclonal antibody.

Table 2. Use of induction therapy with triple immunosuppression (CyA, Aza, and prednisolone)

Graft no.	N	MP	ATG	MP + ATG	OKT3	Total
1	624	50 (8.0%)	6 (0.9%)	6 (0.9%)	–	62 (9.9%)
2+	155	39 (25.1%)	16(10.3%)	10 (6.4%)	5(3.2%)	70 (45.1%)
Total	779	89(11.4%)	22 (2.8%)	16 (2.0%)	5(0.6%)	132 (16.9%)

(MP), 500 mg/day for three days, anti-thymocyte globulin (ATG) or OKT3 for a 7–10 day course, or MP with ATG. Induction therapy was used in those patients deemed high risk, as a result of sensitization, previous immunological graft loss, historical positive crossmatch or HLA mismatches. Thus, the use of induction therapy may be responsible for the good graft survival in the retransplant population (Figure 3).

Acute rejection

Interestingly, the rate of treatment for acute rejection of patients within 3 months of receiving a first or subsequent graft, is equivalent (65.5 vs 67% respectively), which again may reflect the more aggressive initial immunosuppression in many of the regraft patients. The use of MP, ATG or OKT3 to treat acute rejection is very similar in both first grafts and regrafts, which suggests the rejection episodes in regrafts are no more severe than with first grafts (Figure 4).

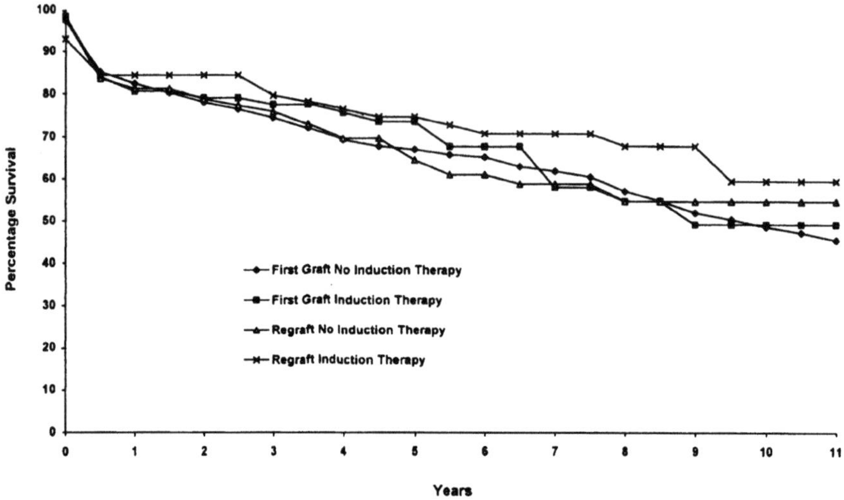

Fig. 3. Survival of cadaveric first or regrafts and the use of induction therapy in Oxford.

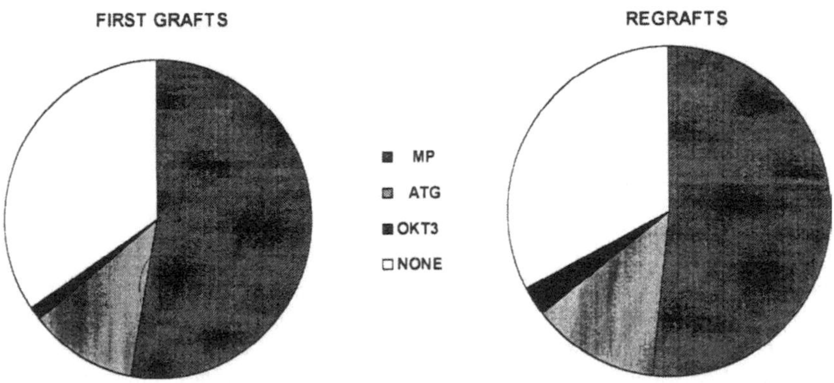

Fig. 4. Treatment of acute rejection within 3 months of transplantation in cadaveric first and regrafts.

Sensitization and HLA matching

Sensitization, for the purposes of this analysis, was defined as reactivity of the patients' serum with 85% or greater of a panel of chronic lymphatic leukaemia (CLL) cells selected for the expression of the commonly recognized HLA antigens of both class I and II. Of the 624 first grafts, 25 were highly sensitized (CLL > 84), 147 were moderately sensitized (CLL > 10 and < 85), and 452 were non-sensitized (CLL < 11). Of the 123 second grafts, 34 were highly sensitized, 60 moderately sensitized and 29 were non-sensitized (Table 3).

Table 3. Sensitization of first graft and second graft recipients

Sensitization		First graft	Second graft
Highly sensitized	CLL > 84	25 (4.1%)	34 (27.6%)
Sensitized	CLL > 10 and <85	147(23.6%)	60 (49.1%)
Non-sensitized	CLL < 11	452(72.3%)	29 (23.3%)
Total		624	123

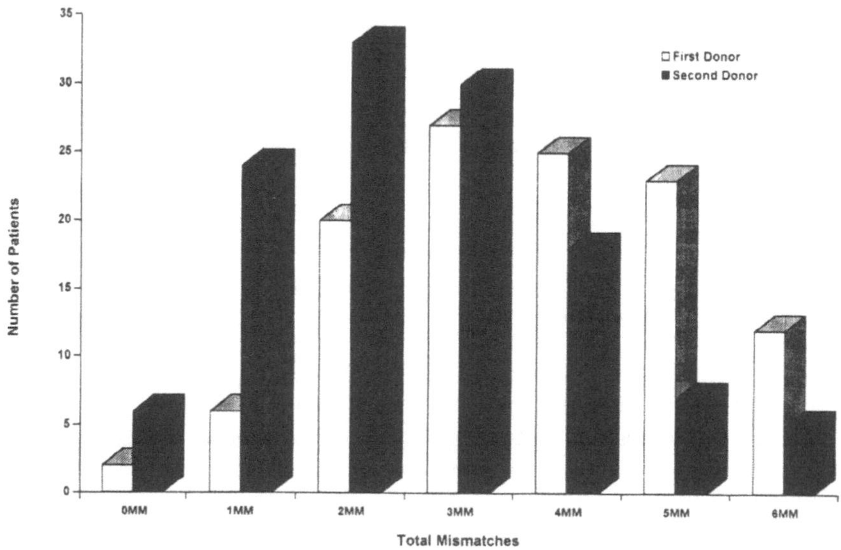

Fig. 5. The number of patients with the number of HLA mismatches (0 to 6) between donor and recipient for first and second cadaveric grafts.

Repeated HLA mismatches between first and second donors of retransplanted patients are uncommon in our unit and were only performed in the presence of negative historical and current crossmatches. Of 123 second transplants, there was one patient with a repeat DR mismatch, three patients with repeated HLA-A mismatches, three with repeated HLA-B and 5 with repeated HLA-C mismatches. Two patients had repeats of both HLA-B and C mismatches. Only one of the patients with a repeat mismatch (DR) has lost his graft, and this was at five days from a non-immunological cause. The remainder of these patients have functioning grafts.

HLA matching of second transplants in our unit appears to be better than matching of the first graft. This may be the result of greater organ sharing across the UK in recent years or because an even greater effort is made to find a well matched kidney for second transplants (Figures 5 and 6). HLA-DR matching, in particular, is better for the second transplant than the first and

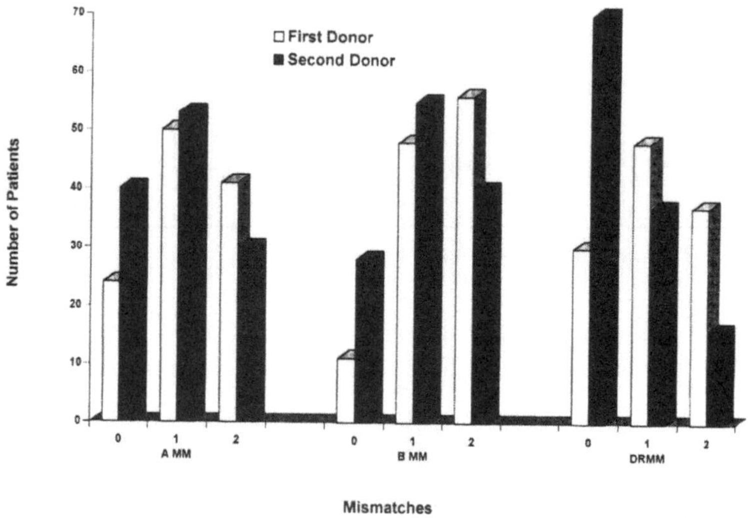

Fig. 6. The number of patients with the number of HLA mismatches at the HLA-A, B and DR loci for first and second cadaveric grafts.

again is probably a contributory factor for good graft survival in this retransplant population, as shown previously from our unit [10].

There is little difference in the current cytotoxic crossmatch results of patients receiving a first cadaveric transplant compared with those receiving a second transplant. Both the B and T cell cytotoxic crossmatch was negative in 90.3% of first grafts and 87.1% of second grafts. However, the peak historical crossmatch was negative in 82.6% of first grafts but in only 46.6% of second graft recipients, indicating significant foreign antigen exposure in the past.

Early graft failure

Of the 123 second cadaveric transplants, 17 (13.8%) failed less than 90 days from the time of transplant. Of the early failures, 10 were due to immunological cause and 7 due to technical causes (renal vein thrombosis or primary non-function or death with functioning graft). Of the 624 first graft recipients receiving triple therapy, 82 patients (13.1%) lost their graft within 90 days of transplantation, 28 from rejection and 54 from non-immunological causes. Many of the first grafts would have been immunosuppressed with azathioprine and prednisolone, with correspondingly poorer graft survival. Of the ten regrafts losing a second graft in less than 90 days due to rejection, 8/10 had also lost the first graft in <90 days. The majority (9/10) of these regrafts with early graft loss were highly sensitized and of these 4 received ATG and one received OKT3 in addition to standard triple therapy. Of the early regraft losses due to rejection, there were 4/10 with no DR mismatch and 4 with one DR mismatch with the second donor. The primary grafts of these patients were slightly less well matched, with 2/10 complete DR mismatches, 4 single DR mismatches, two with no mismatch and two patients in whom the DR typing of the donor was not performed.

Discussion

Data from the United Kingdom Transplant Service Support Authority (UKTSSA) does show that retransplantation of kidneys, livers and hearts is not as successful as first grafts [11]. Since 1988, UNOS data has shown an improvement in one year survival of renal regrafts from 66 to 75% ($p < 0.0001$) and from 67 to 70% in the UCLA Registry [12]. This improvement may be due to better patient selection, better screening for preformed antibodies, more sensitive crossmatch techniques and better immunosuppression. The cost of retransplanation of renal transplants is only slightly higher than for first grafts in the USA (US$41 000 vs $38 000 in 1993), in contrast to liver retransplantation which is almost 3 times the cost of primary grafts [13], and these comparisons are probably similar in Europe.

The apparent reduction in second renal graft survival in Registry data is probably related to sensitization, with peak antibody reactivity being most predictive of graft outcome [14], although this is disputed by others [9]. In addition, factors such as the source of both the first and second graft, the cause of graft loss and the duration of first graft [1] may influence regraft outcome. Loss of a first graft within the first few months from rejection worsens the outcome of a second graft, but if the first graft survives longer, then a second graft has an equal chance of doing well, at least in the azathioprine era [15–18]. In the cyclosporine era, second transplants with a first graft duration less than 3 months were found to have 57% one year graft survival, whereas those with first graft duration of more than 12 months, had 75% one year survival [4]. For patients receiving immunosuppression with azathioprine, prednisolone and ALG (antilymphocyte globulin), risk factors for second renal allograft survival included primary graft loss caused by rejection after 6 months, use of cadaver donors, and an interval between primary graft loss and retransplantation of greater than or equal to 6 months. With CyA based immunosuppression, risk factors for second graft survival were primary graft loss due to rejection in under 6 months, non-CyA based immunosuppression for the primary graft and peak PRA (panel-reactive antibody) of >21. By avoiding these risk factors, survival of a second graft can be similar to primary graft survival [19]. Importantly, loss of the primary graft from non-immunological causes does not compromise second graft survival [5, 19].

Many transplant centres do not alter immunosuppression regimens for second and subsequent transplants. However, some centres suggest that induction with OKT3 or ATG may result in better regraft survival [19–21] and should be used for 'high risk' recipients. There is some evidence that ALG, used for induction in sequential therapy, may improve second graft survival [6]. Studies have suggested that additional immunosuppression, such as intravenous immunoglobulins, may be associated with longer graft survival in retransplanted patients, as a result of suppressing anti-HLA antibodies [22]. Induction therapy using MALG or OKT3 for pediatric regraft recipients has not been shown to improve graft survival [23]. Similarly, quadruple therapy, using MALG in addition to cyclosporine, azathioprine and prednisolone, has not improved graft survival for black or white adult recipients [24]. FK506 when used for primary grafts or regrafts results in similar one year graft survival (89 vs 84%), respectively [25] but has no advantage in survival over standard triple therapy.

In the azathioprine era, patients with a good HLA match for the primary transplant were more likely to be regrafted than those with a poor match. They were also more likely to receive the second transplant within two years of the first graft failure because PRA levels were lower than those with a poorly matched first graft [26].

Retransplantation using kidneys with repeated HLA mismatches is avoided at most centres, although provided no relevant antibody response to repeat mismatches has been detected (permissible mismatches) this should not be a barrier [9, 27]. However, there may be a slightly increased risk of primary non-function if this is performed [28]. More specifically, repeated HLA-DR mismatches do seem to result in significantly reduced graft survival and should be avoided [29]. HLA-DR matching is associated with increased graft survival in retransplants [20, 24, 30, 31], particularly on long term regraft survival as opposed to short-term survival [29]. Matching for HLA-A or -B appears to have no beneficial effect on second graft survival [32]. Graft survival in renal retransplantation is improved by identifying donor-directed HLA class 1 antibodies with flow cytometry cross-matching (FCXM), and by avoiding recipients with a IgG positive crossmatch. Positive FCXM is a risk factor for early graft loss, while a negative FCXM is associated with reduced risk of graft loss [24]. These results are independent of a negative cytotoxic crossmatch. Second transplants with positive FCXM have been found to have 61% 3 month survival and those with a negative crossmatch 82% 3 month survival [4]. One study found that flow cytometric crossmatch (FCXM) is a predictor of kidney regraft survival only when correlated with first graft survival time [9]. For patients with primary graft survival of >3 months, FCXM can be positive or negative without influencing second graft survival. However, there is greater impact on patients with primary graft survival of less than 3 months, in whom FCXM positive T and/or B cell, is a predictor of early regraft loss. Primary graft survival <3 months but with a negative FXCM is not a risk factor for second graft loss.

Use of a living donor for regrafting results in superior survival compared to the use of a cadaveric graft for retransplantation, regardless of the source of the previous donor or primary graft outcome [31]. There is some evidence that sex of the donor can affect the outcome of regrafts, with female donors being a risk factor for early graft loss [24, 33]. Older donors (>60 years) are also associated with worse retransplant outcome, and especially in those recipients with a previous nephrectomy [19]. Patients younger than 10 and older than 60 years may be less suitable for retransplantation with graft survival rates of 46.1% and 51.7%, respectively, compared with 66.1% for all cadaveric regrafts, according to one study [33]. Paediatric retransplantation does not yet result in graft survival that is equivalent to first grafts. Paediatric regraft survival rates are 8% lower than primary grafts at one year, except for living related donor retransplants where the outcome is identical to primary transplants [23]. In this population, the main risk factor for early graft loss is the use of cadaver donors less than 6 years of age.

Early graft function is an important predictor of subsequent graft survival of patients undergoing retransplantation. Urine production on the first day post transplant correlates well with graft outcome. Failure to diurese on the first day resulted in second graft survival of 60% at one year, compared with 80% for those who diuresed on the first day. Similarly, if dialysis was required following a second graft, one year survival was 63%, compared with 84% if no dialysis was needed [7].

Recipients of a third renal graft can also have very good graft survival (74% at one year). Survival is best in those patients who kept their second graft more than one year, and in those who received a third graft more than one year after second graft failure. There was also a trend to better graft survival following the use of a living related donor [34]. Indeed, the two longest surviving fifth cadaveric renal transplants in the world (8 years and 6 years respectively) are patients of the Oxford unit, both having rejected earlier grafts quite soon after transplantation.

The effect of nephrectomy of the primary renal allograft on subsequent retransplantation in the cyclosporine era is not clear. Primary allograft nephrectomy is associated with higher preformed antibody levels but is said to have no effect on frequency of acute rejection or graft outcome after retransplantation [35] at least out to 3 years post-transplant [36]. There may be a higher incidence of delayed graft function in those patients who underwent nephrectomy of the first graft [36] but this is disputed by others [35]. Pre-cyclosporine, there appeared to be an advantage for second graft survival to leave the primary graft *in situ* [37]. With cyclosporine use this may still be the case, as demonstrated by one study where transplant nephrectomy resulted in worse outcome of regrafts than those who kept their failed grafts. This may be improved by minimizing the time between nephrectomy and regraft and by using antilymphocyte globulin at induction [19]. Another important factor is maintenance of the failed graft with low dose immunosuppression which may prevent sensitization and high PRA developing in the potential recipient of a second transplant. Retransplantation prior to nephrectomy or return to dialysis can also significantly improve regraft survival [19].

Conclusion

It would seem that recipients of second cadaveric transplants treated with cyclosporine based triple therapy have equivalent graft survival to recipients of first grafts. There are a number of risk factors that may negatively influence regraft survival and these include first graft survival of 12 months or less, high PRA, positive FCXM, DR mismatch and first graft nephrectomy prior to retransplantation. By identifying such factors, additional immunosuppression with an antilymphocyte agent such as ATG or OKT3, can be given as induction therapy, resulting in no greater risk of acute rejection and an equivalent graft survival, compared with first cadaveric renal grafts. However, overall the accurate definition of the antibody status of the recipient and the accuracy of the crossmatch are probably the most important factors determining the outcome of regrafts.

Acknowledgement

Mr A. McLaren and Ms C. Gray for the database and graphs.

References

1. Morris PJ. Results of renal transplantation. In: Morris PJ (ed.), Kidney Transplantation Principles and Practice. W.B. Saunders, 1994.
2. Opelz G. Collaborative Transplant Study – 10th Anniversary, 1993, p. 1.
3. Terasaki PI, Cecka JM, Gjertson DW, Cho Y, Takemoto S, Cohn M. A ten-year prediction for kidney transplant survival. In: Terasaki PI, Cecka JM (eds.), Clinical Transplants. U.C.L.A. Tissue Typing Laboratory, Los Angeles, 1992, p. 501.
4. Ogura K, Cecka JM. Cadaver retransplants. Clin. Transplant. 1990; 471–483.
5. Hiesse C, Neyrat N, Busson M, Bensadoun H, Lantz O et al. High rate of success in kidney cadaveric retransplantation with optimal matching and potent immunosuppression. Transplant. Proc. 1990; 22: 1909–1910.
6. Fasola CG, Fryd DS, Fischel RJ, Ascher NL, Payne WD et al. Adult kidney retransplantation: evolution of treatment and results over 25 years at the University of Minnesota. Transplant. Proc. 1989; 21: 2165–2167.
7. Hirata M, Terasaki PI. Renal retransplantation. Clin. Transplant. 1994; 419–433.
8. UNOS. 1993 Annual report of the U.S. Scientific Registry of Transplant recipients and the organ procurement and transplantation network. Richmond, VA: UNOS, and Bethesda, MD: Division of Organ Transplantation, Health Resources and Services Administration.
9. Mahoney RJ, Norman DJ, Colombe BW, Garovoy MR, Leeber DA. Identification of high and low risk second kidney grafts. Transplantation 1996; 61: 1349–1355.
10. Taylor C, Welsh K et al. Clinical and socioeconomic benefits of serological HLA-DR matching for renal transplantation over three eras of immunosuppression regimens in a single unit. In: Terasaki PI (ed.), Clinical Transplants 1993; U.C.L.A. Tissue Typing Laboratory, Los Angeles.
11. UK National Transplant Database: a digest of published audit material. UKTSSA National Transplant Database. Clin. Transplant. 1995; 91–110.
12. Mitsuishi Y, Cecka JM. Recent improvements in cadaver-donor kidney retransplantation. Clin. Transplant. 1991; 281–291.
13. Evans RW, Manninen DL, Dong FB, McLynne DA. Is retransplantation cost effective? Transplant. Proc. 1993; 25: 1694–1696.
14. Ogura K. Sensitisation. In: Terasaki PI, Cecka JM (eds.), Clinical Transplants 1992. U.C.L.A. Tissue Typing Laboratory, Los Angeles, 1993, p. 357.

15. Kountz SL, Thibault PM, Endo T, Margules R, Balzer O. Results of immediate and delayed retransplantation. Transplant. Proc. 1972; 4: 739.
16. Husberg BS, Starzl TE. The outcome of kidney transplantation. Arch. Surg. 1974; 108: 584.
17. Opelz G, Gustafsson LA, Terasaki PI. Influence of interval between first graft removal and retransplantation on outcome of second cadaver kidney grafts. Transplantation 1976; 22: 521.
18. Ascher NL, Ahrendolz DH, Simmons RL, Najarian JS. 100 second renal allografts from a single transplantation institution. Transplantation 1979; 27: 30.
19. Abouljoud MS, Deierhoi MH, Hudson SL, Diethelm AG. Risk factors affecting second renal transplant outcome, with special reference to primary allograft nephrectomy. Transplantation 1995; 60: 138–144.
20. Schweizer RT, Bow L, Roper L, Hull D, Bartus SA. Renal transplantation at Hartford Hospital. Connecticut. Clin. Transplant. 1988; 147–158.
21. Gaber AO, Thistlewaite JR, Haag BW, Stuart J, Mayes J et al. Transplant. Proc. 1987; 19: 1915–1916.
22. Peraldi MN, Akposso K, Haymann JP, Flahaut A, Marlin C et al. Long-term benefit of intravenous immunoglobulins in cadaveric kidney retransplantation. Transplantation 1996; 62: 1670–1673.
23. Tejani A, Sullivan EK. Factors that impact on the outcome of second renal transplants in children. Transplantation 1996; 62: 606–611.
24. Gaston RS, Shroyer TW, Hudson SL, Deierhoi MH, Laskow DA et al. Renal retransplantation: the role of race, quadruple immunosuppression, and the flow cytometry cross-match. Transplantation 1994; 57: 47–54.
25. Shapiro R, Jordan ML, Scantlebury VP, Vivas C, Fung JJ et al. A prospective randomised trial of FK506-based immunosuppression after renal transplantation. Transplantation 1995; 59: 485–490.
26. Sanfililppo F, Goeken N, Niblack G, Scornik J, Vaughn WK. The effect of first cadaver renal transplant HLA-A, B match on sensitization levels and retransplant rates following graft failure. Transplantation 1987; 43: 240–243.
27. Welsh KI, van Dam M, Bewick ME, Koffman GK, Taube DH et al. Successful transplantation of kidneys bearing previously HLA A and B locus antigens. Transplant. Int. 1988; 1(4): 190–195.
28. Povlsen JV, Madsen M, Birkeland SA, Lokkegaard H, Pedersen EB et al. The impact of repeated HLA mismatches on the outcome of renal allograft retransplantation. Transplant. Proc. 1992; 24: 307–308.
29. Cecka JM, Terasaki PI. Repeating HLA antigen mismatches in renal retransplants – a second class mistake? Transplantation 1994; 57: 515–519.
30. Hendriks GF, de Lange P, Persijn GG and van Rood JJ. Cyclosporine A, hyperimmunized patients and renal retransplantation. Transplant. Proc. 1987; 19: 733–734.
31. Stratta RJ, Oh C-S, Sollonger HW, Pirsch JD, Kalayoglu M et al. Kidney retransplantation in the cyclosporine era. Transplantation 1988; 45: 40–45.
32. Almond PS, Matas AJ, Gillingham K, Troppmann C, Payne W et al. Risk factors for second renal allografts immunosuppressed with cyclosporine. Transplantation 1991; 52: 253–258.
33. Imagawa DK, Cecka JM. Renal regrafts. Clin. Transplant. 1988; 387–398.
34. Fasola CG, Kim YS, Morel P, Dunn DL, Sutherland DER et al. Kidney retransplantation: patients with a failed second kidney transplant should be considered for a third transplant. Transplant. Proc. 1991; 23: 1336.
35. Douzdjian V, Rice JC, Carson RW, Gugliuzza KK, Fish JC. Renal retransplants: effect of primary allograft nephrectomy on early function, acute rejection and outcome. Clin. Transplant. 1996; 10: 203–208.
36. Sumrani N, Delaney V, Hong JH, Daskalakis P, Sommer BG. The influence of nephractomy of the primary allograft on retransplant graft outcome in the cyclosporine era. Transplantation 1992; 53: 52–55.
37. Freier DT, Haines RF, Rosenzweig J, Niederhuber J, Konnak J et al. Sequential renal transplants: some surgical and immunological implications on management of the first homograft. Surgery 1976; 79: 262.

16. Immunological rationale for induction therapy in patients with donor-specific memory T cells

SYLVIE FOURNEL, NATHALIE BONNEFOY-BÉRARD, ROMAIN PAILLOT, OLGA ASSOSSOU, ERIC ROBINET, CAROLE FERRARO, DAVID FEVRE, LAURENT GENESTIER, AICHA DEMIDEM & JEAN-PIERRE REVILLARD

Introduction

The phenomenon of 'second set' or 'accelerated' rejection which characterizes the rapid destruction of a second tissue or organ transplant from the same donor into the same recipient was first described by Medawar and coworkers. Those observations made in untreated recipients were considered as a major evidence for the immunological mechanisms of allograft rejection since such capacity to reject transplants of donor strain origin in an accelerated mode could be transferred to naive recipients by T cells from the presensitized hosts. Cross-reactive grafts from donors sharing MHC class I and/or class II alleles with the sensitizing donor were also rejected in an accelerated fashion, suggesting that accelerated rejection was mediated by sensitized $CD4^+$ and/or $CD8^+$ donor specific alloreactive T cells. The capacity to mount an anamnestic rejection could persist several weeks or months after completion of the first graft rejection, suggesting that memory T cells had been produced following the first transplant. However the mechanisms of memory induction and the phenotypic and functional differences between memory and effector T cells remain controversial. The allograft response entails the clonal expansion of donor MHC class II and MHC class I specific $CD4^+$ and $CD8^+$ T cells, associated with several phenotypic changes, including increased surface expression of CD2 and CD58 (LFA-3), increased affinity of the integrin CD11a/CD18 (LFA-1), *de novo* expression of the integrin $\alpha4\beta1$ (CD29/49d, VLA-4), changes in expression of CD62L and CD44 and decrease of the CD45RA isoform with a compensatory increase of the shorter CD45RO isoform. Some of these phenotypic changes are associated with the acquisition of new homing properties which allow preactivated T cells to infiltrate the transplant. Whether memory T cells are long-lived T cells which remain quiescent in the G0 phase of the cell cycle for long periods of time, or, alternatively, divide following low grade persistent stimulation by donor's antigens (or persisting donor's cells) is unknown.

J.L. Touraine et al. (eds.), Retransplantation, 121–135.

In clinical transplantation, early data showing that retransplantation in patients who had lost their first graft from rejection within one year was associated with a higher rate of graft loss, may represent the human counterpart of experimental second set rejection. However the increased initial loss of second transplants varies depending on the type of organ and the conditions of retransplantation (e.g. minimal in kidney but more important in heart [1]). This may reflect progress in immunosuppressive treatment and cross-matching techniques, although there is no evidence at present that improving cross matching for detection of preformed anti-donor antibodies could substitute for the determination of presensitized or memory T cells. In addition, it should be stressed that early graft failure or delayed function that are more frequent in retransplantation than in primary transplantation often correspond to misdiagnosed cellular acute rejection episodes. This is typically examplified by kidney transplantation, since we reported that delayed graft function (assessed by the number of post-operative dialysis) was markedly reduced by preoperative thoracic duct drainage [2] or prophylactic ATG [3] which are both unlikely to interfere with ischemic damage. Moreover daily monitoring of serum C-reactive protein (CRP) levels allowed us to distinguish between renal insufficiency due to ischemic damage, characterized by a progressive drop in CRP levels, and misdiagnosed acute cellular rejection associated with initial decrease followed by a sustained elevation of serum CRP [4]. Interestingly, graft failure following retransplantation occurs very early, whereas subsequent graft failure rates are identical in primary and secondary transplants [1]. This observation suggests that increased graft failure is associated with recipient's T cell presensitization. Furthermore, the lack of increased risk of graft failure upon retransplantation reported in several recent series (this volume) suggests that regulatory mechanisms occuring during the first transplantation may contribute to restrict clonal expansion and differentiation into alloreactive memory T cells. In this respect, understanding the precise mechanisms of action of each immunosuppressive agent is of utmost importance, in order to select immunosuppressive regimens which would not only prevent or delay initial graft loss but also help to prevent retransplantation failure.

The mixed leukocyte reaction as an in vitro model of allograft reaction

Co-culture of leukocytes from individuals bearing different MHC class II alleles results in clonal expansion of $CD4^+$ alloreactive T cells followed by proliferation of alloreactive $CD8^+$ T cells if there is an associated class I allelic difference between the two cell populations. This mixed leukocyte reaction (MLR) can be made unidirectional by blocking the proliferative but not the stimulating properties of one cell population by irradiation or exposure to mitomycin C. Cell proliferation, as measured by ^{3}H-thymidine incorporation, reaches a maximum at days 5–6 then drop to background level. Such kinetics reflect the expansion of multiple alloreactive T cell clones, followed by activation-induced

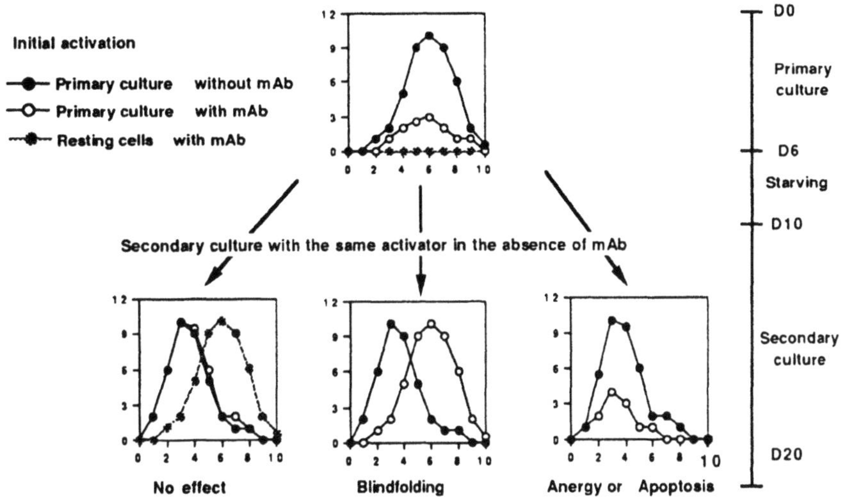

Fig. 1. Protocol used for evaluating the effects of anti-lymphocyte mAbs (or other immunosuppressive agents) on primary MLR and induction of clonal hyporesponsiveness (or enhancement) of subsequent activation measured in the absence of immunomodulating agent.

cell death (AICD, see below) and lysis of stimulating cells by primed alloreactive cytotoxic T lymphocytes (CTL). Upon re-introduction of the same stimulator cells (or cells sharing MHC class II alleles) the secondary MLR is characterized by accelerated kinetics ('primed lymphocyte test': PLT) with a peak of ^{3}H-thymidine incorporation at days 2–3 followed by a rapid drop (Figure 1). Restimulation by third party cells which do not share class I or class II cross-reactive alleles with the first stimulator results in a primary type kinetic. Primary MLR is associated with the differentiation of alloreactive CTL specific for MHC class I (CD8$^+$ CTL) or MHC class II (CD4$^+$ CTL), resulting in the lysis of stimulator cells. At least two mechanisms may account for the accelerated kinetics of secondary MLR: (i) clonal expansion and therefore increased numbers of stimulator-specific alloreactive CD4$^+$ and CD8$^+$ T cells, and (ii) changes in activation requirements (number of engaged TCRs or dependence on costimulatory signals) of pre-activated alloreactive T cells. The question has been addressed by several studies with conflicting results. Using a murine MLR model, with varying ratios of responding/stimulator CD4$^+$ T cells, Constant et al. [5] reported that accelerated kinetics in secondary MLR was exclusively accounted for by clonal expansion during primary MLR, despite the fact that only pre-activated alloreactive T cells could produce detectable levels of cytokines such as interferon γ (IFNγ). Other studies suggested that reactivation of primed T cells (proliferation and IL-2/IL-4 secretion) required TCR occupancy but no other antigen-presenting cell (APC) costimulation derived signal [6, 7]. Using a TCR transgenic model, Van de Velde et al.

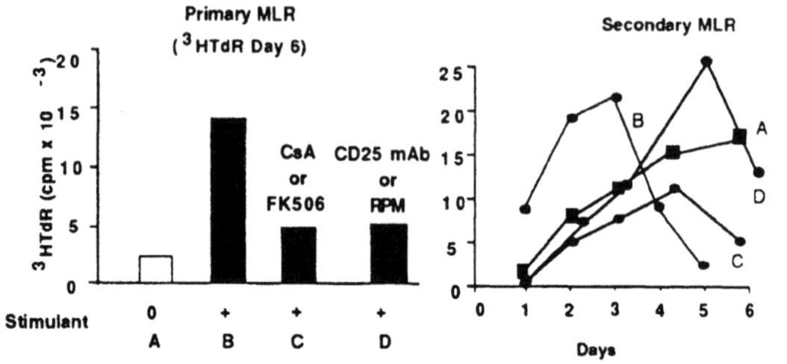

Fig. 2. Immunosuppressive agents which interfere with the IL-2 pathway decrease primary MLR but do not induce clonal anergy and/or deletion.

showed that the costimulatory B7 (CD80) signal could be provided by a third party stimulatory cell and that requirement for costimulation by CD80/CD28 interaction was mandatory for naive T cell but not for pre-activated ($CD45RO^+$) T cell stimulation [8].

The MLR model is pertinent for investigating how alteration of the primary response by immunomodulatory agents will modify the secondary response measured in the absence of the modulating agent.

The immunosuppressive agent may decrease the alloreactive T cell proliferative response and cytokine secretion during the primary response, but also induce specific unresponsiveness as measured in the secondary response, by altering the initial activating signals and inducing clonal deletion (apoptosis of activated T cells) or clonal anergy. Hence, addition of mitogenic or non-mitogenic CD3 antibodies during the primary culture induces clonal anergy [9]. Inhibition of the CD28 costimulatory pathway by soluble CTLA-4 induces a clonal anergy [10] which can be reversed by addition of rIL-2. CD4 antibodies also induce a state of clonal unresponsiveness [11] associated with down-regulation of IL-2 but not IFNγ synthesis [12]. However this type of anergy which can be induced in primed as well as in naive $CD4^+$ T cells is not reversible in the presence of rIL-2 [11] but only by costimulation with CD3 and CD45 RA antibodies [13]. The CD11a antibodies 25.3 and BL5 inhibit the primary proliferative response as well as IL-2 and IFNγ expression but do not induce clonal unresponsiveness (Fournel et al. unpublished data). Similarly, interference with cytokine synthesis by cyclosporin A or FK506 or with IL-2 signaling by CD25 antibodies or rapamycin inhibits the primary response without inducing clonal anergy or deletion (Figure 2). Gupta et al. recently reported that addition of cyclosporin A at low doses (100 ng/ml) during primary culture enhanced the differentiation of memory T cells and the proliferative response in secondary culture [14]. Similarly, addition of pentoxyfilline, a phosphodiesterase inhibitor, inhibits the primary response but enhances the recall response [14]. As discussed below, other antibodies may selectively induce clonal deletion of activated T cells. Interestingly no obvious difference in susceptibility to inhibition by current immunosuppressive agents between primary and secondary MLR has been reported but systematic comparisons have not been performed in this model and further investigations are needed. In preactivated T cells, the transcription enhancer AP-1 is already translocated to the nucleus so that cyclosporin A and tacrolimus are no longer effective. An important issue is whether a similar state of preactivation may exist in alloreactive memory T cells and account for a relative resistance to cyclosporin A, as suggested by Claas and coworkers in this volume.

Activation-induced cell death (AICD)

Several recent studies have demonstrated that clonal expansion of activated T cells can be controlled by induction of programmed cell death of activated lymphocytes. The major pathway of this AICD involves interaction between Fas (CD95, Apo-1) expressed on activated T and B cells and Fas-ligand (Fas-L) on a subset of activated T cells [15]. Fas is a 45–48 kDa cell surface glycoprotein which belongs to the tumor necrosis factor (TNF)/nerve growth factor (NGF) receptor family [16–19]. Fas-L is a member of the TNF family that is expressed by activated T cells [20–22]. Fas-L is a type II transmembrane protein of approximately 40 kDa which can be cleaved from the cell surface by a metalloprotease [23, 24]. The transmembrane protein as well as the soluble factor can induce apoptosis [21]. Mice with mutations in the *lpr* and *gld* loci, which bear defective Fas and Fas-L expression, respectively [25–27], develop a lymphoproliferative disease associated with a systemic lupus erythematosus-like autoimmune disorder. This syndrome is accounted for by the inability of mutant mice to properly delete their activated peripheral T and B lymphocytes [25]. A comparable syndrome has been recently reported in patients with a mutation in the Fas gene leading to defective Fas expression or Fas-mediated signaling [28, 29].

One of the best studied models of in vivo AICD is the superantigen-induced deletion of peripheral T cells in the mouse. Indeed, parenteral administration of the bacterial superantigen SEB (*Staphyloccocus aureus* enterotoxin B) induces proliferation of reactive T cells ($V\beta8^+$ T cells) followed by a phase of deletion of activated T cells [30]. Lenardo [31] reported that IL-2 may control SEB-induced AICD. Indeed, an antibody which blocks the binding of IL-2 reversed the clonal deletion of lymph node $V\beta8^+$ T cells seen in mice exposed to SEB.

Fas-mediated apoptosis may be controlled at various levels, including Fas-L synthesis, Fas expression and acquisition of cell susceptibility to Fas-induced apoptosis. Fas molecules are expressed on T cells after activation by antigens or mitogens. Susceptibility to Fas-mediated apoptosis is progressively acquired during activation and proliferation. For instance, Klas et al. [32] have reported that one day-activated T cells expressed Fas but were resistant to anti-Fas-mediated apoptosis whereas six day-activated T cells were sensitive. We have

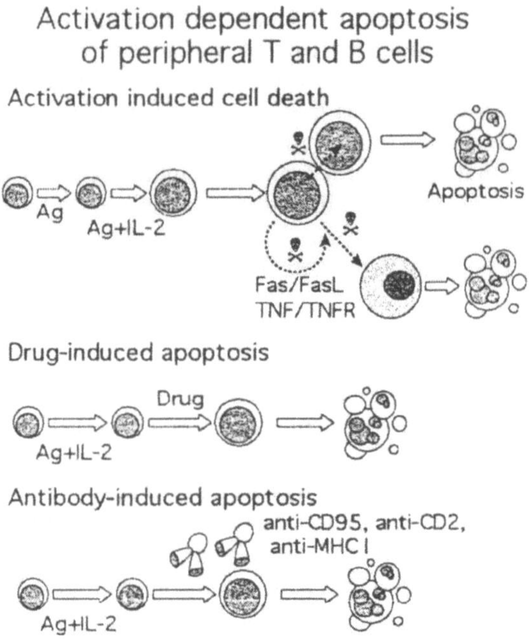

Fig. 3. Activation-induced cell death, antibody-induced cell death and drug-induced cell death.

investigated the kinetics of expression of Fas, Fas-L, and the susceptibility of Fas positive cells to Fas-mediated apoptosis. Following mitogenic activation of human peripheral blood lymphocytes the expression of CD45RA progressively declines whereas that of CD45R0 increases. At day 3 after PHA-activation, most blast cells express a mixed $CD45RA^+R0^+$ phenotype and at day 4–6 nearly all blast cells are $CD45RA^-R0^+$ (Figure 4). CD95 is expressed early after activation and throughout the culture period. However the susceptibility to Fas-mediated apoptosis, measured by the number of cells undergoing apoptosis in the presence of an agonist anti-Fas mAb (CH 11), develops slowly and follows the kinetics of CD45RO expression (Figure 4). When the IL-2 pathway is inhibited by addition of cyclosporin A, FK506, rapamycin or CD25 mAbs, activated T cells are arrested in the G1 phase of the cell cycle and remain resistant to Fas-mediated apoptosis, despite the fact that they strongly express Fas [33]. Acquisition of sensitivity to Fas-dependent apoptosis requires an IL-2 signal, whereas transition from G1 to S phase of the cell cycle, which can be achieved by IL-4, IL-7, or IFNγ, failed to restore apoptosis in the presence of anti-Fas antibodies. Moreover these data suggest that the β chain of IL-2 receptor rather than the common γ chain is involved in delivering the signal(s) necessary to the acquisition of sensitivity to Fas dependent apoptosis. Similar conclusions were reached by *in vitro* studies in mice [34]

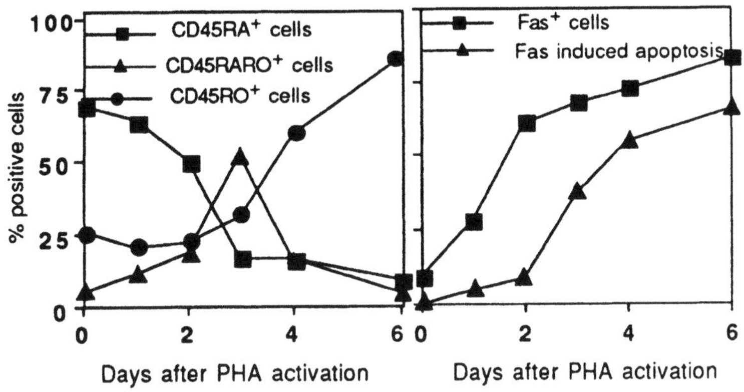

Fig. 4. CD45 isoforms, Fas expression and Fas-mediated apoptosis following human peripheral blood T cell activation.

and supported by the development of lymphoproliferative disorders in mice genetically deficient in IL-2 [35, 36] or IL-2 receptor α or β chains [37, 38].

By extrapolating these data to clinical transplantation, one may assume that restriction of alloreactive T cell clonal expansion by Fas/Fas-L interactions seems to be limited to a subset of preactivated T cells which express the $CD45RO^+$ phenotype. Conventional immunosuppressive treatments which interfere with the IL-2 pathway inhibit Fas-L expression [39] and prevent the development of sensitivity to Fas-mediated apoptosis without impairing Fas expression [33]. It is likely that drugs or mAbs that induce apoptosis of activated T cells through a Fas dependent pathway may be antagonized by conventional immunosuppressive agents. Conversely drugs or mAbs which do not depend on Fas-L for their apoptotic activity could target early activated T cells ($CD45RA^+$ and $CD45RA^+RO^+$) and therefore display a broader spectrum of activity.

Activation dependent antibody-induced cell death

Some antibodies to lymphocyte surface molecules may induce apoptosis of activated but not resting T (and B) lymphocytes and therefore be considered for therapeutic applications in clinical transplantation. Indeed such antibodies, if administered during the period of *in vivo* donor specific T cell activation, could induce peripheral T cell clonal deletion while leaving non-activated T cells unharmed. Such antibodies may induce apoptosis by Fas-dependent or Fas-independent pathways.

The veto phenomenon is characterized by clonal deletion of activated T helper and cytotoxic T cell precursors following interaction of their MHC class I molecules with CD8 on allogeneic antigen presenting cells [40]. In a search for a human equivalent of the veto effect, we tested a series of anti-HLA class

I mAbs for their capacity to delete activated but not resting T cells. We found that two mAbs which recognize an epitope of the $\alpha 1$ domain of HLA-A, -B, -C and -G molecules (mouse mAb90, and rat YTH862 from Pr. H. Waldmann's laboratory) could induce apoptosis of activated T cells by a Fas-independent pathway [41, 42]. Cells susceptible to the HLA-class I mediated apoptosis expressed the $CD45RA^+$ RO^+ phenotype and appeared earlier following activation than those susceptible to anti-Fas.

Interestingly the same mAbs induced apoptosis of CD40-activated B cells but engagement of the B cell receptors (mIgM) protected B cells against this type of apoptosis [43].

Some co-mitogenic CD2 mAbs were reported by Mollereau et al. to induce apoptosis of T cells that had been preactivated by a pair of CD2 mAbs, and strong evidence against a contribution of the Fas pathway was documented, but the precise phenotype of the target cells was not studied [44]. We analyzed the effects of another non-comitogenic CD2R mAb (YTH 655.5 from Pr. Waldmann's laboratory) and we showed that this mAb induced Fas-L expression and triggered apoptosis of activated T cells by a Fas dependent pathway, since apoptosis was completely inhibited by addition of an antagonist anti-Fas mAb (Figure 5). Interestingly, the CD2R mAb YTH 655.5 was found to activate $p56^{lck}$, in keeping with the recent demonstration by Gonzalez-Garcia et al. [45] that expression of activated $p56^{lck}$ in transfected cells was required and sufficient to induce Fas-L expression. However, CD4 mAbs which also activate $p56^{lck}$ induced IL-2 resistant anergy but did not trigger apoptosis (S. Fournel et al., unpublished data). CD4 mAbs rather decreased AICD in solid phase OKT3 stimulated T cells by inhibiting IL-2 synthesis. Indeed, cells activated in presence of CD4 mAbs down-regulate their IL-2 synthesis and therefore lack the IL-2-dependent signal which permits the acquisition of susceptibility to Fas-L-lysis during T cell activation.

Polyclonal ATG are potent inducers of Fas-L expression even when used at submitogenic concentrations. At high doses they activate the classical complement pathway and opsonize circulating lymphocytes irrespectively of their activation status. At low doses however, they trigger Fas-L expression (Figure 5) and destroy activated (Fas-sensitive) but not resting (Fas negative) T lymphocytes through the predominant but not exclusive use of the Fas pathway (L. Genestier et al., submitted). This property, so far only demonstrated *in vitro*, could be evaluated in clinical trials in which low doses of ATG given after transplantation or during rejection episodes would target activated but not resting T cells. Quite likely other mAbs may share with the former the capacity to delete activated T cells. Possible candidates from *in vitro* studies include anti-CTLA4 [46], CD30 [47], CD45 [48], CD43 [49] and CD40 [50].

Activation dependent drug-induced cell death

Knowing that some mAbs can induce apoptosis of activated T (and B) cells, we investigated whether similar effects could be achieved by drugs. As already

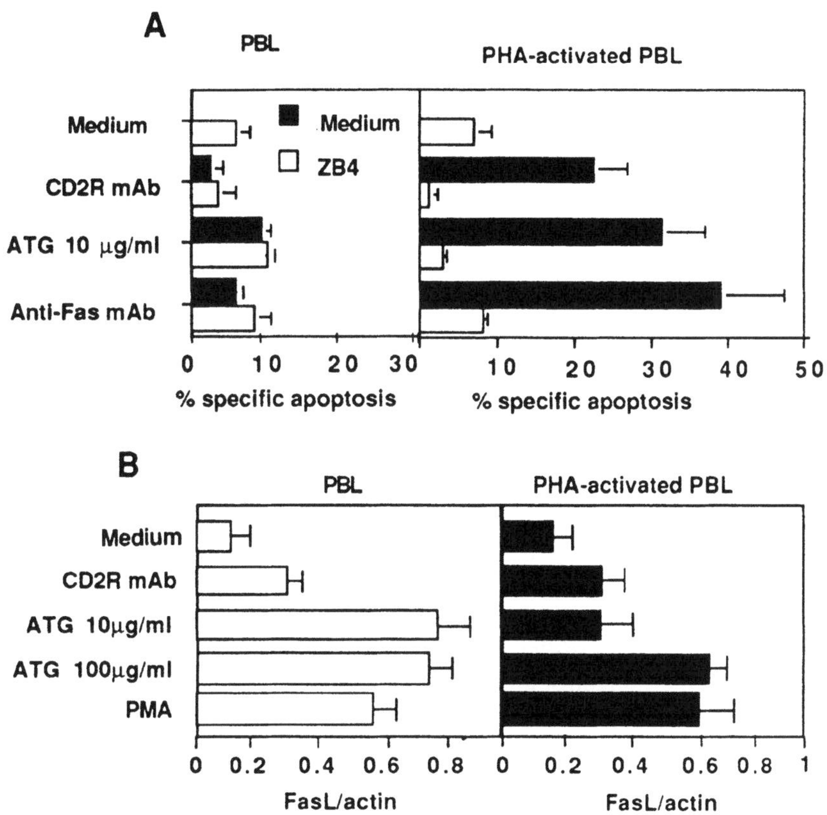

Fig. 5. Fas-dependent apoptosis induced by CD2R mAb and ATG. ATG: Anti-thymocyte globulins, ZB4: Fas specific antagonist mAb, PMA: Phorbol Myristate Acetate. A: specific apoptosis, B: Fas-L mRNA as determined by RT-PCR.

mentioned, cyclosporin A, tacrolimus (FK 506) and rapamycin lack such activity at concentrations corresponding to the peak of plasma levels during treatment. However the dihydrofolate reductase inhibitor methotrexate (MTX) was found to induce apoptosis of up to 80% of PHA-blasts at concentrations within the μM range which are achieved *in vivo*, for instance in rheumatoid arthritis patients who are given 10–15 mg I.M. at weekly intervals (Figure 6). MTX is actively taken up by resting as well as by activated lymphocytes, but only activated cells in the S/G2 phases of the cell cycle are signalled to apoptosis. Interestingly, at higher concentrations which are used for oncologic applications, MTX still inhibits T cell proliferation but no longer induces apoptosis. Although MTX may exert other biological activities (e.g. anti-inflammatory effects through stimulation of adenosine synthesis – see ref 51) the demonstration of its apoptosis inducing capacity provides a rationale for intermittent administration in allografts and auto-immune diseases. Moreover this new end-

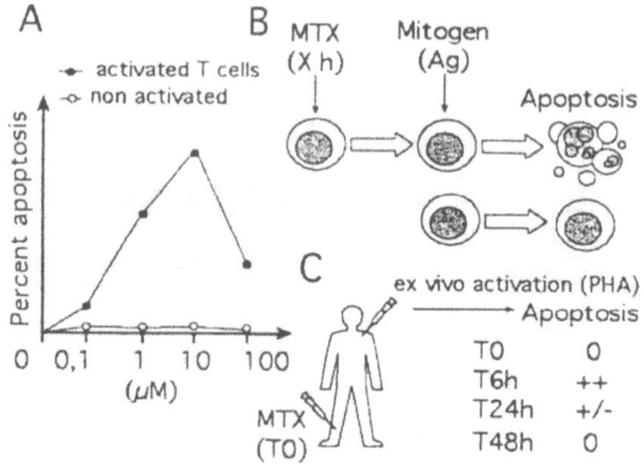

Fig. 6. *In vivo* and *in vitro* apoptosis of activated T cells induced by MTX.

point could be used as a read-out assay for individual adjustment of doses and intervals between injections.

It was suggested in a recent report that MTX could stimulate Fas-L expression in cell lines and use the Fas pathway to achieve apoptosis [52]. In our experiments, the antagonist anti-Fas mAb ZB4, which completely inhibits anti-Fas or Fas-L-mediated apoptosis, did not decrease MTX-induced lysis. Furthermore susceptibility to MTX can be demonstrated within 24 h of stimulation by PHA, at a time when T cells are still resistant to anti-Fas (see Figure 4).

Knowing that many immunosuppressive agents were initially developed for cancer chemotherapy, we initiated a systematic screening of antimitotic agents for their capacity to induce apoptosis of activated but not resting T cells. Such effect measured *in vitro* on peripheral blood T cells may be associated with a selective ability to induce clonal deletion of activated T cells *in vivo*, providing that the active concentrations were below toxic levels. Preliminary experiments from our group demonstrate that the topoisomerase II inhibitor, etoposide (VP 16), and the topoisomerase I inhibitor, camptothecin may have such activity whereas the intercalating agent daunorubicin induces apoptosis of resting as well as activated T cells at concentrations much higher than those required for killing the CEM T cell line (Figure 7). An important issue is whether such drugs induce apoptosis by a Fas-dependent pathway as suggested by a recent report [53]. Actually such drugs would seem to induce Fas-L mRNA expression but their apoptotic activity is not antagonized by the anti-Fas antibody ZB4 and apply to both Fas-susceptible and Fas-resistant subsets of PHA-activated blasts (Figure 8) (C. Ferraro et al., manuscript in preparation). Experiments in progress investigate whether such agents may induce clonal deletion of activated T cells in murine models.

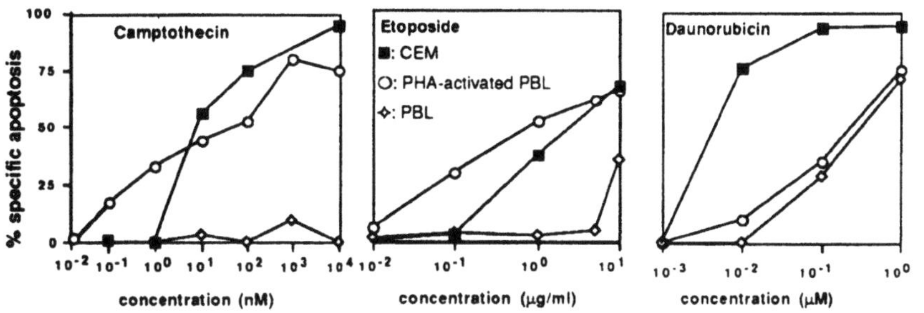

Fig. 7. Apoptosis of activated and resting T cells induced by topoisomerase inhibitors. The intercalating agent daunorubicin used as control induces apoptosis of both resting and activated T cells.

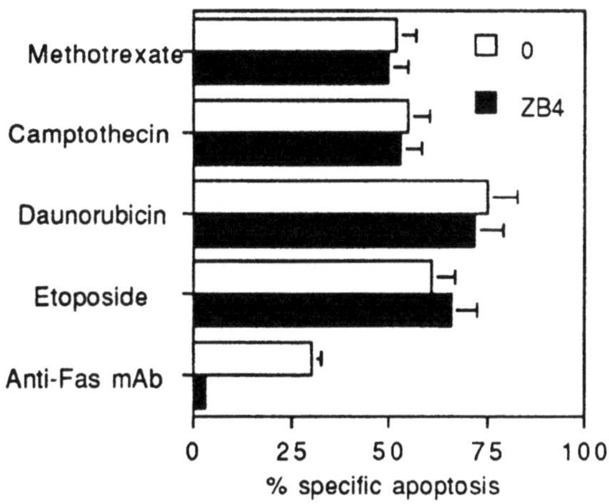

Fig. 8. Activation-dependent drug-induced apoptosis of human peripheral T cells does not involve the Fas pathway. ZB4 is a Fas specific antagonist mAb (see Figure 5).

Prospects for clinical applications

The recently discovered homeostatic mechanisms of AICD accounting for the clonal deletion of some activated peripheral T cells may be relevant to the *in vivo* regulation of the allograft reaction. However converging evidence supports the view that currently used immunosuppressive agents, which interfere with the IL-2 pathway and prevent T cell activation, inhibit both Fas-L expression and the aquisition of sensitivity to Fas-mediated apoptosis. Therapeutic application of AICD would require application of a 'minimal window' of therapeutic abstinence followed by Fas-dependent deletion of *in vivo* alloreactive T cells. Such strategy is at high risk of inducing early irreversible rejection, despite the fact that long-term clonal deletion may be beneficial for tolerance induction.

Clinical observations showing that a single acute rejection crisis does not *per se* entails further risk of graft loss are in keeping with the hypothesis that deletion of alloreactive T cells may contribute to graft acceptance. The use of mAbs or drugs which selectively delete activated T cells by a Fas-independent pathway may represent an improvement in the clonal deletion strategy, as exemplified by MTX. Their mechanism of action is compatible with intermittent or short term (e.g. induction therapy) administration and their selectivity relies exclusively on the timing of administration versus *in vivo* activation. When used during a viral infection, such agents could have long-lasting effects preventing recovery, by deletion of virus specific T cell lines.

T cell activating antibodies (e.g. high dose ATG or OKT3) may prime T cells for Fas-L expression upon subsequent antigenic stimulation. In this respect they are likely to induce sustained non-specific immunosuppression with increased risk of viral infections and virus-associated tumors (lymphomas, skin and cervix cancers). However low doses of ATG given immediately after transplantation may selectively delete *in vivo* activated donor specific T cell clones, and clinical trials based on this mechanism may be warranted.

Whether immunological monitoring could provide a rationale for induction therapy remains highly controversial because of the lack of simple and reliable assessment of anti-donor preactivated or memory T cells. To our knowledge systematic investigation of T cell presensitization by short term donor-recipient MLR (equivalent of an *ex vivo* secondary MLR) has not been performed. Detection of anti-donor CTL frequency, as performed for allogeneic non HLA-identical stem cell transplantation, requires *ex vivo* expansion of CTL precursors. Therefore, such assay may be suited for the detection of minor incompatibilities recognized by the recipient's TCR repertoire, but it is not applicable to the screening of presensitized recipients in organ transplantation. Detection of anti-donor cell CTL that are not inhibited by anti-CD8 mAbs clearly deserves further evaluation, as it might indicate the presence of memory T cells that do not require co-activation signals for differentiating into effector CTL. Further studies should focus on highly sensitive and quantitative detection of activation makers (e.g. CD69 or CD95 mRNA by RT-PCR) in unidirectional donor-recipient MLR.

In conclusion, induction therapies aimed at deleting donor specific peripheral alloreactive T cells could represent a major improvement over current strategies based on blocking T cell activation (cyclosporin, tacrolimus, rapamycin, CD25 mAbs) or deleting a great part of peripheral T cells (high dose ATG, OKT3, Campath or other depleting mAbs). The selectivity of such treatments would rely on the timing of their administration. Possible candidates for such activity may be methotrexate, topoisomerase inhibitors, low dose ATG or mAbs such as CD2R or anti-HLA class I $\alpha 1$ domain.

Acknowledgements

Supported in part by Région Rhône-Alpes H098730000.

References

1. Etablissement Français des Greffes. Annual report from the Conseil Medical et Scientifique, 1996.
2. Traeger J, Touraine JL, Malik MC, Revillard JP, Laville M. Antilymphocyte globulin and thoracic duct drainage in renal transplantation. Kidney Int. 1983; 23 (Suppl. 14); S74–S81.
3. Touraine JL, Traeger J, Bétuel H et al. Antilymphocyte globulin in renal transplantation. Transplant Clin. Immunol. 1983; 15: 41–47.
4. Revillard JP, Laville M, Vincent C. Serum C-reactive protein assay in renal transplantation. In: Allen R, Bienvenu J, Laurent P, Suskind R (eds.), Marker Proteins in Inflammation. Walter de Gruyter, Berlin, 1982, pp. 509–510.
5. Constant S, Zain M, Pasqualini T, Ranney P, Bottomly K. Are primed $CD4^+$ T lymphocytes different from unprimed cells? Eur. J. Immunol. 1994; 24: 1073–1079.
6. Luqman M, Bottomly K. Activation requirements for $CD4^+$ T cells differing in CD45R expression. J. Immunol. 1992; 149: 2300–2306.
7. Johnson JG, Jenkins MK. Monocytes provide a novel costimulatory signal to T cells that is not mediated by the CD28/B7 interaction. J. Immunol. 1994; 152: 429–437.
8. Van de Velde I, Lorré K, Bakkus M, Thielemans K, Ceuppens L, de Boer M. $CD45RO^+$ memory T cells but not $CD45RA^+$ naive T cells can be efficiently activated by remote co-stimulation with B7. Int. Immunol. 1993; 5: 1483–1487.
9. Anasetti C, Tan P, Hansen JA, Martin PJ. Induction of specific nonresponsiveness in unprimed human T cells by anti-CD3 antibody and alloantigen. J. Exp. Med. 1990; 172: 1691–1700.
10. Tan P, Anasetti C, Hansen JA, Melrose J, Brunvand M, Bradshaw J, Ledbetter JA, Linsley PS. Induction of alloantigen-specific hyporesponsiveness in human T lymphocytes by blocking interaction of CD28 with its ligand B7/BB1. J. Exp. Med. 1993; 177: 165–173.
11. Vincent C, Fournel S, Wijdenes J, Revillard JP. Specific hyporesponsiveness of alloreactive peripheral T cells induced by CD4 antibodies. Eur. J. Immunol. 1995; 25: 816–822.
12. Fournel S, Vincent C, Assossou O et al. CD4 mAbs prevent progression of alloactivated $CD4^+$ T cells into the S phase of the cell cycle without interfering with early activation signals. Transplantation 1996; 62: 1136–1143.
13. Robinet E, Fournel S, Fatmi A, Revillard JP. IL-2-resistant hyporesponsiveness induced by CD4 mAbs in OKT3-activated human T cells is reversed by CD45RA triggering. Cell Immunol. 1996; 167: 1–7.
14. Gupta M, Satyaraj E, Durkik JM, Rath S, Bal V. Differential regulation of T cell activation for primary versus secondary proliferative responses. J. Immunol. 1997; 158: 4113–4121.
15. Lynch DH, Ramsdell F, Alderson MR. Fas and Fas-L in the homeostatic regulation of immune responses. Immunol. Today 1995; 16: 569–574.
16. Trauth BC, Klas C, Peters AMJ, Matzku S, Möller P, Falk W, Debatin KM, Krammer PH. Monoclonal antibody-mediated tumor regression by induction of apoptosis. Science 1989; 245: 301–305.
17. Itoh N., Yonehara S, Ishii A et al. The polypeptide encoded by cDNA for human cell surface antigen Fas can mediate apoptosis. Cell 1991; 66: 233–243.
18. Smith CA, Farrah T, Goodwin RG. The TNF receptor superfamily of cellular and viral proteins: activation, costimulation and death. Cell 1994; 76: 959–962.
19. Armitage RJ. Tumor necrosis factor receptor superfamily members and their ligands. Curr. Opin. Immunol. 1994; 6: 407–413.
20. Suda T, Takahashi T, Golstein P, Nagata S. Molecular cloning and expression of the Fas ligand, a novel member of the tumor necrosis factor family. Cell 1993; 75: 1169–1178.
21. Suda T, Nagata S. Purification and characterization of the Fas-ligand that induces apoptosis. J. Exp. Med. 1994; 179: 873.
22. Suda T, Okazaki T, Naito Y et al. Expression of the Fas ligand in cells of T cell lineage. J. Immunol. 1995; 154: 3806–3813.

23. Kayagaki N, Kawasaki A, Ebata T et al. Metalloproteinase-mediated release of human Fas ligand. J. Exp. Med. 1995; 182: 1777–1783.
24. Mariani SM, Matiba B, Baümler C, Krammer PH. Regulation of cell surface APO-1/Fas (CD95) ligand expression by metalloproteases. Eur. J. Immunol. 1995; 25: 2303–2304.
25. Watanabe-Fukanaga RC, Brannan I, Coneland NG et al. Lymphoproliferation disorder in mice explained by defects in Fas antigen that mediates apoptosis. Nature 1992; 356: 314–317.
26. Ramsdell, F, Seaman MS, Miller RE, Tough TW, Alderson MR, Lynch DH. gld/gld mice are unable to express a functional ligand for Fas. Eur. J. Immunol. 1994; 4: 928–933.
27. Takahashi T, Tanaka M, Brannan CI et al. Generalized lymphoproliferation disease in mice, caused by a point mutation in the Fas ligand. Cell 1994; 76: 969–976.
28. Rieux-Laucat F, Le Deist F, Hivroz C et al. Mutations in Fas associated with human lymphoproliferative syndrome and autoimmunity. Science 1995; 268: 1347–1349.
29. Fisher GH, Rosenberg FJ, Straus SE et al. Dominant interfering Fas gene mutations impair apoptosis in a human autoimmune lymphoproliferative syndrome. Cell 1995; 81: 935–946.
30. MacDonald HR, Baschieri S, Lees RK. Clonal expansion precedes anergy and death of $V\beta 8^+$ peripheral T cells responding to staphylococcal enterotoxin B *in vivo*. Eur. J. Immunol. 1991; 21: 1963–1966.
31. Lenardo MJ. Interleukin-2 programs mouse $\alpha\beta$ T lymphocytes for apoptosis. Nature 1991; 353: 858–861.
32. Klas C, Debatin KM, Jonker RR, Krammer PH. Activation interferes with the Apo-1 pathway in mature human T cells. Int. Immunol. 1993; 5: 625–630.
33. Fournel S, Genestier L, Robinet E, Flacher M, Revillard JP. Human T cells require IL-2 but not G1/S transition to acquire susceptibility to Fas-mediated apoptosis. J. Immunol. 1996; 157: 4309–4315.
34. Wang R, Rogers AM, Rush BJ, Russel JH. Induction of sensitivity to activation-induced death in primary $CD4^+$ cell: a role for interleukin-2 in the negative regulation of response by mature $CD4^+$ cells. Eur. J. Immunol. 1996; 26: 2263–2270.
35. Kneitz B, Herrmann T, Yonera S, Schimpl A. Normal clonal expansion but impaired Fas-mediated cell death and anergy induction in interleukin-2-deficient mice. Eur. J. Immunol. 1995; 25: 2572–2577.
36. Kündig, TM, Schorle H, Bachmann MF et al. Immune responses in interleukin-2-deficient mice. Science 1993; 262: 1059–1061.
37. Willerford DM, Chen J, Ferry JA et al. Interleukin-2 receptor α chain regulates the size and content of the peripheral lymphoid. Immunity 1995; 3: 521–530.
38. Suzuki H, Kündig TM, Furlonger C et al. Deregulated T cell activation and autoimmunity in mice lacking interleukin-2 receptor β. Nature 1995; 268: 1472–1476.
39. Anel A, Buferne M, Boyer C, Schmitt-Verhulst A-M, Golstein P. T cell receptor-induced Fas ligand expression in cytotoxic T lymphocyte clones is blocked by protein tyrosine kinase inhibitors and cyclosporin A. Eur. J. Immunol. 1994; 24: 2469–2476.
40. Sambhara SR, Miller RG. Programmed cell death of T cells signaled by the T cell receptor and the $\alpha 3$ domain of class I CMH. Science 1991; 252: 1424–1427.
41. Genestier L, Paillot R, Bonnefoy-Berard N, Waldmann H, Revillard JP. T cell sensitivity to HLA class I-mediated apoptosis is dependent on IL-2 and IL-4. Eur. J. Immunol. 1997; 27: 495–499.
42. Genestier L, Paillot R, Bonnefoy-Berard N et al. Fas independent apoptosis of activated T cells induced by antibodies to the HLA class I $\alpha 1$ domain. Blood 1997; 90 (in press, Nov. issue).
43. Genestier L, Meffre G, Garrone P et al. Antibodies to HLA class I $\alpha 1$ domain trigger apoptosis of CD40-activated human B lymphocytes. Blood 1997; 90: 726–735.
44. Mollereau B, Deckert M, Déas O et al. CD2-induced apoptosis in activated human peripheral T cells: A Fas-independent pathway that requires early protein tyrosine phosphorylation. J. Immunol. 1996; 151: 3184–3190.
45. Gonzalez-Garcia A, Borlando L, Leonardo E, Mérida I, Martinez A, Carrera AC. Lck is necessary and sufficient for Fas-ligand expression and apoptotic cell death in mature cycling T cells. J. Immunol. 1997; 158: 4104–4112.

46. Gribben JG, Freeman GJ, Boussiotis VA et al. CTLA-4 mediates antigen-specific apoptosis of human T cells. Proc. Natl. Acad. Sci. USA 1995; 92: 811–815.
47. Lee SY, Park CG, Choi Y. T cell receptor-dependent cell death of T cell hybridomas mediated by the CD30 cytoplasmic domain in association with Tumor Necrosis Factor receptor-associated factors. J. Exp. Med. 1996; 183: 669–674.
48. Klaus SJ, Sidorenko SP, Clark EA. CD45 ligation induces programmed cell death in T and B lymphocytes. J. Immunol. 1996; 156: 2743–2753.
49. Brown TJ, Shuford WW, Wang W-C et al. Characterization of a CD43/leukosialin-mediated pathway for inducing apoptosis in human T-lymphoblastoid cells. J. Biol. Chem. 1996; 271: 27686–27695.
50. Hess S, Engelmann H. A novel function of CD40: induction of cell death in transformed cells. J. Exp. Med. 1996; 183: 159–167.
51. Cronstein BN, Eberle MA, Gruber HE, Levin RI. Methotrexate inhibits neutrophil function by stimulating adenosine release from connective tissue cells. Proc. Natl. Acad. Sci. USA 1991; 88: 2441–2445.
52. Friesen C, Herr I, Krammer P, Debatin K-M. Involvement of the CD95 (APO-1/Fas) receptor/ligand system in drug-induced apoptosis in leukemia cells. Nature Med. 1996; 2: 574–577.
53. Müller M, Strand S, Hug H et al. Drug-induced apoptosis in hepatoma cells is mediated by the CD95 (APO-1/Fas) receptor/ligand system and involves activation of wild-type p53. J. Clin. Invest. 1997; 99: 403–413.

PART FOUR

Allo-antibody positive recipient

17. Therapeutic intervention on preformed anti-HLA antibodies

FAYÇAL KRIAA, CHRISTIAN HIESSE, SYLVIE MARCHAND, CHRISTOPHE GOUPY, HOSSEIN FARAHMAND, ALAIN BISMUTH, GÉRARD BENOIT & BERNARD M. CHARPENTIER

Introduction

The presence of broadly reactive antibodies directed at allogeneic lymphocytes is a major and increasing cause of delay in transplantation of patients with end-stage renal disease. In addition, hyperimmunized status is associated with a lower graft success rate that non-immunized status, unless patients were transplanted with excellent matched graft. Hyperimmunized patients represent an increasing proportion of graft waiting list, caused by previous graft failure, pregnancies and blood transfusions.

Currently, a sizeable proportion of the 4000 patients awaiting transplantation in France are sensitized [1], of which 9–15% are defined as hyperimmunized (PRA $\geq$ 80%). Although the French organization has developed a special organ-sharing program for this population, only 12% of the total number of transplants performed in France in 1995 have been done in highly sensitized recipients. The magnitude of this problem, similar in Europe and North America [2], explains why more active strategies for managing hyperimmunized patients have been introduced during the past decade.

Document sensitization

The human kidney expresses class I and variably, class II MHC antigens [3]. Thus, it is not surprising that anti-HLA antibodies, present in the circulating vascular compartment after HLA sensitization, might damage grafts expressing the appropriate HLA antigens. This fact, known in the early time of transplantation, and inducing 'hyperacute' or humoral rejection, lead to the discovery of the cross-matching technique. Anti-graft antibodies are detected by complement-dependent cytotoxicity test (CDC) just before transplantation, using donor's lymphocytes as source of target cells and current and historical samples of recipient's sera. On the other hand, sera from patients awaiting transplantation are screened regularly with panels of HLA typed lymphocytes, selected for the representation of the maximum of defined class I and II HLA molecules. The proportion of the panel cells that an individual patient serum kills is expressed at the percentage reactivity. Moreover, the specificities recognized

J.L. Touraine et al. (eds.), Retransplantation, 139–149.

by the antibodies is determined from the HLA types of killed donor lymphocytes. Patients with >75% of PRA are called highly sensitized.

The notion of allosensitization is associated with several immunological problems.

Targets of alloreactivity: HLA molecules

Recent advances in the crystallographic and functional structures of the HLA molecules led to better understanding of recognized epitopes [4]. First, serologic determinants are not the same that cellular determinants which are detected by anti-HLA cytotoxic T cells (CTL). This notion is based, at least in class I molecules, by epitopic peptides taken part in the conformation of the antigen groove determined by helices and β sheet. Most of the epitopes recognized by antibody are located outside the groove, mostly on the border of the groove, since peptides of the wall or the bottom side are not reached by antibodies. Moreover there are clearly also non dominant or cryptic determinant, in this sense HLA molecules are similar to other protein antigens which contain both dominant and cryptic determinant regions.

The HLA antibodies, usually IgG, are mainly directed against class I HLA antigens [5]. Two types of HLA antibodies are found in sensitized patients. Most patients have antibodies directed against cross-reactive groups of HLA class I antigens similar to those detected in the sera of multiparous women. These antibodies are directed against shared public determinants on the HLA class I heavy chain. The public epitopes are shared by several HLA antigens: therefore an antibody directed against one ot these antigens can cause a high percentage of panel reactivity. Individuals can have one of 3 different antibodies recognizing different groups of HLA antigens, thus causing very high percentage reactivities. The degree of cross-reactivity depends on the titer of antibody. This can be shown by the use of mouse monoclonal antibody generated against class I HLA antigens or by the examination of sera at different dilutions from highly sensitized patients. The presence of cross-reactive group antibodies is associated with an increased rate of early graft loss and certain cross-reactive groups have a high rate of rejection. Patients also can have high percentage reactivity because they have multiple antibodies directed against private determinants on different HLA class I molecules. Non HLA lymphocytotoxic autoantibodies [5], which are usually IgM, cause high broadly reactive percentage reactivities and occur in 10% of sensitized patients awaiting renal transplantation. It has long been recognized that these antibodies do not cause hyperacute rejection and that transplantation across a positive IgM cross-match is associated with good graft survival. These antibodies are now inactivated by pretreating sera with dithiothreitol which does not modify IgG. These antibodies can be found in systemic lupus erythematosus patients and after viral infections.

Since the discovery of the complement-dependent microdroplet cytotoxicity test in 1964, several modifications have been described such as a precomplement wash step and the use of antihuman immunoglobulin. Nevertheless, unpredicted early graft losses still occur in CDC negative cross-matches. A recent analysis of 7788 renal allografts demonstrated that 6% of first grafts, 12% of second grafts and 18% of third regrafts never functioned [6]. The standart CDC crossmatch test was negative, and technical failures were excluded from the analysis. The flow cytometric cross-match test (FCXM), developped in 1983, has proven to be a very sensitive (quantitative) method for detecting T and B cell bound class-specific antibody [7]. Several retrospective studies have reported that a positive FCXM, CDC negative is associated with rejection episodes and graft failure. Other studies have shown that a positive FCXM is not predictive of graft loss. It has been suggested that the lower graft outcome in highly sensitized patients is only in small part related to vascular rejection and results mainly from accelerated cellular rejection. In these circumstances the PRA activity is merely a reflection of a 'high responder' state for enhanced cellular immunity. Pretransplant identification of renal allografts that will undergo acute irreversible rejection remains an unresolved crossmatch problem.

Management of sensitized patients

Prevention

By far, the best approach to sensitization is the prevention of such a state in potential transplant recipients. Recent major improvements in immunosuppression and in management of transplant recipients will decrease the number of immunological graft failure, thus a strong cause of allosensitization. On the other hand, nothing can be done on sensitization secondary to pregnancies. Thus, efforts must be concentrated on the role of blood transfusions (BT). BT are needed in ESRD patients because of blood loss (hemorrhage, anemia) and in pre-transplant BT protocols in order to improve graft survival. Since several years, recombinant human erythropoietin (rHu EPO) has been introduced in ESRD patients and currently fully controlled anemia, whereas it disclosed some well-known side effects such as HBP and thombosis of dialysis fistulae. There are some controversies regarding the decrease of PRA in previously sensitized patients. A variable numbers of sensitized patients substentially reduces HLA antibody titers, and to some extent, in percentage reactivity. One certainly would hope that the use of rHu EPO will have a major impact on the sensitization of ESRD patients induced by regular blood transfusions.

Attempts at extinguishing the antibody-secreting B cell clone

One direct approach of allogeneic sensitization would lie in the directed killing of the secreting B cell clones. Since most of the humoral response to allogeneic molecules is T-cell dependent, it was tempting to destroy particular T and B cell having the memory and the specificity of the allogeneic responsiveness.

Since memory B and T cells are long lived, most of them are homing in the spleen, lymph-nodes, liver and the thoracic duct and one physical approach would be treating patients with either splenectomy, or total lymphoïd irradiation, or immunosuppressive drugs. Few data are reported in the literature and currently there are only reports dealing with patients transplanted in ABO group incompatibility through the natural anti A anti B antibodies [8]. It is worth to say that the results were mitigated with some cases of hyperacute or accelerated rejection. It is a good proof that the secreting clones are particularly difficult to be localized and destroyed.

Attempts at the regulation of the antibody secreting clones

Two approaches can fit with this chapter, namely hypertransfusions and the use of polyclonal immunoglobulin. The first approach is the use of frequent small-aliquot blood transfusions [9]. This methodology is based upon the immunological phenomenon of B cell tolerance to high dose of antigens. Unfortunately, few data in human are available in the literature.

The use of repeated injection of intravenous polyclonal immunoglobulin, which may be of benefit in certain immunoregulatory disorders, has complex interactions with antibody synthesis immune complexes and the reticuloendothelial system. It has recently been used with success in sensitized renal transplant recipients [10], further work is needed for better definition of this therapeutic agent.

Removal of anti-HLA antibodies

Since Cardella et al. [11] reported in 1982 that a positive crossmatch with historic sera, but negative with current serum was not an absolute contraindication to renal transplantation, one of the most attractive approaches has been the removal and prevention of resynthesis of anti-HLA antibodies. Conventional plasma exchanges were extensively carried out to remove antibodies [12], but with controversial results [13], and with the disadvantages of side-effects, and the introduction of the risk of infections if freshly frozen plasma is used as substitution fluid.

The immunoadsorption (IA) system with Sepharose-bound staphylococcal protein, which interacts with high affinity with IgG [14] was developed to remove IgG in a variety of immune disorders, and since 1986 has been utilized for anti-HLA alloantibody removal. Controversial experiments from different groups have been published recently [15, 20], and most reports deal with pooled multicentric cases. Here, we report our experience with IA before planned renal transplantation in 15 hyperimmunized ESRD patients.

Selection criteria and patient characteristics. From 1987 to 1996, 15 hyperimmunized ESRD patients awaiting graft (12 females and 3 males), were selected to undergo the IA protocol to enable renal transplantation. The patients were enrolled in the study if they had a persistent historical PRA level of ≥80% for a minimum of one year, except for one patient whose peak PRA was of 65% (mean peak PRA 89 ± 9%). Patients whose PRA determined immediately before starting the IA protocol exhibited a transient decrease were not excluded from the study. Four patients with immediate pre-IA PRA < 50% were also immunoadsorbed (mean immediate pre-IA PRA ± 29%). PRA was determined by standard complement lymphocytotoxicity testing, using dithiothreitol to exclude IgM-dependent lymphocytotoxicity. Serial dilution (1:1–1:1256) for pre-IA sera was performed to determine the antibody titration. Patients whose pre-IA antibody titer was > 1:128, in which IA was expected to be unsuccessful were excluded from the study. Dilutions were also used to determine the pre-IA antigen specificities of anti-HLA antibodies.

All the selected patients had in the past received multiple transfusions, 9 of the 12 women had previous pregnancies. Four patients had received a previous graft, lost by hyperacute rejection in three. The patients had been on hemodialysis awaiting a cadaveric transplant for an average of 95 months, and 3 had vascular access problems. Finally, all patients had positive crossmatches with potential donors (total number of crossmatches performed = 33).

Immunoadsorption protocol. Immunoadsorption treatment for selected hyperimmunized patients was performed alternatively with hemodialysis. The extracorporeal treatment consists first of a conventional plasmapheresis to obtain plasma, which is pumped over the IA system. A plasma flow monitor (CITEM 10R, Excorim, Lund, Sweden) controls the plasma and elution solution flows, alternatively, over two parallel columns of sepharose-bound staphylococcal protein A (Immunosorba protein AR, Excorim). The elution fluids are directed to the waste, while treated plasma is returned to the patient after reconstitution with the blood cells. Each 4 h procedure treats two or three plasma volumes.

All the patients underwent a course of 3–7 alternate-day IA treatments, according to the tolerance and the degree of decrease in the anti-HLA antibody titers. From January 1990, the patients underwent a minimum of 6 treatments for the IA procedure. No additional courses were performed in our patients.

To prevent anti-HLA antibody resynthesis, the patients received an immunosuppresive protocol from the day before IA, consisting of prednisolone (0.5 mg/kg/day with a reduction of 10 mg/day per 15 days to a baseline of 10 mg/day), and cyclophosphamide. The cyclophosphamide was administered orally (2.5 mg/kd/day) to the first 9 patients. From September 1990, in order to improve tolerance and efficiency, 6 patients received cyclophosphamide boluses (10 mg/kg) every 3 weeks. After the IA course, the patients received one infusion of human polyclonal IgG (1.5 × 0.03 × body weight × IgG initial level) to restore serum IgG levels, and to potentially interfere with the immunological idiotypic network. To prevent infectious complications, patients received oral cotrimoxazole for a period of 2 months from the start of IA.

All the patients were routinely followed by clinical examination and WBC counts, and sera were checked for anti-HLA antibody titers after each procedure, and the PRA level every week after the end of treatment. Only the most recent post-IA serum, and the serum of the day of transplantation were used to perform T and B crossmatches. The transplantation was accepted on the basis of negative T and B crossmatches using the post-IA sera. Crossmatches with historical and pre-IA sera were preformed retrospectively.

For posttransplant immunosuppression, patients received a quadruple sequential protocol including a prophylactic 14-day course of 15 ml of horse polyclonal anti-lymphocyte globulins (ALG, lymphoglobulines, Institut Mérieux, Lyon, France), cyclosporine (CsA) 8 mg/kg/day, prednisolone 2 mg/kg/day and azathioprine 1 mg/kg/day introduced at day 45 posttransplant. Maintenance immunosuppression was the triple association of CsA, prednisone and azathioprine. Acute rejection episodes were treated by Methylprednisolone boluses (10 mg/kg for 3 days), and a 7-day course of 15 ml of polyclonal rabbit antithymocyte globulins (ATG thymoglobulines Mérieux).

Effect of immunoadsorption. A dramatic decrease of more than 90% in serum IgG levels was obtained in all patients. (Mean IgG level before IA: 12.3 ± 3.2 g/l, and after IA: 0.54 ± 0.2 g/l). However, each immunoadsorption course induced variable changes in the percentage PRA. The mean percentage PRA in the whole group decreased from $59 \pm 29\%$ before IA, to $22 \pm 25\%$ immediately after the last treatment, but individual responses varied considerably: in four patients, post-IA PRA was not detectable, and in 3 others, the magnitude of decrease of PRA was highly significant (>70%). In two patients, the effects of IA on the percentage PRA was intermediate (50–70% decrease), and it was only mild (<50%) in two others. Finally, there was no effect, and even an increase in the percentage PRA in the four remaining patients. For the subgroup of seven patients who had a highly significant or complete response, the mean pre-IA level was $60 \pm 24\%$, identical to the mean pre-IA PRA level in the 8 patients for whom IA was less effective ($59 \pm 34\%$). This parameter, was clearly not predictive for the success of the method. The mean percentage PRA remained stable until day 14, and then returned to pre-IA values at day 30 post IA. Individual responses also varied considerably, but in the majority of patients, the post-IA rebound was observed between day 14 (3 patients out of 14 awaiting transplantation) and day 30 (all 10 patients awaiting transplantation). In this subgroup of 10 patients not transplanted at day 30, PRA levels remained stable at pre-IA values, and the transplantation performed in 7 patients did not influence the percentage PRA. In the subset of 5 patients who were transplanted during the first month post-IA (four following a successful IA course, and one following a less effective treatment, but with a low pre-IA titer), transplantation was performed in one patient while PRA level had raised to pre-IA value. In this patient, the percentage PRA remained at pretransplant high values following transplantation. Finally, among the subgroup of 4 patients who where promptly transplanted after IA, and with low pretransplantation PRA levels, the percentage PRA rose significantly after transplantation in 2 patients, and remained at low levels in 2 others.

After the last IA treatment, we observed an uniform significant decrease in anti-HLA titers from 2 to 7 dilutions, except for 2 patients in whom the titers increased. This was observed regardless of the initial anti-HLA antibody titer, including patients whose initial titer was >1:64.

However, neither the magnitude of the decrease of PRA after IA, nor the initial pre-IA titers of the antibodies nor the presence of antibody specificity against crossreacting antigenic groups, were clinically predictive for the subsequent chances for getting any individual patient transplanted.

Crossmatching and transplantation. Twelve of our sensitized ESRD patients were able to receive a cadaver transplant following the IA procedure. However, only 9 were transplanted during the 2-month period after the last treatment. Furthermore, only five patients had negative crossmatch with post-IA serum, and positive with pre-IA sera. Seven patients (including 2 immediately after IA) were transplanted with negative crossmatches with both pre and post-IA sera. In these patients, transplantation was performed with highly compatible kidney donors (mean number of HLA A-B-DR mismatches between donor and recipient: 2.86 ± 0.8), while compatibility was poorer in positive crossmatch patients (mean number of A-B-DR mismatches: 4.2 ± 1.4). The subgroup of 6 patients for whom IA was unable to allow transplantation during the 2 month post-IA period (3 were not transplanted, and 3 received a compatible graft 233–701 days post-IA) included the patient in which IA was stopped because of his poor tolerance although the procedure had been highly effective, 4 patients for whom IA had been only slightly effective in decreasing percentage PRA, and finally a patient who was of B blood type, for which we were unable to find an ABO-matched donor before PRA increased at day 14 post-IA. Among the historical positive subgroup of 5 patients, the IA course had been highly effective for 2 for the percentage PRA, but in the 3 others, IA had induced only moderate decreases in PRA levels (70%, 43% and 0% respectively). This group of successful IA and graft included a patient who had a low pre-IA percentage PRA, and in whom PRA remained at the same level after IA, while the antibody titer increased from 1:2 to 1:8. These results indicate that while an effective IA course, as defined by as a greater than 70% in PRA, is able to enhance the opportunity for transplantation, also mild changes in percentage PRA may produce a significant effect in some individuals.

In the five patients with historical positive crossmatches with the donors, one died at day 29 from myocardial infarction after an initial tubulonephritis. A renal biopsy performed at day 14 in this patient showed the absence of rejection features. Two grafts were lost by hyperacute rejection at day 2 and day 10, respectively. Microscopic transplant nephrectomy examination showed vascular lesions, intraglomerular thrombosis and fibrin deposits in the vessel wall and the glomeruli. Two grafts are still functioning from 4 to 8 months post transplant, and the actuarial graft survival rate is only 40% at 6-months posttransplant. One surviving patient had an uneventful course after transplantation except for a mild cellular rejection at day 15, reversed by antirejection therapy. The other had an immediately favourable outcome with a decrease in serum creatinine from 640 μmol/l before grafting to 98 μmol/l at day 7. On day 20, serum creatinine suddenly rose to 350 μmol/l, and urine output was reduced. A transplant biopsy was performed and showed intraglomerular thrombi with endarterial proliferation but without cellular infiltration, compatible with humoral rejection. Antirejection treatment was started, together with an infusion of polyclonal IgG. We also decided to start a second course of 5 IA treatments. Under this therapy, renal function progressively improved (2 haemodialyses were required), and returned to pre-rejection values at day 40. Weekly infusions of polyclonal IgG were contined for 1 month, and no rebound rejection has been observed. Neither the pre-IA PRA levels, nor the effectiveness of IA on PRA levels were predictive for the success of the transplantation in this group. However, the 3 patients who had high pretransplantation PRA levels (two had a post-IA antibody resynthesis, and one an uneffective IA course) were those who experienced graft failure (including 2 hyperacute rejections). On the other hand, among the 2 patients who had low pretransplant PRA levels was the patient who had an uneventful posttransplant course. The PRA levels remained during the posttransplantation period at low values in this patient. Finally, the last patient with low pretransplant PRA level experienced reversible humoral rejection at day 10. The PRA level rose to 95% at day 17, and then decreased to pretransplant values (8%). Retrospective crossmatches were performed with posttransplant sera in the 3 patients experiencing vascular rejections. Only one had a positive posttransplantation crossmatch, the one whose graft failed at day 2 by an immediate hyperacute rejection.

In the group of 7 patients transplanted with negative historical peak and pre-IA crossmatches, one graft never functioned but transplant nephrectomy examination excluded rejection. The 6 other patients are surviving with a functional graft 7–39 months posttransplant. No humoral rejection was observed. Acute cellular rejection was histologically documented in 3, and successfully treated by 1 or 2 (one patient) antirejection courses. In one patient, renal function at 39 months posttransplant is impaired, and chronic rejection is histologically proven. In this group, the actuarial graft survival rate is 86% at 3-year posttransplant.

For the whole group of 12 transplants, the actuarial graft survival rate is 66% from 3 months to 3 years post transplant. Severe infection did not develop in any patient including those transplanted within 2 months post-IA. Only four patients (33%) developed mild CMV infection that was in all cases responsive to a 14-day IV ganciclovir course. Leucopenia < 3000 WBC was observed in 3 patients who had previously received oral cyclophosphamide.

This side effect did not occur in the five patients who received IV cyclophosphamide boluses.

Discussion

The present results confirm that IA, with the selectivity of sepharose-bound protein A columns for IgG, was a highly effective method for reducing more than 90% of IgG in our patients awaiting transplantation. Probably as a result of avoiding repeated courses, giving prophylactic antibiotherapy and stopping immunosuppressive drugs two months following the end of the last treatment, the hematologic and clinical tolerances were good.

Although no patient was transfused, and immunosuppressive treatment with prednisolone and cyclophosphamide was administered, we did not observe any uniform effect of IA in decreasing percentage PRA levels. The total removal of antibodies was observed only in 4 (26.7%) patients, and IA had no effect in 4 others. In all the responding patients, as defined by more than 70% reduction in percentage PRA, the antibodies returned to pre-IA values within the first month post IA when transplantation was not performed. As previously reported [14, 17, 19], our data confirmed that initial titers in anti-HLA antibodies were predictive for the success of the method. Indeed in our experience, among the 6 patients for whom titers were $\leq 1:64$, 3 had no response, and in the 3 others PRA rose to initial levels at day 14 post-IA. One was transplanted, and lost his kidney through hyperacute rejection. Since crossreactivity may be titer dependent, it has been suggested [19, 20] that antibody removal should depend upon the presence of crossreactive groups. However, neither the peak PRA level, nor the pre-IA PRA level, nor the presence of crossreactive group antibodies were predictive for IA effectiveness in our study. Indeed, one of the major concerns of the IA procedure is still the defining criteria for selecting patients, but it is also finding an effective method to limit antibody rebound. Six patients in our sample received IV instead of oral cyclophosphamide, but with no detectable effects on resynthesis. Further trials should be conducted using other agents which interfere with the immunological idiotypic network such of the repeat administration of intravenous immunoglobulins, or specific drugs active against cells responsible for antibody production such as anti-B lymphocyte monoclonal antibodies.

Paradoxically, our results with transplantation in IA patients demonstrate firstly that the method of choice for managing hyperimmunized patients is still to find a compatible donor and to perform transplantation with both negative historical and current sera. Seven patients received a graft within such conditions (three had an ineffective IA course, no kidney was found before PRA rebound in 3 others, and a compatible graft became available by chance in 2 patients). One graft failure was caused by a perservation injury of non immunological origin. These patients had no major complications, with only reversible mild cellular rejection occuring in 3, and the graft survival is currently excellent (86% at 3 year posttransplant).

For the 5 patients transplanted with a similar heavy immunosuppressive regimen including prophylactic ALG, but with positive peak and pre-IA crossmatches, the outcome has been much poorer. An increased incidence of acute humoral rejection was observed, leading to graft loss in 2 patients Interestingly, we are able to reverse the humoral rejection in one patient with standard antirejection therapy in association with retreatment by IA and IV polyclonal immunoglobulins. No rebound rejection was observed by continuig weekly infusions of human immunoglobulins. This suggests that such an additional treatment might be helpful to prevent resynthesis during both the post-IA and the immediate posttransplant periods. Although comparisons between subgroups should be cautiously viewed because of the small number of patients and the shortness of the follow-up time, our study confirms that transplantation with historical positive crossmatch carries an increased danger of hyperacute rejection, and that graft survival is far lower (40%) than in transplantations performed with full-negative crossmatch. Finally, only two patients from our initial group of 15 (13.3%) who had successful transplantation with positive pre-IA crossmatch clearly benefited from the method. Their immunological patterns were different. In one, IA was able to totally remove the anti-HLA antibodies, but in the other, IA had no apparent effect, this case suggesting that an undetectable amount of monospecific antibodies responsible for the pre-IA positive crossmatch may have been removed by IA. Both patients, however, had low pre-IA percentage PRA (9% and 29%, respectively), and low anti-HLA antibody titers (1:2 and 1:16).

Considering the decreasing availibility of cadaveric donor organs, and the poor results of special organ sharing programs for hyperimmunized patients, we can expect a build-up in renal transplantation waiting lists. Grafts in hyperimmunized transplant candidates may be required in social or medical emergencies. In such patients IA is a safe method that may offer an unique opportunity for rapid transplantation. This benefit may outweight the disadvantages of the irregular efficacy, and of the high risk of hyperacute rejection.

Acknowledgements

This work was supported by grants from INSERM/CNAMTS, ARC, DRED/MEN and DRC/AP-HP. The skillfull assistance of Mrs LEVILLAIN was highly appreciated.

References

1. Etablissement Français des Greffes, Rapport Annuel, 1995. Le prélèvement et la greffe en France en 1995.
2. Keown PA. The highly sensitized patient: aetiology, impact and management. Transplant. Proc. 1987; 19: 74–78.

3. Fuggle SV, Errasti P, Daar AS, Fabre JW, Ting A, Morris PJ. Localisation of MHC (HLA-ABC and DR) antigens in 46 kidneys. Differences in HLA-DR staining of tubules among kidneys. Transplantation 1983; 35: 385–390.
4. Robinson MA, Kindt TJ. Major histocompatibility complex antigens and genes. In: Paul WE (ed.), Fundamental Immunology. New York, Raven Press, 1989, p. 489.
5. Chapman JR, Taylor CJ, Ting A, Morris PJ. Immunoglobulin class and specificity of antibodies causing positive T cell cross-matches. Transplantation 1986; 42: 608–613.
6. Iwaki Y, Terasaki PI. Primary nonfunction in human cadaver kidney transplantation: evidence for hidden hyperacute rejection. Clin. Transplant. 1987; 1: 125–131.
7. Mahoney RJ, Ault KA, Given SR, Adams RJ, Breggia AC, Paris PA, Palomaki GE, Hitchcox SA, White BW, Himmelfarb JJ, Leeber DA. The flow cytometric crossmatch and early renal transplant loss. Transplantation 1990; 49: 527–535.
8. Alexandre GPJ, Squifflet JP, De Bruyere M, Latinne D, Moriau M, Carlier C, Pirson Y, Lecomte C. ABO-incompatible related and unrelated living donor renal allografts. Transplant. Proc. 1986; 18: 1090–1092.
9. Ferrara GB, Tosi M, Azzolina G, Carminati G, Longo A. HLA unresponsiveness induced by weekly transfusions of small aliquots of whole blood. Transplantation 1974; 17: 194–198.
10. Rondeau E, Fournier A, Kanfer A, Sraer JD. Polyvalent immunoglobulins in sensitised renal transplant recipients. Nephrol. Dial. Transplant. 1991; 6: 675–676.
11. Cardella CJ, Nicholson MJ, Falk JA, Harding M, Cook GT. Successful renal transplantation in patients with T-cell reactivity to donor. Lancet 1982; 2: 1240–1242.
12. Taube DH, Welsh KI, Kennedy LA. Successful removal and prevention of resynthesis of anti-HLA antibody. Transplantation 1984; 34: 254–255.
13. Hillebrand G, Castro LA, Samtleben W. Removal of preformed cytotoxic antibodies in highly sensitized patients using plasma exchange and immunosuppression therapy, azathioprine or cyclosporine prior to renal transplantation. Transplant. Proc. 1985; 17: 2501–2504.
14. Gjorstrup P, Watt RM. Therapeutic protein A immunoadsorption. A review. Transfus. Sci. 1990; 11: 281–302.
15. Palmer A, Taube D, Welsh K. Removal of anti-HLA antibodies by extracorporeal immunoadsorption to enable transplantation. Lancet 1989; 1: 10–12.
16. Gjorstrup P for the Collaborative Study Group on Anti-HLA removal. Anti-HLA antibody removal in hyperimmunized ESRF patients to allow transplantation. Tranpslant. Proc. 1991; 23: 392–395.
17. Esnault V, Bignon JD, Testa. Effect of protein A immunoadsorption on panel lymphocyte reactivity in hyperimmunized patients awaiting a kidney graft. Transplantation 1990; 50: 449–453.
18. Brocard JF, Farahmand H, Fassi S. Attempt at depletion of anti-HLA antibodies in sensitized patients awaiting transplantation using extracorporeal immunoadsorption, polyclonal IgG and immunosuppressive drugs. Transplant. Proc. 1989; 21: 733–734.
19. Kupin WL, Venkat KK, Hayaski H. Removal of lymphocytotoxic antibodies by pretransplant immunoadsorption therapy in highly sensitized renal transplant recipients. Transplantation 1991; 51: 324–329.
20. Hakim RM, Milford E, Himmelfarb J. Extracorporeal removal of anti-HLA antibodies intransplant candidates. Am. J. Kidney Dis. 1990; 16: 423–432.

18. Role of anti-HLA antibodies in allograft rejection

HONG BIAN, PAUL E. HARRIS & ELAINE F. REED

Introduction

It is well recognized that pre-existing antibodies to HLA antigens expressed by the allograft is detrimental to survival of kidney allografts and results in hyperacute and accelerated rejection [1]. Furthermore, it has been shown that heart and liver transplant recipients with pre-existing anti-donor HLA antibodies experience lower graft survival than patients without anti-donor anti-HLA antibodies [2, 3]. In hyperacute rejection, the injury occurs immediately, and the classical pathological features are infiltrating neutrophils, fibrinoid necrosis, and platelet thrombi. Fortunately, the occurrence of this type of rejection has been largely reduced by performing a pretransplant cross-match with the donor. The role of anti-HLA antibodies in chronic rejection is less well understood. Chronic rejection is the major limiting factor to long-term survival of organ allografts [4–6]. It is responsible for the loss of 50% of kidney allografts and 45% of cardiac allografts by 5 years after transplantation. The graft survival rates for other organ transplants generally show comparable results, with the exception of liver, which seems somewhat better tolerated. Chronic rejection, is defined as progressive functional deterioration of transplanted tissue occurring months or years after engraftment. The hallmark of chronic rejection is accelerated graft atherosclerosis which is characterized by diffuse, concentric, intimal occlusive lesions leading to gradual fibrosis of the transplanted organ [4–6]. The vascular narrowing results from infiltration of the intima by vascular endothelial cells, smooth muscle cells and fibroblasts, and intimal deposition of extracellular matrix material. The pathogenesis of accelerated graft vasculopathy has not been elucidated but several mechanisms may contribute to the development of the disease, including immunosuppressive agents, hyperlipidemia, viral infections and ischemic injury occurring at the time of engraftment [4–6]. There is substantial evidence indicating that humoral immunity to the allograft contributes to the development of chronic rejection. In the following we will discuss the prognostic importance of post-transplant monitoring of anti-HLA antibodies for identification of patients at risk of chronic rejection. Furthermore, we will present data showing that anti-HLA antibodies contribute to the development of chronic rejection by binding to HLA class I molecules on endothelial and smooth muscle cells and transducing signals which induce tyrosine phosphorylation of intracellular proteins, inositol phosphate generation and cell proliferation.

J.L. Touraine et al. (eds.), Retransplantation, 151–158.

Post-transplant monitoring of soluble donor HLA alloantigens and anti-HLA alloantibodies identifies patients at risk of chronic rejection

Humoral immunity has long been considered the immunological mechanism that causes chronic vascular rejection as both immunoglobulin and complement deposits have been shown in areas of intimal thickening [4–6]. In addition, the vascular remodeling associated with chronic rejection can be experimentally induced by intra-arterial infusion of donor-specific antisera [7, 8]. In studies from our laboratory, we have found that the development of anti-HLA antibodies following transplantation is positively associated with chronic rejection of heart and renal allografts [9–13]. Based on these findings we postulated that chronic rejection is mediated by T helper cells, which recognize processed forms of soluble HLA alloantigens released from the graft in context of self MHC. Such Th cells, engaged in the indirect recognition pathway, produce the lymphokines required for the growth and maturation of alloantibody producing B cells. To further explore this hypothesis we have analyzed the impact of chronic alloantigenic stimulation, anti-HLA antibody production and acute rejection on the development of chronic rejection [13]. Heart transplant patients ($n = 274$) were monitored by angiogram for the development of transplant associated coronary artery disease (T-CAD). The incidence of T-CAD was 2%, 18%, and 42% at 1, 2 and 3 years following transplantation, respectively. Multivariate analysis of risk factors associated with T-CAD such as recipient gender, age, race, number of HLA mismatches between the recipient and donor, frequency of acute rejection episodes and production of anti-HLA antibodies indicated that T-CAD was strongly associated with the occurrence of multiple rejection episodes and anti-HLA antibody production (Table 1). Univariate analysis showed that heart recipients with more than two episodes of acute allograft rejection had a much earlier onset of T-CAD than patients with less-frequent rejection (Table 1). Patients developing anti-donor HLA antibodies following transplantation also displayed an earlier onset of T-CAD than patients without anti-donor HLA antibodies (Table 1).

To determine whether soluble donor HLA class I antigens (sHLA) are released into the recipient's circulation following transplantation, we tested sequential sera ($n = 594$) from 24 recipients who received heart allografts mismatched for HLA-A2. Ten of the patients were diagnosed with T-CAD, while 14 patients were free from T-CAD. Sera were tested for the presence of donor-derived soluble HLA-A2 antigens using a quantitative sandwich ELISA assay. Fifty-eight percent of the sera from patients with T-CAD showed soluble HLA-A2, compared to only 23% of sera from patients without T-CAD. The soluble alloantigens from the graft persisted in the patient's circulation for varying lengths of time ranging from 1 week up to 351 weeks following transplantation. The median time of sHLA-A2 persistence was 106 weeks in patients with T-CAD and only 16 weeks in patients without T-CAD.

To determine if chronic antigenic stimulation with soluble HLA alloantigens is associated with the development of T-CAD we divided the patients into two

Table 1. Analysis of risk factors associated with the development of chronic rejection

	Multivariate analysis		Univariate analysis	
Factor	SE	*p* value	Median time to onset of T-CAD (months)	*p* value
Number of acute rejection episodes	0.290	0.001		0.0001
0/year			64.5	
1/year			38.7	
≥2/year			12.5	
Anti-HLA antibody production	0.256	0.001		0.03
Nonproducer			81.4	
Producer			61.5	

groups. Group 1 included patients whose sera contained sHLA-A2 antigens throughout a period of up to 26 weeks following transplantation ($n = 8$). Group 2 consisted of patients whose sera showed no detectable sHLA-A2 antigens during this time ($n = 16$). Patients with persistent HLA-A2 antigens in the circulation for more than 26 weeks had a significantly earlier onset of T-CAD ($p = 0.008$) compared with patients with a shorter exposure to sHLA-A2 antigens. The median time to onset of T-CAD was 137 weeks in patients with chronic exposure to sHLA-A2 antigens compared to 205 weeks in patients with short-term exposure to donor soluble alloantigens. These results indicate that patients with persistent donor alloantigens in their circulation are at increased risk of chronic rejection.

The chronic release of donor alloantigens might stimulate the production of anti-HLA antibodies through the indirect recognition pathway. To determine whether continuous stimulation by soluble alloantigens is accompanied by the development of anti-HLA antibodies we analyzed the relationship between the length of antigen release and that of antibody production. Linear regression analysis indicated that the time span of alloantigen release and of anti-HLA antibody production were highly correlated ($p < 0.0002$).

The data presented above indicate that patients at risk of chronic rejection can be identified by monitoring the release of soluble HLA antigen from the graft and the development post-transplant of anti-donor HLA antibodies.

Anti-HLA antibodies transduce signals in endothelial cells

Complement-fixing antibodies which bind to the endothelial cells (EC) of a newly transplanted allo- or xenogeneic graft cause hyperacute rejection, an explosive phenomenon which has been extensively described. Although the alloantibodies developing during chronic rejection are also complement fixing, the EC alterations which they cause are of a subtle and progressive nature. Anti-HLA antibodies may act as an initiator of the chains of events that culminate in vascular lesions by altering the surface of the endothelium. We have postulated that anti-HLA antibodies contribute to the development of chronic rejection by binding to class I molecules on the endothelium and smooth muscle of the graft and transducing signals which ultimately result in cell proliferation. To determine whether ligation of HLA class I molecules on the surface of EC by anti-HLA class I antibodies transduces signals by stimulating tyrosine phosphorylation of intracellular proteins we performed Western blot analysis [14]. EC-pSV1, a stable human SV40 transfected endothelial cell line carrying the HLA-A2 antigen was used for these studies. EC-pSV1 cells were treated with the anti-HLA class I mAb W6/32 alone, or in conjunction with, a secondary cross-linking antibody for various periods of time. Cell lysates were electrophoresed and immunoblotted with the anti-phosphotyrosine mAb PY20. Treatment of EC with W6/32 resulted in an increase in tyrosine phosphorylation of cellular proteins at approximate molecular masses ranging from 66 kDa to 80 kDa. This effect was seen after treatment of the cells with the primary antibody (W6/32) alone, and was further enhanced upon cross-linking with the secondary antibody. Increased tyrosine phosphorylation was not observed when the cells were incubated in isotype control mAb or in anti-CD31 mAb.

To determine if anti-HLA class I antibodies stimulate the release of calcium from intracellular stores of EC through the generation of inositol trisphosphate ((1,4,5)$InsP_3$) we measured its production following antibody ligation [14]. EC-pSV1 cells were deprived of endothelial cell growth factors for 18 h, and then treated with mAb W6/32 or isotype matched control mAb for various times. As a positive control, EC-pSV1 cells were exposed in parallel cultures to endothelial growth factors in EGM medium. Treatment of EC-pSV1 with W6/32 lead to the generation of 3 and 4 pmoles of [(1,4,5)$InsP_3$]i at 3 and 7 min, respectively. Media containing endothelial cell growth factors also stimulated the generation of (1,4,5)$InsP_3$, whereas, (1,4,5)$InsP_3$ release was unaffected by reacting the cells with isotype control antibodies. These data demonstrate that binding of anti-HLA antibodies to HLA antigens on by EC results in release of (1,4,5)$InsP_3$ from phosphatidyl inositol stores.

Anti-HLA alloantibodies present in a transplant recipient's serum transduce signals in endothelial cells

To determine if anti-HLA alloantibodies are also able to transduce signals in EC we determined if anti-HLA-A2 antibodies obtained from a transplant recipient were capable of stimulating tyrosine phosphorylation of intracellular proteins in EC. Prior to testing, the IgG fraction of the alloantiserum was isolated on a Protein G column. Following treatment of EC-PSV1 (HLA-A2+) with anti-HLA-A2 IgG, cell lysates were electrophoresed and immunoblotted with the anti-phosphotyrosine mAb PY20. Treatment of EC-PSV1 with recipient anti-HLA-A2 antibodies alone (Figure 1, Lane 3) or in the presence of a

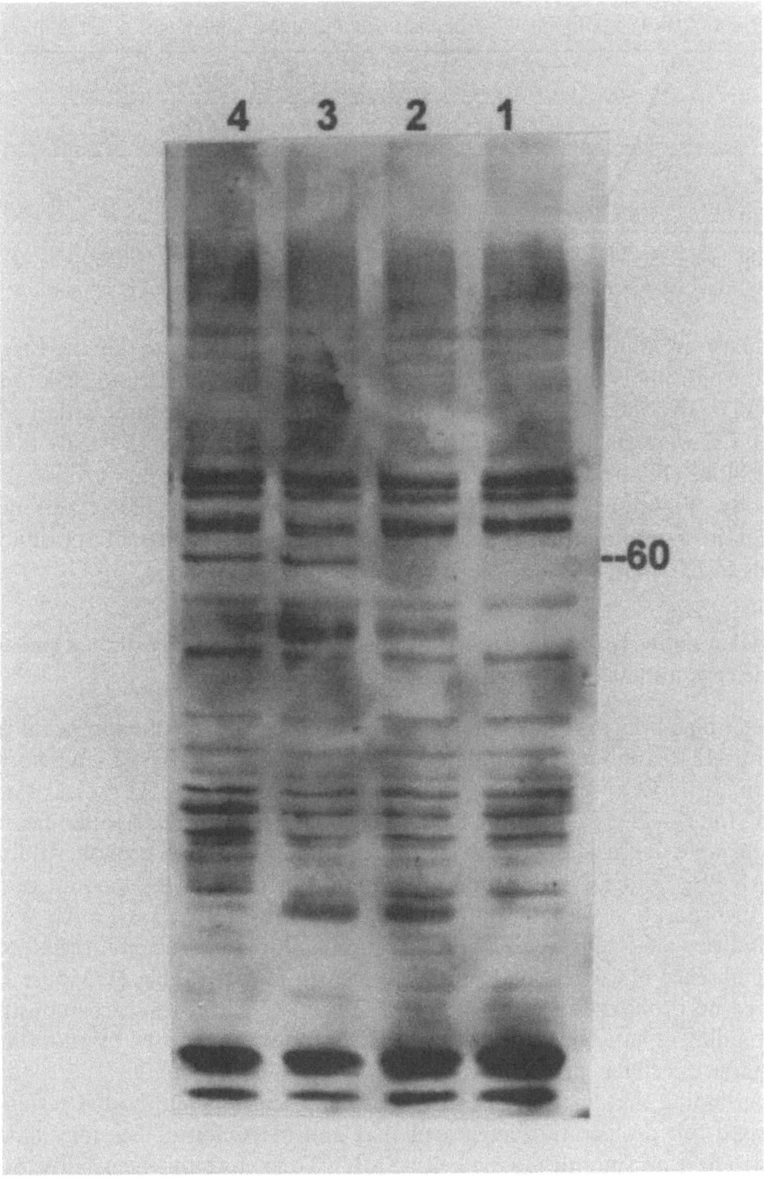

Fig. 1. Phosphotyrosine blot after incubation of endothelial cells with human anti-HLA-A2 IgG alloantibodies: (Lane 1) EC-pSV1 treated with 10 μg/ml human IgG from non-sensitized male for 10 min; (Lane 2) EC-pSV1 cells treated with 10 μg/ ml human IgG from non-sensitized male for 10 min followed by cross-linking with 10 μg/ml goat anti-human Ig for 10 min; (Lane 3) EC-pSV1 treated with 10 μg/ml anti-HLA-A2 IgG for 10 min; (Lane 4) EC-pSV1 treated with 10 μg/ml anti-HLA-A2 IgG for 10 min followed by cross-linking with 10 μg/ml goat anti-human Ig for 10 min. A representative experiment is shown.

Table 2. Anti-HLA class I antibodies stimulate endothelial and smooth muscle cell proliferation

	[^{3}H]TdR incorporation[a] (cpm)		
Stimulus	EC-PSV1	Aortic EC	SMC
mIgG (10 μg/ml)	1102	2110	989
W6/32 (10 μg/ml)	15 510	12 100	5689

[a] ^{3}H-TdR incorporation was measured 24 h after anti-HLA antibody stimulation. Data are the mean of triplicate determinations (SD was <10%). A representative experiment is shown.

secondary crosslinking antibody (Figure 1, Lane 4) lead to an increase in tyrosine phosphorylation of cellular proteins at an approximate molecular mass of 60 kDa. In contrast, there was no increase in tyrosine phosphorylation when donor EC were treated with IgG from a non-sensitized healthy male donor, either alone (Figure 1, Lane 1), or in the presence of a secondary cross-linking antibody (Figure 1, Lane 2). These results show that anti-HLA antibodies present in a serum from a transplant recipient are capable of transducing signals in EC.

Anti-HLA antibody ligation to class I molecules on endothelial cells and smooth muscle cells stimulates cell proliferation.

To determine if ligation of class I molecules on the surface of endothelial cells by anti-HLA antibodies stimulates cell proliferation, EC-pSV1 and normal human aortic ECs were cultured in the presence of the anti-HLA class I mAb W6/32 for 24–72 h [14]. Prior to the addition of monoclonal antibodies, the cultures were deprived of growth factors for 24 h to arrest cell growth. Addition of mAb W6/32 to EC-pSV1 induced a 14-fold increase in the amount of ^{3}H-TdR incorporation within 24 h (Table 2). The anti-MHC class I mAb W6/32 also induced a 6-fold increase in proliferation of normal aortic endothelial cells, in the absence of exogenous endothelial growth factors (Table 2). Mouse IgG induced no proliferation of EC-pSV1 or aortic EC. These results demonstrate that binding of anti-HLA antibodies to HLA antigens expressed by endothelial cells induces cellular proliferation.

The finding that ligation of HLA class I molecules by antibodies results in increased cell proliferation suggested that anti-MHC antibodies may have a similar effect on smooth muscle cells (SMC). To explore this possibility, SMC were cultured in the presence of mAb W6/32 for 24–72 h (Table 2). Prior to the addition of monoclonal antibodies, the cultures were deprived of growth factors for 24 h to arrest cell growth. The addition of anti-HLA class I mAb to SMC induced a five-fold increase in the amount of ^{3}H-TdR incorporation after 24 h of culture whereas, isotype control antibodies had no effect on SMC growth. These results demonstrate that binding of anti-HLA antibodies to HLA antigens expressed by SMC induces proliferation.

Table 3. W6/32 induced endothelial cell proliferation is inhibited by neutralizing antibodies to basic fibroblast growth factor

Stimulus	Neutralizing antibodies (concentration)	[^{3}H]TdR incorporation[a] (cpm)
Mouse IgG	none	1196
W6/32 IgG	none	7397
	Anti-bFGF (1 μg/ml)	1592
	Anti-PDGF (10 μg/ml)	7422
	Anti-TGFβ (10 μg/ml)	7159

[a] ^{3}H-TdR incorporation was measured 24 h after anti-HLA antibody stimulation. Data are the mean of triplicate determinations (SD was < 10%). A representative experiment is shown.

Anti-HLA antibodies alter FGF receptors on EC

To investigate the mechanism of W6/32 induced EC proliferation we evaluated the ability of W6/32 to stimulate EC growth in the presence of neutralizing antibodies to basic fibroblast growth factor (bFGF). The addition of anti-bFGF neutralizing antibodies effectively blocked W6/32 induced cell proliferation (Table 3). In contrast, neutralizing antibodies to other growth factors produced by EC, such as TGFβ and PDGF showed no inhibition of W6/32 induced EC proliferation. These studies suggest that ligation of class I molecules by anti-HLA antibodies stimulates EC proliferation by stimulating bFGF synthesis and/or by increasing FGF utilization.

To determine if class I ligation leads to an increased production of bFGF the amount of bFGF present in the culture supernatant was measured. Supernatant from EC monolayers incubated with mAb W6/32 contained a similar amount of bFGF (40 $\pm$ 2 pg/ml) compared to EC treated with mIgG. This suggested that class I ligation leads to an increased utilization of bFGF by EC, rather than an increased synthesis of bFGF. Scatchard analysis of ^{125}I-bFGF binding to anti-HLA class I antibody treated EC showed that when ECs were treated with mAb W6/32, the affinity of ^{125}I-bFGF binding increased significantly. The observed changes in bFGF binding were not related to an increase in the total number of fibroblast growth factor (FGF) receptors, as the Scatchard analysis indicated the number of bFGF binding sites per cell to be similar for both W6/32 and isotype control treated EC. These results suggest that anti-HLA antibody binding to class I molecules on EC transduce signals that lead to an increase in the affinity of FGF receptors and enhance the EC proliferative response to bFGF.

Summary

Our studies indicate that patients at risk of chronic rejection can be identified by monitoring the release of soluble HLA antigens from the graft and monitoring the production of anti-HLA antibodies following transplantation. Anti-HLA antibodies are likely to be the primary mediators of chronic rejection by binding to the endothelium and smooth muscle of the graft and transducing signals which increases the affinity of the FGF receptors thereby enhancing the ability of the cell to respond to bFGF and grow. Proliferation of ECs and SMCs has serious implications for overall growth of the atherosclerotic plaque since every new mesenchymal cell formed represents a source of collagen and other extracellular matrix proteins which will increase the size of the atherosclerotic plaque. Furthermore, increased responsiveness of EC to bFGF represents a potential mechanism to stimulate neovascularization of atherosclerotic plaques. Elucidation of the mechanism through which anti-HLA antibodies transduce signals resulting in EC and SMC cell proliferation is crucial for the future development of therapeutic modalities for the treatment and prevention of chronic rejection.

Acknowledgements

This work was supported by NIAID grant RO1AI33699.

References

1. Patel R, Terasaki PI. Significance of the positive crossmatch test in kidney transplantation. N. Engl. J. Med. 1969; 280: 735–739.
2. Takaya S, Bronsther O, Iwaki Y et al. The adverse impact on liver transplantation of using positive cytotoxic crossmatch donors. Transplantation 1992; 53: 400–406.
3. Ratkivec RM, Hammond EH, O'Connell JB et al. Outcome of cardiac transplant recipients with a positive donor-specific crossmatch – preliminary results with plasmapheresis. Transplantation 1992; 54: 651–655.
4. Paul LC, Fellstrom B. Chronic vascular rejection of the heart and the kidney – have rational treatment options emerged? Transplantation 1992; 53: 1169–1179.
5. Tilney NL, Whitley W, Diamond JR, Kupiec-Weglinski JW, Adams DH. Chronic rejection – an undefined conundrum. Transplantation 1991; 52: 389–398.
6. Ewel CH, Foegh ML. Chronic graft rejection: accelerated transplant arteriosclerosis. Immunol. Rev. 1993; 134: 21–31.
7. O'Connel TX, Mobray JF. Arterial intimal thickening produced by alloantibody and xenoantibody. Transplantation 1973; 51: 262–263.
8. Russel PS, Chase CM, Winn HJ, Colvin RB. Coronary atherosclerosis in transplanted mouse hearts. II. Importance of humoral immunity. J. Immunol. 1994; 152: 5135–5141.
9. Fenoglio J, Ho E, Reed E et al. Anti-HLA antibodies and heart allograft survival. Transplant. Proc. 1989; 21: 807–809.
10. Suciu-Foca N, Reed E, D'Agati V et al. Soluble HLA antigens, anti-HLA antibodies and anti-idiotypic antibodies in the circulation of renal transplant recipients. Transplantation 1991; 51: 593–601.
11. Suciu-Foca N, Reed E, Marboe C et al. Role of anti-HLA antibodies in heart transplantation. Transplantation 1991; 51: 716–724.
12. Cherry R, Nielsen H, Reed E, Reemtsma K, Suciu-Foca N, Marboe CC. Vascular (humoral) rejection in cardiac allograft biopsies: relation to circulating anti-HLA antibodies. J. Heart Lung Transplant. 1992; 11: 24–29.
13. Reed EF, Hong B, Ho E, Harris PE, Weinberger J, Suciu-Foca N. Monitoring of soluble HLA alloantigens and anti-HLA antibodies identifies heart allograft recipients at risk of transplant-associated coronary artery disease. Transplantation 1996; 61: 566–572.
14. Bian H, Harris PE, Mulder A, Reed EF. Anti-HLA antibody ligation to HLA class I molecules expressed by endothelial cells stimulates tyrosine phosphorylation, inositol phosphate generation, and proliferation. Human Immunol. 1997; 53: 90–97.

19. Antibody screening and crossmatching in retransplantation

PHILIP A. DYER, SUSAN MARTIN, JUDITH WORTHINGTON & STEPHEN SHELDON

The risk of immediate rejection in retransplantation

Classical immunological dogma stipulates that reexposure to antigen results in an immediate and forceful response by the adaptive immune system. In the context of organ retransplantation this response is influenced by several factors, including antibody specificity of the primary response [1], affinity and isotype of preformed antibody, dose and immunogenicity of the antigen, immune responsiveness and health of the recipient. The pioneering work of Kissmeyer–Nielsen in Europe and Terasaki in the USA in the mid 1960s established that kidney transplants could be rejected hyperacutely by thrombosis of the transplant due to binding of preformed recipient antibody to donor antigen. It is now accepted that the most frequent target antigens in such instances are HLA antigens, coded for by the class I (HLA-A, -B, -Cw) or class II (HLA-DR, -DQ) genes of the major histocompatibility complex. Primary sensitization in transplant recipients usually occurs by one of three routes: blood transfusions, pregnancy and organ transplantation [2].

It is universally accepted that before any kidney transplant proceeds a crossmatch between recipient serum and donor lymphocytes must be negative. For other organs it is highly advisable that such a crossmatch be performed when the potential recipient has been shown to have produced antibody detected in screening assays. In retransplantation crossmatching is essential for all recipients because of previous exposure to alloantigen [3] when the risk of immediate organ failure is increased.

Screening and crossmatching procedures are intimately linked

If results from an acute crossmatch are unpredictable or unexpectedly positive then recipient work-up has probably been inefficient since prior to crossmatching, all potential recipients should be screened for potentially harmful antibodies. After initial sample testing, serum must be screened following each potential sensitizing event such as blood transfusions. Infectious events may non-specifically stimulate appearance of alloantibodies in patient serum and samples taken shortly after such episodes should also be screened. At the time of crossmatch all patients should therefore have a detailed antibody profile

J.L. Touraine et al. (eds.), Retransplantation, 159–166.

which will be an essential aid to interpreting crossmatching data. This intimate link between antibody screening and acute crossmatching can be extrapolated so that the need for any crossmatching at all following efficient screening may be debated.

Techniques currently available

Until recently, the complement dependent cytotoxicity assay developed by Terasaki over 30 years ago was the sole technique in widespread use for detection of sensitization to alloantigens. There have been many modifications of this assay to improve its sensitivity including isolation of pure target cell preparations with immunomagnetic beads but there are still drawbacks, not least that non-complement fixing antibodies (IgG2 and 4) cannot be detected [4]. Binding assays such as those using fluorochrome labels and detection by flow cytometry (FC) [5] or enzyme linked immunosorbent assays (ELISA) [6] are now available and can be applied both to screening and crossmatching testing. The principle advantages of FC and ELISA assays are standardization and quantitation although there is the need to comprehend and interpret the data from such assays rather than to expect concordance with previously used assays such as CDC. In most cases new assays will not be directly comparable with previous experience so specificity, sensitivity and clinical relevance of antibodies detected must be addressed.

Which antibody detection techniques are essential for retransplantation

In essence, techniques used for screening and crossmatching prior to retransplantation need not differ from those for primary transplantation. There is little evidence that sensitive techniques should not be applied to first transplants, particularly if patient immunization history and screening data is incomplete. A possible exception is the use of FC crossmatching tests which are probably of no additional benefit to CDC crossmatching for unsensitized first transplant recipients [7]. Due to the generally increased immune response seen in paediatric recipients and the need to ensure successful long term outcome in young patients FC crossmatching for children is advisable.

The need to define 'sensitization'

It is becoming increasingly important to quantify recipient sensitization. In CDC screening patient serum samples are tested against a panel of lymphocytes from donors unrelated to the patient to give a score for reactivity which can be expressed as a percentage of panel reactive alloantibodies (PRA). The clinical relevance of '% PRA' and sensitization detected by that method is, therefore, influenced by antibody present in the circulation, the size of the screening panel, the frequency of alloantigens in the panel/selection of panel cells, the isotype (IgG1,3 or IgM) of the antibody, the specificity of the antibody, the sensitivity of the assay.

A patient with circulating monospecific cytotoxic antibody to the most frequent HLA-A specificity, A2, should give a PRA of approximately 50% with screening panels reflecting the frequency of this specificity in a random population. However a small panel of 20 cells selected to cover most HLA specificities in suitable combinations could give a much lower reaction frequency for the same antibody. Should the antibody be the of IgG2 or 4 isotype, which do not bind complement, then a negative result could occur. Perhaps the time has come to abandon use of the term '%PRA'. Use of suitably designed FC and ELISA assays allows definition of specificities to which the patient is sensitized giving more useful information for the acute crossmatch. One commercially available ELISA (PRASTAT, Sangstat) uses HLA antigens from cultured cell lines as targets allowing standardization between assays by the use of a permanent panel and thus assignment of a true percentage of reactivity. Comparison of percentage reactivity detected by PRAStat with other techniques is therefore not valid. Furthermore, it is unwise to compare percentage reactivity between cell panels and between laboratories when standardization of CDC assays is not done.

The sensitization status of any potential recipient must be clinically relevant to be useful and at present there is consensus that the following antibodies are damaging to transplanted organs and are thus a contraindication to successful transplant function: all HLA specific IgG subtypes detected at any time prior to transplantation, cytotoxic IgG alloantibodies with undefined specificity, and HLA specific IgM detected less than six months prior to transplantation.

There is debate as to the relevance of some antibodies, such as HLA specific IgM in historical samples. The post transplant outcome following a positive crossmatch due to historical IgM antibody is influenced by the immunosuppressive regime used. For example, use of induction therapy with high drug doses including anti thymocyte/lymphocyte globulins may facilitate early function in the face of low levels of antibody mediated rejection. Thus local policies on relevant antibodies detected by crossmatching should be established.

In all cases it is quite clear that an understanding of 'sensitization' in the context of the local unit policy and local laboratory screening and crossmatching techniques used must be established based on past experience as well as on published data [8]. A clear aim must be to define reactivity to HLA specificities in patient serum samples.

A protocol for antibody screening

Over the past 15 years we have assembled a group of techniques for antibody screening which have enabled comprehensive identification of clinically relevant antibodies and which provide information to support efficient crossmatching. Currently all newly referred potential transplant recipients and all patients on kidney transplant waiting lists on a bimonthly basis are screened for sensitization status using the following protocol: (1) ELISA assay 'GTI Quikscreen', (about 30% positive); (2) Positives from (1) screened by CDC using 40 random, 20 B-CLL and 10 HLA phenotype selected cells, (about 80% positive); (3) Negatives from (1) screened by FC using 2 pools of LCLs, (about 10% positive). If negative, serum reported as screened negative for relevant antibodies; (4) Positives from (3) screened by CDC as in (2) to assign specificity; (5) Negatives from (2) screened by PRASTAT ELISA, (about 20% positive). Positives assigned specificity and reported.

Antibodies which are IgM but have no HLA specificity can be due to false positive reactivity with carbohydrate residues found on the surface of lymphocyte targets. Such antibodies appear to be related to immune stimulatory episodes such as infection but their production is a nonspecific response. They react with most panel lymphocytes but not with B-CLL cells and they are weakly cytotoxic so their presence can be speculated on following CDC screening. Their presence can give a pattern of repeated positivity in crossmatching [9]. Experience has shown that these antibodies usually react with a patient's own lymphocytes and have no clinical relevance following positivity in a crossmatch. Whilst such antibodies can be removed by digestion with dithiothreitol it is essential that autoreactivity is established by performing an auto crossmatch during screening procedures since HLA specific IgM antibodies do occur. In our current screening procedure outlined above we are now able to clearly identify HLA specific IgM antibodies by their reactivity in the GTI Quikscreen ELISA.

The fundamental aim of this approach is to define clinically relevant sensitization which in our experience is chiefly HLA specific.

A protocol for matching and crossmatching

The aim of crossmatching is to avoid transplantation which will lead to early failure. In our centre good results in cadaveric kidney transplantation, in heart transplantation and in lung transplantation have been achieved (Table 1) and efficient crossmatching and antibody screening have played their part.

Crossmatching for thoracic organ transplants is usually restricted to cases where potential recipients have been identified as having clinically relevant antibodies at the time of pretransplant screening. All thoracic organ recipients should be crossmatched on a retrospective basis but we find an absolute correlation with screening data in that no recipient who was negative on screening had a positive crossmatch. Prospective crossmatch results for sensitized thoracic organ recipients also correlate well with pretransplant screening data and patients having a positive prospective crossmatch should not be transplanted because of the greatly increased risk of early rejection. If a potential thoracic organ donor possesses HLA specificities to which a possible recipient has been shown to be sensitized then we have not considered that patient for

Table 1. Survival of organ transplants in the NW of England at 1 and 5 years of follow-up

Organ transplanted	Experience (years)	Number of cases	% transplant survival at 1 year	% transplant survival at 5 years
First cadaver kidney	1989–1996	868	85.9	76.1
Repeat cadaver kidney	1989–1996	144	84.9	72.2
Heart	1987–1996	248	78.4	68
Single lung	1987–1996	51	73.8	51.9
Double lung	1987–1996	25	61.3	45.3
Heart and lung	1987–1996	35	65.7	33.8

transplantation. This clearly illustrates the intimate relationship between efficient HLA phenotyping of organ donors and pretransplant screening data. Prospective crossmatching for thoracic organ transplants will usually use donor peripheral blood lymphocytes as targets so there is potential for false negative results.

There is ongoing debate as to the relevance of crossmatching for liver transplantation and at least for first transplants a crossmatch seems unnecessary [10] but the situation in sensitized retransplant liver recipients might be different.

Regrafting of corneas is not infrequent but few centres HLA type cornea donors and recipients, which makes useful crossmatching difficult. There are ongoing studies to evaluate the role of HLA matching but not crossmatching, for cornea regrafts. It is widely considered that the cornea is not strongly immunogenic although there is mounting evidence to the contrary [11].

In kidney transplantation two filters exist to reduce the number of potential recipients: ABO blood group compatibility (preferably identity), and HLA-A, -B, -DR mismatches. It is our own experience with a waiting list of almost 500 potential recipients that no mismatch for HLA-DR can be achieved in 60% of cases. Between 1989 and 1996 we performed 144 repeat kidney transplants and no mismatch for HLA-DR was achieved in 63.9% of cases leading to a transplant survival at five years of 73.5% in contrast to 68.4% for DR mismatched retransplants.

Sensitization to HLA-A, -B, -Cw, -DR or -DQ specificities present in the donor and identified in *any* patient sample over time through screening excludes that recipient from crossmatching and thus from further consideration for transplantation of kidneys from that donor. Retransplantation candidates will probably have been exposed to HLA mismatches at the time of first transplantation and so will be ineligible to receive some kidneys, accepting that repeated HLA mismatching is undesirable leading to aggressive rejection [12]. Some centres claim that reexposure to mismatched HLA antigens does not reduce outcomes in retransplantation [13] but there are two influences: recipient response to mismatched antigens, and use of immunosuppression.

It has been claimed [14] that recipients who do not produce antibodies to the mismatched antigens can safely be reexposed to the same mismatches. Efficient sampling and crossmatching are clearly essential before such decisions can be made. There is no doubt that use of high dose multiple immunosuppressive drug therapy can reduce recipient responses to mismatched antigens but there are accompanying significant risks of increased morbidity and mortality [15].

Selection of serum samples for crossmatching is important and whenever possible all available samples should be used. If many samples are available careful selection of antibody positive sera may have to be made for logistical reasons. Some centres restrict crossmatching to peak reactive samples and samples collected in the six months prior to crossmatching. If this is practised then it must be realized that not all samples may have the same antibody specificity and this approach must be considered a high risk practice which must be accompanied by a very comprehensive screening programme. The importance of regular sampling is also evident at this time since long periods without samples having been screened indicate potential loss of vital information; this is a particular problem for repeat transplantation when sampling following first transplantation is often infrequent. For those patients with autoreactive IgM antibodies, crossmatching in parallel using DTT to digest IgM antibodies is good practice.

Patients treated with antibodies such as ATG, ALG and OKT3 at the time of acute rejection can have these antibodies in their serum and if such samples are received in the laboratory then false positive screening and crossmatch reactivity may result since these antibodies are cytotoxic. They will not be detected in ELISA and flow cytometry assays when antibody binding is detected by specific anti-human second antibody. The laboratory should be made aware of anti-rejection treatment for all patients. This is a particular risk for retransplant candidates and especially for thoracic organ recipients who may be referred for retransplantation and crossmatching whilst undergoing aggressive anti-rejection therapy.

Potential recipients with negative CDC crossmatches may proceed for transplantation but it is now increasingly accepted that some patients continue to be at high risk of rejection. Experience has shown that high risk recipients are: patients shown to be highly sensitized on screening, retransplant candidates, paediatric patients, and those with poorly defined sensitization. Whilst FC crossmatch protocols have been developed in several centres, in the UK there is an evolving consensus on the most relevant technique [16]. Variables which demand standardization included positivity as defined by channel shift, best negative control serum and detection antibody, and use of multiple detection antibodies.

Centres must define local policies on what constitutes a positive FC result. Based on our own experience we choose a highly conservative approach and proceed with transplantation for high risk candidates only when there is complete absence of reactivity of recipient serum with donor T and B cell targets.

Summary

To attain successful retransplantation of kidney recipients the laboratory must contribute and adopt efficient methods for antibody screening, HLA phenotyping and crossmatching. These procedures are intimately linked. The data from these assays must be interpreted by experts who are aware of the clinical needs of patients and of the risks involved. Retransplantation of thoracic organs is largely unsuccessful in the short and long terms [17] and most centres now regard such procedures as ineffective and unacceptable.

Donated cadaver organs remain in restricted supply throughout the world and it is in the best interests of *all* organ transplant candidates that the most efficient use of this rare resource be made. Lowered survival rates for retransplantation are therefore unacceptable.

Acknowledgement.

We are grateful to members of this laboratory who have contributed to the technical development of the procedures described in this paper. In particular we thank Helen Liggett and Amanda Robson.

References

1. Halloran PF, Schlaut J, Solez K and Srinivasa NS. The significance of the anti-class I response. Transplantation 1992; 53: 550–555.
2. Sanfilippo F, Goeken N, Niblack G, Scornik J and Vaughn WK. The effect of first cadaver renal transplant HLA-A, B match on sensitization levels and retransplant rates following graft failure. Transplantation 1987; 43: 240–244.
3. Harmer AW, Koffman GC, Heads AJ,and Vaughan RW. Sensitization to HLA antigens occurs in 95% of primary renal transplant rejections. Tranplant. Proc. 1995; 27: 666–667.
4. Zachary AA, Klingman L, Thorne N, Smerglia AR and Teresi GA. Variations of the lymphocytotoxicity test. Transplantation 1995; 60: 498–503.
5. Harmer AW, Sutton M, Bayne A, Vaughan RW and Welsh KI. A highly sensitive, rapid screening method for the detection of antibodies directed against HLA class I and II antigens. Transplant. Int. 1993; 6: 277–280.
6. Zaer F, Metz S and Scornik JC. Antibody screening by enzyme-linked immunosorbent assay using pooled soluble HLA in renal transplant candidates. Transplantation 1997; 63: 48–51.
7. Scornick JC, Brunson ME, Schaub B, Howard RJ and Pfaff WW. The crossmatch in renal transplantation; evaluation of flow cytometry as a replacement for standard cytotoxicity. Transplantation 1994; 57: 621–625.
8. Hirata M and Terasaki PI. Renal retransplantation. Clinical Transplants 1994: 419–433.
9. Ting A and Morris PJ. Successful transplantation with a positive T and B cell crossmatch due to autoreactive antibodies. Tissue Antigens 1983; 21(3): 219–226.

10. Donaldson PT, Thomson LJ, Heads A et al. IgG donor-specific crossmatches are not associated with graft rejection or poor graft survival after liver transplantation; as assessment by cytotoxicity and flow cytometry. Transplantation 1995; 60: 1016–1023.
11. Vail A, Gore SM, Bradley BA, Easty DL, Rogers CA and Armitage WJ. Influence of donor and histocompatibility factors on corneal graft outcome. Transplantation 1994; 58: 1210–1217.
12. Opelz G. Repeated HLA mismatches increase the failure rate of second kidney transplants. Tranplant. Proc. 1995; 27(1): 658–659.
13. Senitzer D and Matas AJ. Transplantation Proc. 1988; 20: 34.
14. Welsh KI van Dam M, Bewick ME, Koffman GC, Taube DH, Raftery MJ and Rigden S. Successful transplantation of kidneys bearing previously mismatched HLA-A and -B locus antigens. Tranplant. Intl. 1988; 1: 190–195.
15. Opelz G, Schwarz V, Wujciak T, Schnobel R, Henderson R and Grayson H. Analysis of non-hodgkin's lymphomas in organ transplant recipients. Transplantation Reviews 1995; 9(4): 231–240.
16. Harmer AW, Garner S, Bell AE et al. Evaluation of the flow cytometric crossmatch; preliminary results of a multicentre study. Transplantation 1996; 61: 1108–1111.
17. Ensley RD, Hunt S, Taylor DO et al. Predictors of survival after repeat heart transplantation. J. Heart & Lung Transplantation 1992; 11:S142–S148.

20. Retransplantation following AHG-negative crossmatches

RONALD H. KERMAN, BRIAN M. SUSSKIND, JOEL SLATON, RICHARD M. LEWIS, ABBAS HEYDARI, JIM RUTH, JACKIE WILLIAMS, CHARLES T. VAN BUREN, STEPHEN M. KATZ & BARRY D. KAHAN

Introduction

Retransplant patients are an immunologically unique group since they have already experienced graft loss and have been exposed to a bolus of alloantigen. Having previously lost a transplant, these patients are often sensitized and have poorer early graft function resulting in patient management problems [1, 2]. Survival rates for cadaveric retransplantations have been consistently lower than those for primary grafts [3–6]. Some of the risk factors associated with poor retransplantation outcome include patient high PRA, recipient-donor HLA mismatches, positive flow cytometry crossmatches and, perhaps the most important, previous graft survival time less than 3–6 months [3, 4, 7–9]. Since the introduction of cyclosporine based immunosuppressive protocols in 1983, the one year regraft survival rate of second cadaver donor renal allografts has remained relatively constant, whereas that of first transplants has significantly improved [9]. However, since 1988 survival rates for retransplant cadaver-donor grafts have improved each year with the difference between first and second transplant one year survival rates decreasing from 8% in 1988 to 2% in 1991 [10]. These recent improvements may reflect the impact of more efficacious immunosuppression and more sensitive and informative crossmatching [6, 11]. However, data from the UNOS Registry suggests that a decreasing number of high-risk patients, especially reTx patients with short previous graft survival times, have been retransplanted in recent years and that selection of more low-risk reTx candidates may be an important contributing factor in explaining improved regraft survivals [8]. While this policy may result in improved reTx graft outcome, it also results in high-risk reTx patients accumulating on the transplant patient waiting list.

In a preliminary study, we reported that improved regraft survivals can be accomplished when patients were transplanted following negative AHG-XMs [5]. In the current study, we herein report on the improved regraft survivals of 100 reTx recipients following negative AHG-XMs. Importantly, we saw no

J.L. Touraine et al. (eds.), Retransplantation, 167–177.

Table 1. Patient demographics

	NIH XM-NEG ($N = 120$)	AHG XM-NEG ($N = 100$)
Male (%)	71	75
Female (%)	29	25
Caucasian (%)	69	57
Black (%)	17	15
Hispanic (%)	6	25
Other (%)	26	3
Age (years)	37 ± 9	39 ± 11
Diabetics (%)	30	25
ATG/OKT-3 Rx (%)	19	27
T-cell Rx loss (%)	39	40

impact of PRA, HLA matching or previous graft survival time as risk factors that influenced regraft outcome.

Materials and methods

Patients

We analyzed the impact of pretransplant donor-specific crossmatching results on the graft survivals of 220 retransplant recipients of cadaveric donor allografts. There were 120 reTx recipients transplanted from 1981 to 1989 following a negative NIH-XM and 100 reTx recipients transplanted from 1989 to 1994 following a negative AHG-XM. In both instances, negative XMs included testing historical, high-PRA and preTx sera. Table 1 describes the patient demographics of the NIH-XM negative and the AHG-XM negative groups. Patients were reasonably well matched for all categories except that there were more Hispanics in the AHG-XM negative group and more recipients of other racial origins in the NIH-XM negative group. Recipient immunosuppressive protocols have been previously described [12–14]. From 1980 to December 1988, recipients began their CsA at 14 mg/kg orally on day 0 and during the first week posttransplant. Recipients were usually given CsA i.v. at 3–5 mg/kg on days 0, 1 and 2, and when gastrointestinal malabsorption was suspected. The doses were tapered to 12 mg/kg during weeks 2–3; and 10 mg/kg weeks 3–12; the dosage was then individualized in an effort to keep 24-h serum trough levels at 100–200 ng/ml by radioimmunoassay. Prednisone was initiated at the time of transplant (2 mg/kg), with tapered dose reduction to a maintenance dose of 10–15 mg/day. The diagnosis of rejection was based upon clinical and biochemical data and confirmed by biopsy in most cases. Rejection episodes were treated using i.v. pulse therapy with methylprednisolone and followed by temporary elevation and recycling of oral prednisone [12]. The pharmacokinetic strategy was implemented in late 1988 and early 1989 [13, 14]. Data derived for primary cadaveric allograft survival from the two immunosuppressive regimen periods were not statistically different from each other and therefore the change in 1988 did not influence the re-Tx graft outcome.

Transfusion history

All retransplant recipients had received transfusions prior to their reTx. Transfusion information on all recipients was obtained from the patient, the dialysis unit, and/or from hospital records. Transfusions were generally of packed erthyrocytes without leukocyte depletion by washing or freezing procedures, and were only occasionally of whole blood.

Histocompatibility testing

All donors and recipients were ABO-compatible. HLA A, B, C and DR tissue typing was performed using the microlymphocytotoxicity technique utilizing commercially available tissue typing trays [16]. All recipients displayed a negative donor-specific crossmatch for both their historical-high PRA and preTx sera.

The standard NIH visual lymphocytotoxicity crossmatch was performed by incubating patient sera and donor target cells at room temperature for 120 min (long incubation) followed by a 60-min incubation with complement. Since the antibody concentration is unknown, sera were diluted (1 μl serum plus 1, 2, 3, 4, 5, or 6 μl of McCoy's or increasing amounts of sera were added to reaction wells (1 μl serum plus 1, 2, 3, 4, 5, or 6 μl sera to each well) to test for either high or low levels of antidonor antibody. After the incubation with complement, eosin was added to each well, and the trays were subsequently covered and read using an inverted phase microscope; and each well was scored for the extent of cell death.

The antihuman globulin crossmatch procedure was performed by incubating patient sera and donor target cells at room temperature for 60 min. Sera were added in triplicate wells to a volume of 1 μl and 2 μl or diluted 1:2 and 1:4. In all sera tested, positive (POS) and/or negative (NEG) reactions were always seen with these combinations. Following the incubation, barbital buffer was used to wash the cells. The buffer was removed by flicking the tray with a quick motion. The wash step was repeated once. The antihuman globulin reagent (antihuman kappa light chain, Sigma) in a dilution of 1:256 was added in a volume of 1 μl and incubated for exactly 1 min at room temperature. Thereafter, 5 μl of rabbit complement was added and the tray incubated for 60 min at room temperature. Eosin dye and formalin were added, the trays covered with a glass slide and allowed to settle for 10 min before reading under an inverted phase microscope to determine cell lysis. Cytotoxicity was determined by employing the standard American Society of Histocompatibility and Immunogenetics scoring code. Negative controls included normal AB (+) serum and McCoys (with 5% fetal calf serum). Positive controls consisted of triplicate wells utilizing antithymocyte globulin from Ortho Pharmaceuticals [16].

Dithioerythritol (DTE) treatment of recipient sera was accomplished by setting up a standard NIH visual crossmatch tray, except that recipient sera were added into triplicate wells at dilutions of 1:2 and 1:4 only. To each serum well was added 1 μl of 25 mM DTE for 20 min at 37°C. Donor target cells (1 μl) were then added (as described above) and incubated for 30 min at room temperature. Following these incubations the cell-serum mixtures were washed 2x with barbital buffer and the excess wash fluid removed by hand flicking. Rabbit complement (5 μl) was added to the wells and incubated for 60 min. After the complement incubation, eosin was added and the trays were read as described above. Control wells consisted of either McCoys, normal AB (+) serum, and an IgG or IgM source. Patient sera were tested by the AHG procedure with and without DTE treatment [17]. Patient sera were tested for percent reactive antibody (PRA) against a 60-member donor panel representing HLA A, B, C and DR specificities, utilizing an NIH (up to 1989) and thereafter an AHG procedure.

Flow cytometry crossmatching (FCXM) was performed with a FACSCAN flow cytometer (256 channel resolution) from Becton Dickinson and modified from a protocol of Garovoy [18, 19]. Donor peripheral blood lymphocytes were isolated by the Ficoll-Hypaque density centrifugation technique, washed once with RPMI and brought to a concentration of $2–4 \times 10^6$ PBL/ml. Donor target PBL ($2–4 \times 10^5$ in a 0.1 ml volume) were added to 0.1 ml of recipient test serum and the mixture incubated for 30 min at room temperature. Thereafter, the cells were washed three times with 10% FCS-PBS, the supernatant was discarded, and the cell pellet was resuspended in 0.05 ml of fluoresceinated goat F (ab)2 anti-human IgG (1:50) or IgM (1:300) immunoglobulin and 0.01 ml of PerCP-conjugated anti-CD3 (Leu 4) or PE-conjugated anti-CD19 (Leu 12) antibodies and incubated for 20 min at 5°C, then the cells are washed once with 10% FCS-PBS. If necessary, following the incubation, 1.0 ml of lysing reagent was added for 4 minutes to remove any RBC contamination. The mixture was then centrifuged at 250 × g for 5 minutes, the supernatant was discarded, and the cells were resuspended in 0.4 ml of 1% paraformaldehyde and then read by the FACSCAN for analysis. Background controls consisted of cells with media control FCS-PBS, and the anti-human immunoglobulins, cells with AB+ sera and the anti-human immunoglobulins, cells with pooled high PRA sera ($\geq$ 95–100% PRA), and finally a normal member of our panel (with the same ABO as the recipient) and the human immunoglobulins. A positive FCXM was defined as a shift in the mean channel of fluorescence of $\geq$ 20 channels to the right for IgG or IgM anti-T cell and a 30 channel shift to the right for IgG or IgM anti-B cells. Data processing was done by means of the Consort 32 computer program (Becton Dickinson).

Data analysis

Graft and patient survivals were calculated using standard actuarial life table analysis [20]. Graft loss was recorded on the date of transplant nephrectomy,

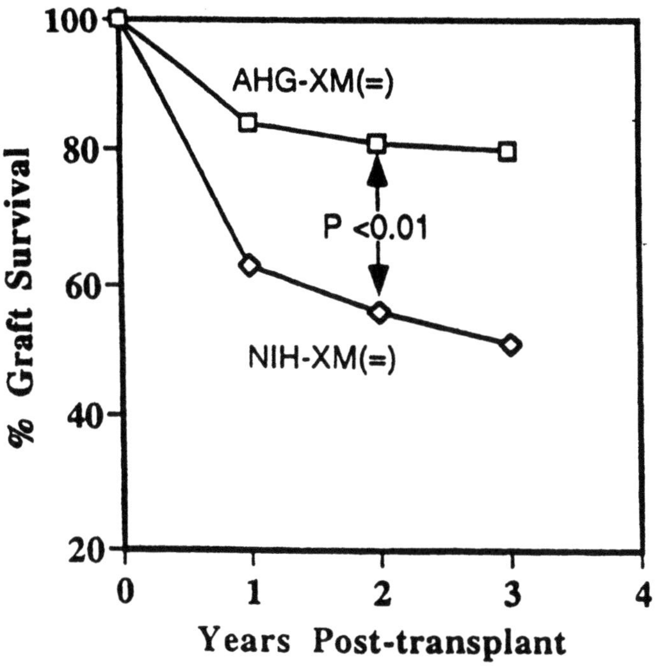

Fig. 1. Retransplant graft survival.

death with a functioning graft, or return to dialysis. The significance of differences between groups was determined by a Wilcoxon rank sum test [21].

Results

The 1, 2 and 3 year graft survivals of 84%, 81%, and 80% respectively were observed for the 100 reTx recipients who had negative AHG-XMs (Figure 1). These results were significantly better than the 1, 2 and 3 year graft survivals of 63%, 56% and 51% respectively for a group of 120 reTx recipients transplanted following only a negative NIH-XM ($p < 0.01$ for each time point vs. the negative AHG-XM recipients). The negative crossmatch results reflected testing of both historical, high-PRA and preTx sera for both NIH and AHG crossmatched groups. Seventy of the 120 NIH-XM negative sera were tested for flow cytometry crossmatch results and the one year regraft survival of 76% for FCXM- negative recipients was significantly better than the 58% survival rate for FCXM-positive regraft recipients $p < 0.01$ (Table 2). However, the flow cytometry crossmatch results for 80 of the tested AHG-XM negative sera revealed identical one-year regraft survivals of 84% for both FCXM-negative ($N = 25$) and positive ($N = 55$) reTx recipients (Table 2). Further investigation of the 55 AHG-XM negative but FCXM-positive sera revealed that 15% (8/55)

Table 2. Re-TX graft outcome: flow cytometry XM results

	NIH XM-NEG ($N = 70$)		AHG XM-NEG ($N = 80$)	
	FCXM (=) ($N = 25$)	FCXM (+) ($N = 45$)	FCXM (=) ($N = 25$)	FCXM (+) ($N = 55$)
12 Month graft survival	76%	58%	84%	84%
	$P < 0.01$		NS	

Table 3. Immunoglobulin reactivity from 55 AHG-XM negative but FCXM positive RETX sera

	One-year graft survival
IgG or IgM anti-T cell only (non-MHC, $N = 8$)	88%
IgM anti-B/T cell (anti-MHC, $N = 18$)	83%
IgG anti-B/T cell (anti-MHC, $N = 15$)	80%
IgG/IgM anti-B/T cell (anti-MHC, $N = 14$)	86%

Table 4. Immunoglobulin and immunoglobulin subclass reactivity of 14 RETX AHG-XM negative but anti-MHC, FCXM positive sera

4 sera were IgM FCXM (+)
3 sera were IgG_3 FCXM (+)
3 sera were IgG_1 FCXM (+)
4 sera were IgG_4 FCXM (+)

of the sera displayed non-MHC antibody reactivity (IgM or IgG anti-T cell only); that 33% (18/58) of the sera displayed IgM anti-B and T cell (anti-MHC) reactivity; that 27% (15/55) of the sera displayed IgG anti-B and T cell (anti-MHC) reactivity; and finally, that 25% (14/55) of the sera displayed both IgM and IgG anti-MHC reactivity (Table 3). Finally, 14 reTx AHG-XM negative but anti-MHC FCXM positive sera were tested for the immunoglobulin and immunoglobulin subclass reactivity against donor T and/or B target cells. Four sera were IgM and 10 sera were IgG reactive. Of the 10 IgG reactive sera 3 were IgG_3, 3 were IgG_1 and 4 were IgG_4 FCXM positive (Table 4).

As previously mentioned, three factors associated with poor retransplant outcome include recipient high PRA, donor-recipient HLA mismatches (MM), and a previous graft survival time of 3–6 months [3, 4, 7–9]. We examined all three parameters in our study. Table 5 shows that the one-year regraft survival outcome for AHG-XM negative recipients was not influenced by percentage PRA since comparable % PRA's were displayed by both regraft successes and losses (when evaluating the impact of historical high-PRA or preTx sera). Figures 2A and 2B illustrate the impact of donor-recipient HLA mismatching on regraft outcome. HLA matching was highly significant for improved regraft

Table 5. PRA and one year graft survival of AHG XM-neg retransplant recipients

	One year graft survival		
	Yes ($N = 84$)	No ($N = 16$)	P value
% PRA Pre-TX	24 ± 14	27 ± 11	NS
Highest-historical	$42 \pm 11\%$	$44 \pm 13\%$	NS

outcome for the 120 recipients transplanted following an NIH-negative crossmatch. Well matched (≤ 2 HLA A, B MM ($N = 63$) and 0–1 DR MMs ($N = 14$), NIH-XM negative regraft recipients had significantly improved 1, 2 and 3 year survivals compared to poorly matched (> HLA 2, A, B MMs ($N = 57$) and 2 DR MMs ($N = 106$) recipients ($p < 0.01$ respectively for each time point and match grade comparison). In contrast, however, no significant difference in regraft survival rates was observed for the 100 well or poorly matched AHG-XM negative regraft recipients. Finally, we also evaluated the influence of previous graft survival time. As seen in Table 6, there was no difference in the one year regraft outcome of 82% for the 44 recipients whose previous graft survival time was less than 3 months compared to the one year outcome of 86% for the 56 recipients whose previous regraft survival time was more than 3 months.

Discussion

Regraft survival rates for cadaveric donor renal allografts, have historically been lower than those of primary allograft recipients [3–6]. Risk factors associated with the poor reTx outcome include recipient high-PRA, donor-recipient HLA mismatches, positive flow cytometry crossmatches and previous graft survival times less than 3–6 months [3–9]. Two of these high-risk factors have led transplant centers to regraft only recipients who display either a negative anti-donor FCXM and/or recipients who retained their previous grafts longer than 3–6 months, or both [3, 4, 7–9, 11, 22, 23]. This is an understandably conservative approach that has led to improved regraft survivals, comparable to primary renal allograft outcomes [10]. However, it has also caused those reTx candidates who display positive anti-donor FCXMs or who lost their first grafts in less than 3–6 months to accumulate on the waiting list for a longer time period before being transplanted. The results of our present study suggest that both of these identified high-risk candidate groups may be successfully retransplanted.

Retransplant candidates, who displayed a negative AHG-XM (testing both historical, high PRA and preTx sera), enjoyed significantly improved 1, 2 and 3 year regraft survivals of 84%, 81% and 80% respectively compared to 63%, 56% and 51% respectively, for NIH-XM negative regraft recipients ($p < 0.01$ for each time point). Whereas, there was an impact of donor-recipient HLA

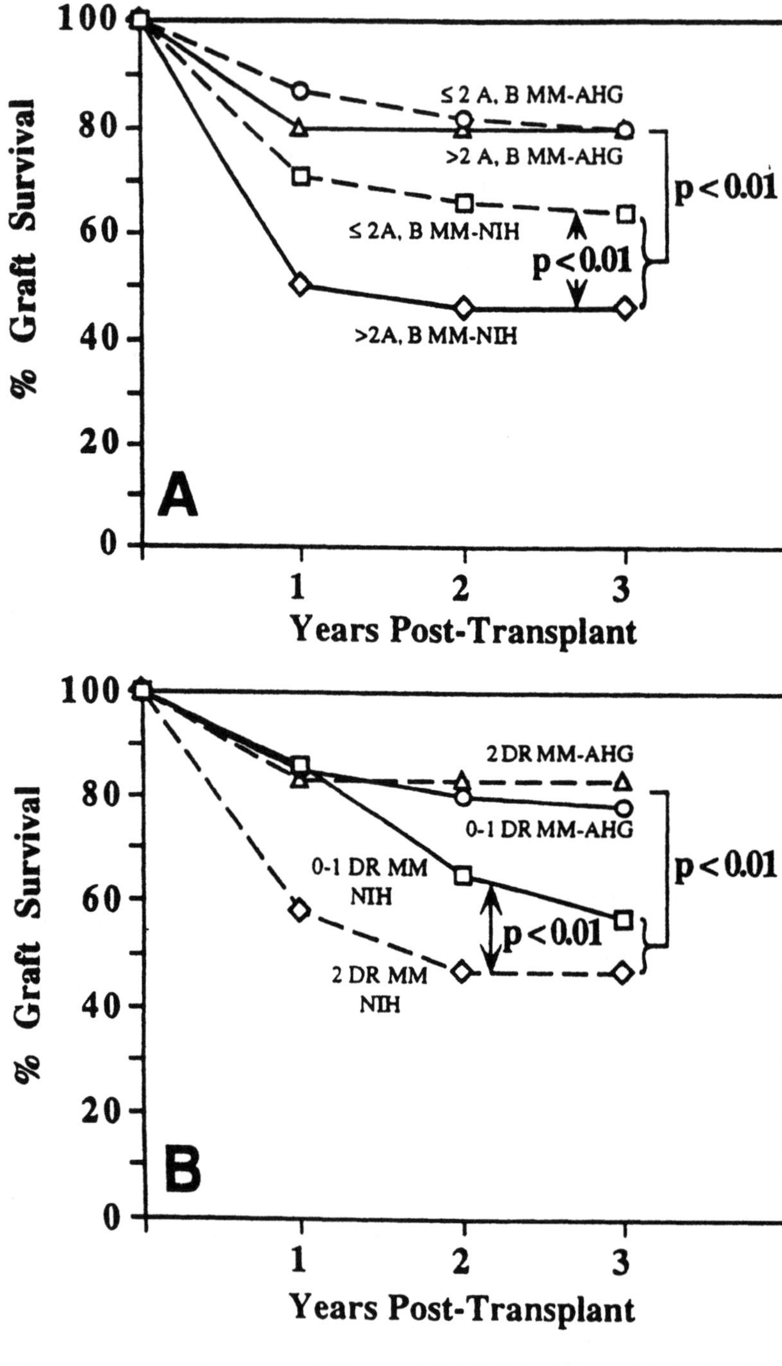

Fig. 2. Retransplant graft survival – NIH vs AHG NEG XMs: HLA, A, B MM (A); HLA-DR MM (B).

Table 6. One year graft survival of AHG XM-neg retransplant recipients based upon previous graft survival time

	Previous graft survival time (months post-TX)	
	<3 ($N = 44$)	>3 ($N = 56$)
One year graft survival	82% (36/44)	86% (48/56)

matching on the regraft outcome of NIH-XM negative recipients none was seen for the AHG-XM negative regraft patients. Similarly, % PRA did not adversely affect regraft outcome for the AHG-XM negative recipient.

Regraft recipients who lost their first transplants in a clinically vigorous fashion early in the post-Tx time period (less than 3–6 months) were identified as high-risk, strong immune responders because they went on to experience poor regraft outcomes [7–9]. It is entirely possible that the preTx XMs performed prior to the first and reTx, coupled with less efficacious immunosuppression, led to the strong-immune responder presentation of these high-risk reTx recipients and their poor clinical outcome. However, utilizing the AHG-XM to identify reTx candidates with no AHG detectable anti-donor reactivity in either historical-high PRA and preTx sera, resulted in appropriate donor-regraft recipient pairings and successful regraft outcomes. This was true for recipients with both short and long previous graft survival times. Therefore, a short previous graft survival time may not be a high-risk factor for an AHG-XM negative reTx candidate.

A number of laboratories, including our own, have reported on the benefit of the flow cytometry crossmatch in delineating appropriate and successful donor-recipient pairings for transplantation [5, 6, 11, 18, 19, 22, 23]. However, care must be taken in the interpretation of the various crossmatch results so as not to be too conservative. Transplanting only FCXM-negative recipients could deny a donor organ to a FCXM-positive recipient who potentially could be successfully transplanted. The AHG-XM negative regraft recipients were devoid of AHG detectable anti-donor reactivity in both high-PRA and preTx sera. However, many of these regraft recipients displayed flow cytometry detected IgM and IgG anti-MHC reactivity including the IgG_3 and IgG_1 complement fixing immunoglobulin subclasses. Yet, these AHG-XM negative, but FCXM-positive anti-MHC recipients, enjoyed an 84% one year graft survival. Therefore, since the sera were devoid of AHG-XM detected anti-donor reactivity the remaining flow identified anti-MHC antibodies were too low in concentration to be clinically deleterious.

Previous reports by many laboratories have suggested that FCXM-negative recipients enjoyed significantly improved graft survivals compared to standard crossmatch negative results [11, 18, 19, 22, 23]. However, these reports compared the least sensitive crossmatch procedures used (NIH and/or Amos-modified) to the most sensitive FCXM procedure without necessarily testing for AHG-detectable antibody reactivity. Therefore, a positive-FCXM result, in this setting, could be due to undetected AHG-reactivity (which might contraindicate a transplant) or to only flow cytometry identified reactivity (which may not be a contraindication to transplant).

Our results suggest that the AHG-XM protocol identifies retransplant recipients with no AHG detectable anti-donor antibodies, but with clinically non-deleterious flow cytometry identified antibodies, who can be successfully retransplanted. HLA mismatching, % PRA, positive-flow cytometry crossmatches and short previous graft survival times are no longer risk factors for AHG-XM negative reTx recipients. Therefore, the AHG-XM protocol would allow us to do the right thing (transplant appropriate donor-recipient pairings) as well as avoid doing the wrong thing (inappropriately deny a donor-organ to a regraft recipient who could be successfully transplanted).

References

1. Cecka JM, Cho L. Sensitization. In: Terasaki PI (ed.), Clinical Transplants 1988. Los Angeles, UCLA Tissue Typing Laboratory, 1989; 365–373.
2. Braun WE. Laboratory and clinical management of the highly sensitized organ transplant recipient. Hum. Immunol. 1989; 26: 245–260.
3. Perdue ST. Risk factors for second transplants. In: Terasaki PI (ed.), Clinical Transplants 1985. Los Angeles, UCLA Tissue Typing Laboratory, 1985; 191–203.
4. Almond PS, Matas AJ, Gillingham K et al. Risk factors for second renal allografts. Transplantation 1991; 52: 253–258.
5. Kerman RH, Van Buren CT, Lewis RM et al. Improved graft survival for flow cytometry and anti-human globulin crossmatch negative retransplant recipients. Transplantation 1990; 49: 52–56.
6. Kerman RH, Kimball PM, Van Buren CT et al. AHG and DTE/AHG procedure identification of crossmatch-appropriate donor-recipient pairings that result in improved graft survival. Transplantation 1991; 51: 316–320.
7. Cabacungan C. Regrafts. In: Terasaki PI, Cecka JM (eds.), Clinical Transplants 1992, Los Angeles, UCLA Tissue Typing Laboratory, 1993, 347–356.
8. Cho YW, Cecka JM. Cadaver-donor renal retransplants. In: Terasaki PI, Cecka JM (eds.), Clinical Transplants 1993, Los Angeles, UCLA Tissue Typing Laboratory, 1994, 469–484.
9. Ogura K, Cecka JM. Cadaver retransplants. In: Terasaki PI (ed.), Clinical Transplants 1990. Los Angeles, UCLA Tissue typing Laboratory, 1991, 471–483.
10. Mitsuishi Y, Cecka JM. Cadaver retransplants. In: Terasaki PI, Cecka JM. (eds.), Clinical Transplants 1991. Los Angeles, UCLA Tissue Typing Laboratory, 1992, 281–291.
11. Cook DJ, Terasaki PI, Terashita GY et al. An approach to reducing early transplant failure by flow cytometry crossmatching. Clin. Transplant. 1987; 1: 253–256.
12. Kahan BD, Van Buren CT, Lin SN et al. Immunopharmacological monitoring of CsA-treated kidney recipients. Transplantation 1982; 34: 36–45.
13. Kahan BD, Grevel J. Overview – optimization of cyclosporine therapy in renal transplantation by a pharmacokinetic strategy. Transplantation 1988; 46: 631–644.
14. Kahan BD, Welsh M, Rutzky L et al. The ability of pretransplant test dose pharmacokinetics to reduce early adverse events after renal transplantation. Transplantation 1992; 53: 345–351.
15. Terasaki PI, Bernoco D, Park MS et al. Microdroplet testing for HLA A, B, C and D antigens. Am. J. Clin. Pathol. 1978; 69: 103–120.

16. Johnson AH, Rossen RD, Butler WT. Detection of alloantibodies using a sensitive antiglobulin microcytotoxicity test: identification of low levels of preformed antibodies in accelerated allograft rejection. Tissue Antigens 1972; 2: 215–226.
17. Barger BO, Shroyer SL, Hudson MH et al. Successful renal allografts in recipients with a positive standard, DTE negative crossmatch. Transplant. Proc. 1989; 21: 746–747.
18. Garovoy MR, Rheinschmidt MA, Bigos M et al. Flow cytometry analysis: a high technology crossmatch technique facilitating transplantation. Transplant. Proc. 1983; 15: 1939–1944.
19. Garovoy MR. Flow cytometry crossmatch testing in renal transplantation. Transplant. Immunol. Lett. 1985; 5: 1–4.
20. Merrele N, Schulman LE. Determination or prognosis in chronic disease. J. Chronic Dis. 1955; 1: 12–18.
21. Mann H, Whitney D. On a test of whether one of two random variables is stochastically larger than the other. Ann. Math. Statis. 1947; 18: 50–59.
22. Scornik JC, Brunson ME, Schaub B et al. The crossmatch in renal transplantation: Evaluation of flow cytometry as a replacement for standard cytotoxicity. Transplantation 1994; 57: 621–625.
23. Ogura K, Terasaki PI, Johnson C et al. The significance of a positive flow cytometry crossmatch test in primary kidney transplantation. Transplantation 1993; 56: 294–298.

PART FIVE

Alternatives to retransplantation

21. Comparison between retransplantation of kidney and chronic dialysis

FRANÇOIS BERTHOUX, ERIC ALAMARTINE, NABIL DIAB
& JEAN-PIERRE DE FILIPPIS

Introduction:

Treatment of end stage renal failure (ESRF) is achieved either by chronic dialysis (haemodialysis or peritoneal dialysis) or by renal transplantation (RTx). The advantages of RTx over dialysis include lower mortality (annual death rate about 1% for transplanted patients, compared with 14% for dialysed patients in year 1995 for France) [1], better long-term rehabilitation of patients, regular improved graft survival (we can expect about 60% at 10 years under triple therapy) and lower cost (on a 10 year basis, the cost of transplantation is 5.5 times less than the cost of hospital dialysis). All these previous demonstrations were made with global data including 85–90% of first grafts.

The question to be answered in this paper is: after a first kidney graft failure, what is the best treatment: a second transplant or chronic dialysis? Specific information in the litterature is clearly lacking on this topic, so we decided to analyse our own results, in order to try to answer this question.

Material and methods

We have analyzed our data obtained during the cyclosporine A era, e.g. from August 1984 (first use of CyA) until december 1996. We performed 683 RTx (582 first graft and 101 second or more graft; the great majority (95%), were cadaver kidneys) in 639 recipients divided into local patients ($N = 241$; first Tx = 209), regional patients ($N = 195$; first Tx = 185), and non-residents ($N = 203$ foreigners; first Tx = 188).

We have collected the data on all patients with a first graft performed in our group, but only for local and regional patients was it possible to obtain good quality, accurate and verified data. We therefore followed 394 recipients (209 local, 185 regional) receiving a first RTx in our center. None of these patients were lost to follow-up.

The results of the first graft were as follows: 290 patients with a functioning graft (74%) and 104 recipients with failure (either death or graft failure).

Our final analyses concerned these 104 local and regional recipients with a first graft failure: 24 deaths and 80 graft failures.

J.L. Touraine et al. (eds.), Retransplantation, 181–183.

Results

The deaths during the first kidney graft

We observed only 24 deaths (6%; 14 males and 10 females; 15 local and 9 regional; 23 cadaver kidneys and one from a living donor). The mean age at death was 56 years (median 59; range 31–66). The distribution of age at death was only 1 in the category 15–39 years, 12 (50%) in the category 40–59 and 11 aged 60 years or more (46%). The timing of death was 6 from 0–3 months, 4 from 3–12 months, 9 from 1–5 years, and 5 after 5 years post-Tx. The causes of death were cardiovascular in 11 (46%), infection in 6 (25%), cancer in 4 (17%), and various in 3. Sixteen recipients died with a functioning graft (2/3).

Outcome of the 80 living recipients with a first renal graft failure

The causes of graft failure were: rejection in 49, *de novo* or recurrent glomerulonephritis in 17, surgical complications in 6, infection in 4, graft cancer in 2, and varied in 2. All these 80 patients returned to chronic haemodialysis and apart from older ($N = 9$) and noncompliant patients ($N = 4$) were registered for a second transplant. These patients were classified in two groups according to final outcome: group I received a second kidney graft ($N = 27$; 34%) while group II remained on chronic haemodialysis ($N = 53$; 66%).

Results of group I with kidney retransplantation [2]

These patients were 20 males and 7 females (16 local and 11 regional). At time of first graft failure, the mean age was 38 years (median 40; range 18–64). The distribution of age was 13 between 15 and 39 (48%); 13 between 40 and 59 (48%) and only 1 over 60 years. The mean interval time between first graft failure and date of second graft (Tx2) was 35.8 months (median 27 months; 5–86). By definition, in order to obtain a second transplant, these patients survived this waiting time and this constituted a major bias in the study (death occurring during this period put the patient in group II).

The mean follow-up for RTx2 was 53 months (median 50; 1–115). The outcome of Tx2 was no death (0%); 4 failures (15%) due to rejection in 3 (10 months, 16 months, 41 months) and to recurrent hemolytic–uremic syndrome (72 months); and 23 are still functioning (85%).

The mean interval time between first renal replacement therapy (RRT) and last follow-up was 118 months (median 113 months; range 34–192 months).

Results of group II, remaining on chronic dialysis

This group comprised 35 males and 18 females (27 local and 26 regional). The mean age at first graft failure was 47 years (median 49; 11–69); making this group nine years older than group I. The age distribution was 1 below 15 years,

12 (23%) between 15 and 39, 31 (58%) between 40 and 59 years, and 9 (17%) aged ≥60 years.

The mean follow-up after Tx1 failure was only 39 months (median 39; 2–128). The final outcome was 12 deaths (23%) and 41 alive patients (77%). The mean interval time between first RRT and last follow-up was 107 months (median 109; range 39–273) and similar to group I.

The mean age at death was 50.5 years (43–70) with 1 in the age group 15–39 years; 7 (58%) in 40–59 years and 4 (33%) aged ≥60 years. The causes of death were unremarkable: cardiovascular in 6; cancer in 5 and suicide in 1. The timing of death was 2 during the first year post-Tx1 failure; 5 during the second year; 1 in the third year; and 4 in the fifth year.

Discussion

Group I with kidney retransplantation and group II with chronic haemodialysis were not exactly comparable. Patients in group I were younger and the waiting time between Tx1 failure and Tx2 was a major bias for the study of mortality. It was therefore necessary to correct mortality in group II by removing the deaths occurring during the first 39 months post-Tx1 failure and the deaths occurring in those aged ≥60 years. If we do that, we remained with only 4 deaths in the category 15–59 years and after 39 months, but the number of patients really exposed to the risk is only 23 in group II. The corrected mortality is therefore 17%. The mortality comparison between group I and group II is 0 out of 27 vs 4 out of 23. The χ^2 is 5.10 and the probability is significant ($P = 0.003$).

Conclusion

In our experience, mortality is lower in group I (regrafting) than in group II (no regraft, but chronic haemodialysis). However, the comparison was difficult mostly because of unavoidable bias than really selection of patients. After a first kidney graft failure, the best option is a second transplant.

References

1. Berthoux F, Bernhein J, Gellert R et al. The project of the European Renal Association (ERA-EDTA) for an European nephrological network. Nephrol. Dial. Transplant. 1997, in press.
2. Mahoney RJ, Norman DJ, Colombe BW, Garovoy MR, Leeber DA. Identification of high and low risk second kidney grafts. Transplantation 1996; 61: 1349–1355.

22. Cardiac retransplantation and mechanical circulatory support

D. LOISANCE

Introduction

Indication for a repeat cardiac transplantation is not an infrequent situation [1]. The risks of the retransplantation are significantly higher than the risk of the first operation [2]. The increasing difficulty for a patient listed for a first transplantation to receive a good donor graft within a reasonable period of time, the attempt in most of the cardiac transplant centers to optimize as much as possible the use of the scarce donor grafts explain the difficulties for a patient selected for a retransplantation to actually receive a graft. This situation justifies an analysis of the real possibilities of mechanical circulation support as an alternative to a retransplantation.

Cardiac retransplantation

Analysis of cardiac transplantation throughout the world may be performed in the Registry of the International Society of Heart and Lung Transplantation [1]. Despite its voluntary nature, this Registry is an unique source of information about activity and results in cardiac transplantation.

The last published data [1] cover 34 326 cardiac transplantations performed in 271 centers. This activity remains steady since 1990, with a peak in 1993, 3546 cases, and a minimum in 1995, 2923 cases. Survival rate at 1 year is 79%, with a 4% mortality per year over the subsequent 11 years. This fall off in survival is almost a straight line from year 1 through year 12 and projected out would represent a maximum survival of approximately 20 years for the entire population.

In the same Registry, 653 retransplantations have been listed, in patients older than 18 years of age: 256 were retransplanted within the first 6 months after the first transplantation, and 334 retransplantations were performed after that first 6-months period. The overall 1 and 3 year survival is respectively 52 and 44% for those patients undergoing retransplantation, the 1-year survival is 39%, whereas those retransplanted after the 6-months period have a 1 year survival of 63%. In the pediatric group, 70 patients have been submitted to retransplantation with a 1 year survival rate of 42%, lower than in the adult population.

J.L. Touraine et al. (eds.), Retransplantation, 185–192.

The causes of retransplantation are of two different natures [3]. In most cases, retransplantation within the first 6-months period, graft failure and early acute uncontrolled allograft rejection are the cause of graft dysfunction and the indication of the retransplantation. Clinical evolution is frequently rapid and cardiogenic shock a frequent complication. In the group of patients retransplanted after this early period, the cause of cardiac failure is mainly related to the allograft arterial vasculopathy. In this group, evolution may be slowly progressive, towards cardiac failure. The exact cause of this vasculopathy is still unclear and its prevention remains an enigma. These causes of allograft failure account to 54% of all deaths after primary graft failure.

One of the major problems of retransplantation is actually the access to the procedure. Beside contraindication related directly to the patients characteristics (hemodynamical stability, immunization, associated infectious complications) which make retransplantation a less than optimal decision, the world wide situation of organ shortage rises major problems. Among those problems, ethical considerations play a major role which finally, lead to refuse to patients candidates to a retransplantation the potential benefit of a reoperation. In the present context evaluation of the real possibilities given by the various methods of mechanical circulatory support deserves some discussion.

Mechanical circulatory support (MCS)

A large variety of mechanical systems is now available to support patients with profound circulatory failure or cardiogenic shock, related to cardiac dysfunction [3]. Their introduction, initiated some 25 years and the development of clinical experience in the past 15 years permit an analysis of the real potential of mechanical support in patients eligible for a retransplantation because of primary allograft failure.

There are different categories of systems. Hemopump type system, based on a catheter technic, allows adequate left ventricular unloading, 1.7–5 l/min bypass flow, temporary (days) circulatory support via a minimal invasive approach (either a percutaneous femoral access or a mediastinal open-chest technic). A second group of systems is based on atrio or ventricular access and aortic or pulmonary reinfusion of the blood. Activation of the blood is obtained either with an axial flow type pump or on occlusive, sac type, pneumatically driven, extracorporeal pump. Pump performance in term of volumic flow rate, head pressure, blood activation is such that clinically the system has been shown acceptable for periods ranging from few days up to few months. The extracorporeal position of the pump, the pneumatic nature of the driving system nevertheless does not allow an acceptable quality of life, since mobilization of the patient out the hospital and autonomy are extremely limited. Consequently such a system can't achieve more than a temporary support, permitting in the best situation either recovery of the native cardiac graft function or optimal conditions for a retransplantation.

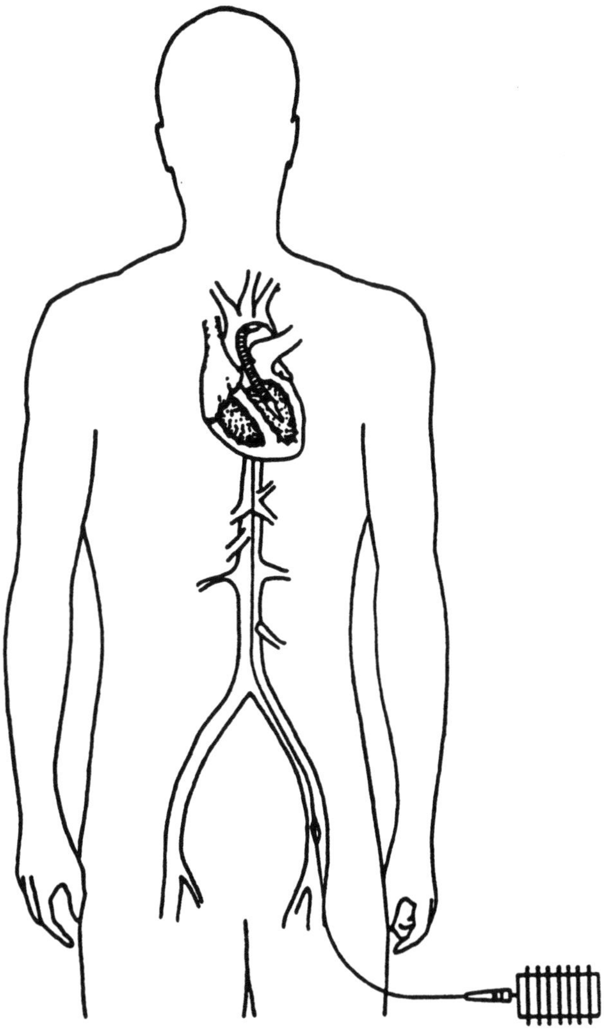

Fig. 1. Intraventricular axial flow pump, permitting minimally invasive left ventricular support.

A third system includes orthotopic artificial ventricles. They are driven pneumatically, the patient being connected to a paracorporeal console. The main advantage of the system is to allow bi-ventricular excision of the failing transplant. The 2 artificial ventricles are then connected to quick connectors sutured to the patient is auriculoventricular annulus. The atrial walls of the transplanted graft are left in place. Because of the nature of the driving force (pneumatic) the method does not allow an acceptable quality of life and

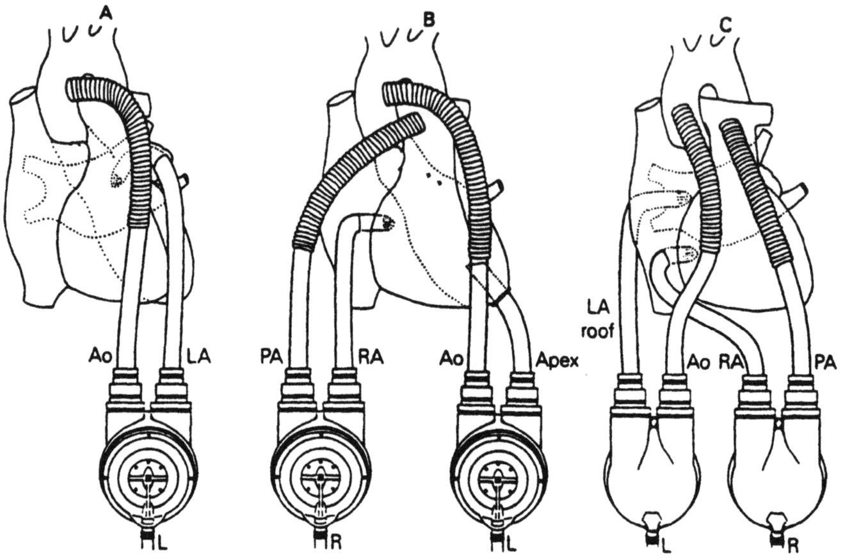

Fig. 2. Various modalities of paracorporeal circulatory support using pneumatically driven pumps. From left to right left ventricular assistance (atrio-aortic); biventricular support: apico aortic left and right ventricular or atrio aortic left and right ventricular support.

consequently the system cannot be considered as an acceptable alternative to retransplantation.

The last group of system includes the implantable devices for left ventricular support. The pump is connected to the ventricle, via an apical conduit. Re-infusion is obtained through an outflow graft, implanted into the ascending aorta, the pump is placed inside the abdominal pump. There are two different types of ventricular pumps: one pneumatically driven, connected to a paracorporeal console, and the other electrically driven. There are two electrically driven pumps: one is based on an electric rotative motor (VE Thermedic); the second one is an electro magnetic device which activates a pump sac (Novacor LVAS). In both cases, the energy source and the controller are portable. In both cases, the system is vented. The basic principle of left ventricular support is to allow a complete left ventricular unloading. The right ventricular function may recover because of the drop in the right ventricular after load. The minimal level of transpulmonary vascular resistance, associated to the recovery of a minimal right ventricular function permit a satisfactory filling of the artificial left ventricle and consequently return to a normal hemodynamical situation. The main advantage of the system is the portability of the subsystems, permitting easy free movement of the patient, long periods of life out of hospital. The system, originally, designed as an alternative to transplantation in the management of patients in profound cardiac failure has been used extensively since

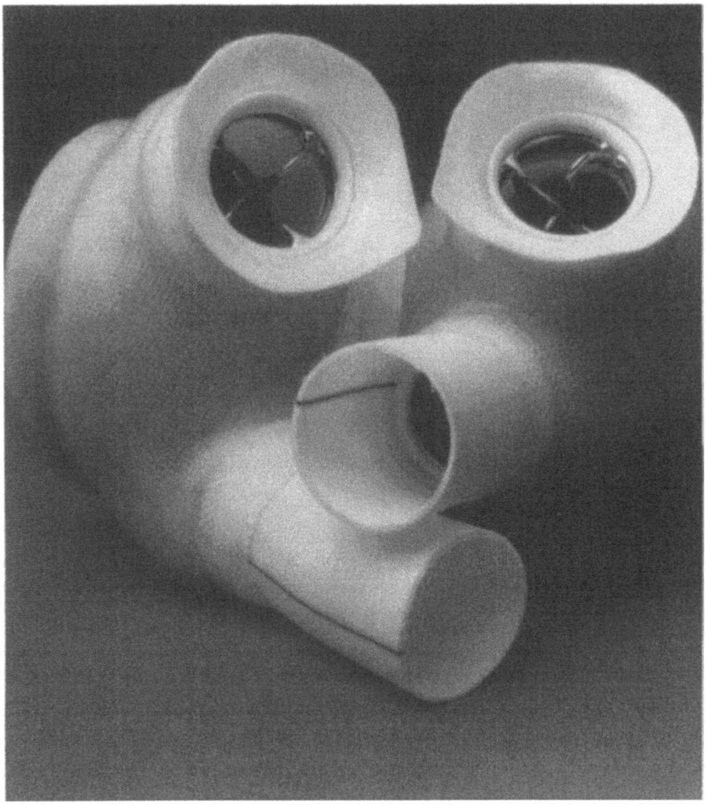

Fig. 3. Orthotopic artificial ventricle, pneumatically driven.

march 1993 both in Europe and in the USA for increasing period of time. In the indication of a bridge to a first transplantation, more than 1000 patients have received such devices, with a full rehabilitation and a possibility of elective transplantation in about 60%. Few patients have received a Novacor LVAS as a definitive treatment of cardiac failure: 18 cases in 11 different centers. None of them has lived more than 2 years. A prospective evaluation has been initiated in the US, in the group of patients with profound cardiac failure, unlikely to be transplanted, receiving an electrically driven vented Thermedic pump. Results are still awaited.

Mechanical bridge to retransplantation

None of the transplant center has an significant experience of MCS support in the patients eligible for a retransplantation. There are only 2 anectodical reports available. One [5] is a case of bridge to a retransplantation, for cardiac failure

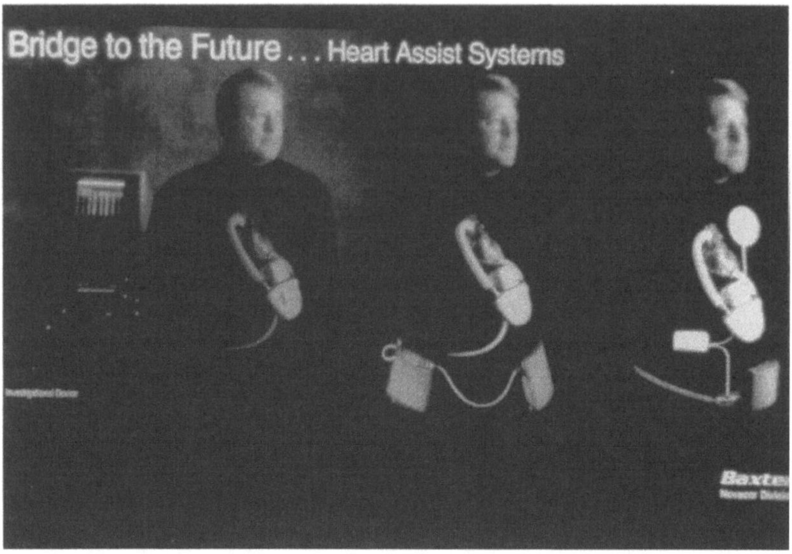

Fig. 4. The implantable left ventricular assist system: from left to right, the console based system, the portable configuration the fully implantable system.

due to an uncontrolled episode of cardiac rejection, treated by a Jarvik implantation. The second [6] reports on a case of cardiac failure, 7 years following a successful primary transplantation listed for retransplantation. A sudden deterioration three week later led to the implantation of a Novacor LVAS for circulatory support and control of the organ dysfunction until a suitable donor could be found. The patient was supported for 95 days. Problems encountered during this period were related to right ventricular dysfunction, successfully treated by temporary mechanical support and pharmacology, to 2 episodes of cardiac rejection, associated with left ventricular arrhythmia. Retransplantation was successful and the patient resumed a normal life.

More cases of temporary mechanical support as a bridge to retransplantation have been analyzed in a study on retransplantation [3] 67% of the patients actually retransplanted were hemodynamically unstable at time of retransplantation, requiring care in intensive care unit, inotropic support. 43% required some type of mechanical circulatory support: intra-aortic balloon pump, total artificial heart, ventricular assist device. In this study, analysis of the risk factors of retransplantation clearly demonstrated that pre-retransplantation mechanical support is the highest risk factor.

The comparison of efficacy of mechanical support as a bridge to transplantation to the experience of mechanical bridge to retransplantation shows the specific problems of mechanical support on a transplanted patients. In case of early graft failure, mechanical support has to be initiated in a patient with a profound circulatory failure, with multiple organ dysfunction. Risk factors in such a life saving setting are maximal. In addition, immunosuppression leads to an increased risk of infectious complications. This situation leads to propose either a very early implantation of a system which will allow a progressive but full rehabilitation, or the selection of a minimal invasive technic and a rapid retransplantation.

In case of late primary graft failure, mechanical bridge to retransplantation should be initiated as early as possible, before multiple organ deterioration, following discontinuation of immunosuppressive therapy, using a system permitting full rehabilitation and autonomy.

Mechanical circulatory support, an alternative to retransplantation?

The real possibility of mechanical circulatory support as a definitive therapy in patients with a failed primary transplantation can be evaluated. Considering the actual performance of each system described previously, the present experience in patients bridged to transplantation and in those bridged to a retransplantation, the unique characteristics of a patient with a failed primary graft, i.e. prolonged immunosuppression, it may be said that the potential of mechanical support as a definitive therapy is not very clear in the patients with a failed transplantation.

Nevertheless, a more optimistic approach might be proposed. Early implantation of a portable implanted left ventricular support system might be a first approach. Problems to be controlled are related to infection, right ventricular function and as in every patient, thrombo embolism. The first and unique reported case [6] suggests that prolongation of the bridge for a much longer period of time might have been possible. The two problems encountered during the 'chronic' phase of this 95 day bridge have been the high level of serum creatinine, related to serum cyclosporin level, and the limited exercise tolerance, in spite of a well functioning device.

A second strategy could be proposed in patients with profound cardiac failure and an adequate indication of cardiac transplantation: the primary implantation, on an elective basis, of an implantable device, followed by a prolonged period, as prolonged as possible of circulatory assist. This strategy based on the primary use of assist devices should allow postponement as much as possible of exposure of the patient to the risk of transplantation and immunosuppression. This strategy, made ethically acceptable by the present and prolonged situation of organ shortage, would in addition allow an evaluation of the role of mechanical support, prolonged or chronic, in promoting left ventricular recovery. This strategy made possible by the recent experience of the Berlin group, would contribute to offer to end stage cardiac failure patients a more flexible long term therapy.

References

1. Hosenpud JD, Novick RJ, Bennett LE, Keck BM, Fiol B, Daily OP. The Registry of the International Society for Heart and Lung Transplantation: Thirteenth Official Report – 1996. J. Heart Lung Transplant. 1996; 15: 655–674.

2. Ensley RD, Hunt S, Taylor DO, Renlund DG, Menlove RL, Karwande SV, O'Connell JB, Barr ML, Michler RE, Copeland JG, Miller LW. The Registry of the International Society for Heart and Lung Transplantation, and contributing investigators. Predictors of survival after repeat heart transplantation. J. Heart Lung Transplant. 1992; 11: S142–S158.
3. Aziz S, McDonalds O, Gohar H. Transplant arterial vasculopathy: evidence for a dual pattern of endothelial injury and the source of smooth muscle cells in lesions of intimal hyperplasia. J. Heart Lung Transplant. 1995; 14: S123–S136.
4. Loisance D. Mechanical circulation support in the 90s. Eur. J. Cardiothoracic Surg. 1992 (Suppl. 1): 2107–2112.
5. Loisance D, Deleuze Ph., Kawasaki K, Hillion ML, Binhas M, Heurtematte Y, Tavolaro O, Léandri J, Cachera JP. Total artificial heart bridge to retransplantation. Journal of Heart Transplantation 1987; 6: 281–285.
6. Jacquet L, Dion R, Noirhomme Ph., VanDijck M, Goenen M. Successful bridge to retransplantation with the wearable Novacor left ventricular assist system. J. Heart Lung Transplant. 1996; 15: 620–622.

23. Pancreas retransplantation or islet transplantation?

A. SECCHI

Islet transplantation can be considered an alternative to pancreas transplantation in two cases: simultaneous islet–kidney transplantation in uremic diabetic patients previously submitted to kidney–pancreas transplantation, who eventually lost the function of the two grafts, and diabetic patients who received kidney transplantation alone.

Simultaneous islet and kidney transplantation

End stage renal failure is a growing problem. Diabetic patients starting renal replacement therapy (dialysis or transplantation) increased from 3.8% (1977) to 17% (1992), as reported by the EDTA Registry. These data were confirmed at a regional level (Lombardy: 7.7% in 1983, 12% in 1992), thus confirming the widespread diffusion of the problem. Furthermore it was shown by the Lombardy Registry that 5 years survival of patients under dialysis are worst in diabetic patients (28%) than in non-diabetic patients (61%). On the contrary diabetic patients receiving kidney transplantation show a higher 5 year actuarial survival rate (75%) than similar patients not submitted to transplantation, but treated with dialysis, being survival rate even higher in case of pancreas/kidney transplantation. From these data it is clear that kidney transplantation must be considered a life-saving procedure in uremic diabetic patients. Metabolic control in diabetic kidney-transplantation patients is difficult, as shown by HbA1c, probably as a consequence of the metabolic effects of immunosuppressive drugs (steroids, Cyclosporin, FK506). In this particular subset of patients pancreas transplantation can be performed simultaneously to kidney transplantation in order to control blood glucose homeostasis, to prevent the deveopment of diabetic nephropathy on the transplated kidney and to improve life quality. This surgical procedure has a 80% success rate at 1 year. Simultaneous kidney/islet transplantation could be an alternative to simultaneous kidney/pancreas transplantation, having the advantage of requiring minor surgery. Furthermore, diabetic patients affected by severe macroangiopathy could be indicated for kidney transplantation, but controindicated for pancreas transplantation for the surgical and perioperative risks related to their clinical conditions. In this case islet transplantation could benefit of the immunological advantages related to the simultaneous kidney transplant, as already described

J.L. Touraine et al. (eds.), Retransplantation, 193–194.

for simultaneous pancreas/kidney transplantations (early detection of rejection, uremia-related immunosuppression). The main advantage of this approach is related to the fact that islet has to be transplanted regardless of the quality of preparation, like is in the case of IAK (see later). In fact these patients cannot wait for the next kidney/islet donor in the case of poor islet preparation due to the long waiting list for kidney transplantation and to the poor survival of diabetic patients in dialysis.

Islet transplantation after kidney transplantation alone (IAK) and after pancreas transplant failure (P failure)

Pancreas transplantation has a 30% probability of failure in case of simultaneous pancreas/kidney transplantation, this probability being higher (50%) in case of pancreas after kidney transplantation, mainly for technical (surgical) or immunological (rejection, recurrence of disease) reasons. It was already shown by the International Pancreas Transplant Registry that pancreas retransplantation has a high rate of failure (50%). As a consequence these patients should not undergo pancreas retransplantation for the low probability of function and the high rate of surgical risks (50% of reoperations). This particular subset of patients could benefit of islet transplantation, like in the case of diabetic patients submitted to kidney transplantation alone. These two groups of patients share the advantage of minor surgical risks, of already established immunosuppression (for the kidney), of an easy post-surgical management (when compared to SIK), of the possibility to select the best islet preparation. The main advantage of these two approaches (P failure and IAK) are the requirement of a second course of ALG (when patients received ALG for the first transplant) and the risk of inducing kidney rejection as a consequence of an immune 'activation' by the antigens presented by the islets, which are different from those of the transplanted kidney.

24. Molecular targets for genetic engineering in pig-to-human vascularized xenotransplantation

BERNARD VANHOVE & JEAN-PAUL SOULILLOU

Introduction

Over the past few years, our understanding of the mechanisms involved in the rejection of discordant xenografts has greatly increased. Several molecules potentially involved in the rejection process have been identified, and the way in which they mediate their pathologic effect largely elucidated. At the same time, improvements in the technology of transgenesis in the pig have made it possible to produce donor animals expressing some of these molecules, particularly on endothelial cells, so that their actual role in the process of pig-to-primate xenograft rejection can be evaluated. One factor limiting genetic manipulation in pigs, however, is that the embryonic stem cells necessary for homologous recombination are currently unavailable, which makes it impossible to knock out a gene in that species. Emerging techniques such as intrabody-mediated phenotypic knockout, overexpression of dominant negative mutants, anti-sense RNA or ribozymes may represent alternatives and result in the production of donor animals with reduced expression of factors that initiate rejection. It is our assumption that combined expression of several protective transgenes associated with reduced expression of some of the endogenous proteins that promote rejection will make it possible to maintain a pig organ in the human body.

This review focuses on those molecules whose involvement in vascular or cellular rejection of pig organs makes them the most relevant for transplantation into humans, identifying them as targets for genetic engineering to modify their expression. In the pig-to-primate combination, the rejection process has been divided into three major stages. First, hyperacute rejection (HAR) is initiated by the recipient's preexisting xenoreactive natural antibodies (XNAs) and complement (C) [1]. It is characterized by interstitial hemorrhage and diffuse thrombosis, and classically leads to graft failure within minutes to hours (although kidneys from piglets can last for several days in Macacus fascicularis – D. White, personal communication). Second, if appropriate treatment leading to C inactivation or XNA depletion, or both, is applied, xenografts may still be rejected after a few days by a process referred to as delayed xenograft rejection (DXR) [2]. This process shares many pathological characteristics

J.L. Touraine et al. (eds.), Retransplantation, 195–208.

with HAR but is believed to be initiated, at least in part, by the induction of anti-pig IgG which activates endothelial cells (ECs) and results in the recruitment of inflammatory cells such as macrophages, PMN and NK cells, as well as procucing several mediators with deleterious effects. Third, and still hypothetical as far as its nature and actual magnitude are concerned, accumulated evidence from *in vitro* experiments suggests that xenografts will elicit a strong direct and indirect T cell mediated response [3]. The extent to which T lymphocytes play a role in the rejection of vascularized xenografts *in vivo*, however, has not been clearly documented.

Identification for genetic manipulation of target factors involved in hyperacute rejection (HAR)

Two primary factors have been shown to be directly responsible for the susceptibility of porcine organs to HAR when transplanted into primates: (1) The binding of recipient XNAs to antigens present on graft ECs, and consisting mainly of the Galα1,3Gal epitopes found on many membrane glycolipids [4] and glycoproteins [5, 6]. Transfer of these carbohydrate moieties takes place in the Golgi compartment in pigs (as well as in lower mammals and New World monkeys) via the enzyme α1,3Galactosyltransferase (α-3-GalT-1), which transfers galactose onto unfucosylated N-acetyllactosamine residues. These residues are not fucosylated because α-2-fucosyltransferase (α-2-FucT) is not expressed in pig endothelium. Galα1,3Gal epitopes will therefore have a dramatic effect on vascularized xenografts, but may have no relevance for pancreatic islet grafts, being expressed on ECs and not on endocrine cells [7]. In man, α-2-FucT is expressed in endothelium and α-3-GalT-1 is not expressed at all. The N-acetyllactosamine structures in man are consequently fucosylated to form the H determinant. (2) The incompatibility of C regulatory proteins (CRPs) on graft ECs with the recipient's C system gives free rein to the uncontrolled activation of C on EC surfaces. Porcine molecules such as DAF (CD55), which inhibits the activation of C3; MCP (CD46), which assists factor I in the cleavage of C3b; CD59, which inhibits C9 polymerization and MAC formation; and CR1 (CD35), which cleaves C3/C5 convertase and assists factor I, have no blocking effect on the corresponding human C factors. Consequently, the binding of anti-Gal XNAs activates the C cascade on ECs.

C activation *per se*, however, does not lead to immediate destruction of the endothelium. While EC lysis would be expected to take place rapidly during HAR [8], it is generally observed late in the rejection process. Platt and colleagues actually reported that porcine ECs challenged with human serum containing active C are not lysed [9] but undergo a reaction called type I activation: within minutes of exposure to XNA and C, most of the heparan sulfate is lost from EC surfaces as a consequence of local C5a production [10]. Heparan sulfate is a surface protein polysaccharide conjugate that functions as a barrier to cell and plasma proteins and anchors molecules that confer anti-coagulant activity (antithrombin III) and protects against oxidation injury (superoxide dismutase). Further down the C cascade, the formation of C5b67 complexes on ECs results in an alteration of cell shape that leads to the formation of intercellular gaps [9], allowing egress of vascular contents and adhesion/activation of platelets through contact with platelet receptor gpIb, collagen and vWf contained in the subendothelial matrix. In humans, shearing stresses are a necessary condition for effective activation of platelets after the interaction of vWF with platelet gpIb. In the pig-to-human combination, porcine vWf interacts strongly with human gpIb and leads to the aggregation of platelets even under static conditions. Platelet activation is accompanied by the release of inflammatory mediators, including complement, platelet-activating factor (PAF), thrombin and leukotrienes, which results in the further recruitment of platelets and in coagulation. The autocatalytic, direct activation of human prothrombin by porcine endothelium has also been observed, leading to the production of thrombin [11]. These situations are likely to contribute to the prothrombotic activity of activated xenogenic endothelium. Type I EC activation also consists in the expression of P-selectin, which mediates the adhesion of neutrophils and monocytes; these, in turn, secrete inflammatory cytokines. Thrombomodulin and membrane ATP/ADPase [12] are also shed from the EC surface, a phenomenon which contributes to thrombus formation by platelets. Under normal circumstances thrombomodulin and thrombin together catalyse the conversion of protein C to activated protein C, a potent anti-coagulant and anti-inflammatory agent.

Several of the molecules described above have been considered for genetic manipulation. First of all, attempts *in vitro* and *in vivo* to express in mice and pigs human CRPs such as CD55 (DAF) [13], CD46, CD59 and CD35 have now been successful. Depending on the level of expression, organs from pigs expressing any of these human CRPs clearly become more resistant to HAR in primates. None of these molecules, however, prevent the first steps in the initiation of C activation, XNA-mediated C1q deposition. This may be of importance because, as pointed out by Bach and colleagues [14], C1q potentially recruits and activates platelets via the platelet GPIIb-IIIa integrin receptor, resulting in the induction of P-selectin and procoagulant activity [15]. Platelets in this state may promote platelet-leukocyte interactions, resulting in the activation of monocytes, the production of superoxide and EC activation with ongoing thrombosis. For this reason, and because XNA may promote EC activation even in the absence of C [16], attempts to reduce or eliminate xenoantigens on pig ECs are likely to be as important as the expression of human CRPs. In 1995, Sandrin and colleagues [17] demonstrated that human α-1,2-FucT expressed in pig cells competes for the same acceptor (N-acetyllactosamine) as α-3-GalT-1 and replaces the Galα1,3Gal xenoantigenic determinant with the non-antigenic universal donor human blood O antigen. Transgenic pigs expressing human α-1,2-FucT have been produced [18] and found to express a greatly reduced level of Galα1,3 Gal epitopes. Alternative techniques with the aim of reducing Gal epitopes are currently under evaluation, for example EC expression of α1,3 Galactosydase or intracellular expression of anti-α1,3Galactosyltransferase ScFv antibodies that reduce enzyme activity in the Golgi compartment (B. Vanhove et al., submitted).

Other molecules could perhaps be pasted into the pig genome, such as anticoagulants (TM, PC, ATIII, TFPI), ADPase, the antioxidant SOD, or PAF acetylhydrolase, which down-modulates the biosynthesis of active PAF [19]. While no conclusive experiments *in vivo* have yet demonstrated the power of these molecules to prevent HAR and EC activation, it is nevertheless reasonable to assume that constitutively expressed anti-coagulant molecules would help to prevent intragraft thrombosis. Pertinent to this idea are recent (at present unpublished) experiments by our group and that of P. Wolf showing that hearts from vWF-deficient pigs, while still hyperacutely rejected in primates, are less infiltrated by host leukocytes. However, the potential advantage of the effect of the vWF-/- phenotype in conditions controlling HAR will require reassessment. Genetic manipulation designed to inactivate the C5a receptor is also likely to confer an advantage, as C5a has been implicated in the shedding of membrane-anchored anticoagulant molecules. The administration of anti-C5a MoAb blocks C-mediated damage and HAR in *ex vivo* pig-to-human heart xenotransplantation [20, 21].

Identification for genetic manipulation of target factors involved in delayed xenograft rejection (DXR)

In pig-to-primate xenotransplantation, when C activation is prevented – for instance by the administration of cobra venom factor or soluble CR1 receptor, or by the expression of CRPs on ECs, or by XNA neutralization – a process of xenograft rejection called DXR may still be observed after a few days or weeks, either before a T-cell based response can be elicited [2] or in addition to such a response. DXR may well be initiated by the same factors that elicit HAR, not totally eliminated but reduced to a level that allows some prolongation of graft survival. Low C levels may trigger the synthesis of IL-1α, a cytokine acting as a paracrine or autocrine factor that stimulates the expression of tissue factor and other coagulation factors [22]. Alternatively, DXR could be elicited by NK cells, which are more numerous in xeno- than in allografts, or by IgM-XNA even in the absence of C, as these factors have been shown to signal directly to and stimulate ECs and the synthesis of genes such as IL-8, PAI-1 and ELAM-1 *in vitro* [16, 23]. In addition, elicited anti-donor high affinity IgG might promote ADCC. While in humans tissue factor pathway inhibitor (TFPI) controls the coagulation cascade by inhibiting factors X and the TF-FVIIa complex, Kopp and colleagues have reported that porcine TFPI does not exert a comparable anti-factor X effect against human C [24]. Consequently, pig endothelium probably does not exert the same anti-coagulant effect on human blood as on autologous blood, and activated platelets in that system may initiate the inflammatory reaction.

DXR is associated with type II EC activation, which means that ECs express de novo genes that will modify the homeostatic properties of the endothelium. Together with activated host monocytes and natural killer cells infiltrating the organ, activated ECs promote inflammation and thrombosis. A very large number of genes (probably more than 50) are expressed or up-regulated in ECs upon activation by agonists such as lipopolysaccharides, inflammatory cytokines (IL-1, TNFα) or oxidation injury. These genes code for molecules involved in functions as diverse as coagulation and C cascades (t-PA inhibitor [25], PAI-1 [26], tissue factor [27], C factors B, H, and I [28]), vasoconstriction (endothelin [29], NO-synthase [30]), chemoattraction (IL-8 [31], RANTES [32], MCP [33]), leukocyte/EC interaction (adhesion molecules like GpIb [34], ELAM-1 [35]), inflammation (IL-1β, IL-6 [36], prostacyclins [37]) and stress (ferritin and heme oxygenase [38],), immunocompetence (MHC I and II [39], B7 [40], CD45RO [41]), growth factors (FGF, PDGF, GM/G-CSF [42]), transcriptional regulation and signal transduction (c-fos and c-myc [43], IκBα[32], Gem [44]), apoptosis regulators (A20 [45]). This list is certainly far from complete. Several other genes to which no function has yet been attributed are also upregulated in activated ECs.

Only the accumulation of *in vivo* experiments, by establishing a hierarchy in the relative importance of these factors, will reveal where potential intervention is necessary. The genes expressed in ECs upon activation can be classified into categories according to the predicted effect mediated by the product they code for. First, there are molecules that clearly favor the outcome of an inflammatory reaction and that obviously contribute to graft rejection. Among these are the adhesion molecules, the cytokines or chemoattractants, the procoagulant factors and vasoconstrictors. Second, ECs up-regulate genes that control and reduce the effect of mechanisms favouring rejection. One instance is the synthesis of C factors H and I [28]: factor H binds to C3b on the membrane allowing factor I to cleave the C3b a chain. C3b then becomes susceptible to degradation by a plasmatic enzyme analogous to trypsin, leaving a small, inactive C3d bound to ECs. The influence of endothelial upregulation of these factors on the control of C activation, however, remains to be demonstrated, as well as its relevance in the xenotransplantation situation. Upon activation ECs also up-regulate IκBα, the inhibitor of the transcription factor NFκB [32]. In resting ECs, NF-κB is retained in the cytoplasm by association with IκBα. After stimulation, IκB$\alpha$is phosphorylated, ubiquitinylated and degraded, and NF-κB can migrate into the nucleus where it binds to the promoter region of the genes controlled by NF-κB. In ECs, most of the inducible genes contain at least one binding site for NF-κB and the expression of several of them is known to be directly NF-κB dependant (for example tissue factor, ELAM-1, IL-8, IL-6 [46] IL1β [47], IκBα[48], P-selectin [49]). As a consequence, ECs expressing IκBα cannot be activated [50]. Recently,

Bach and colleagues have also demonstrated that ECs in hamster hearts, which under certain circumstances are not rejected in rats but rather 'accommodate", expressed A20, Bcl-2 and Bcl-XL, proteins that protect from apoptosis and prevent upregulation of proinflammatory genes such as cytokines, procoagulant and adhesion molecules, probably acting through NF-κB inhibition [51]. It seems that a balance between the expression of genes related to inflammation and thrombosis on the one hand, and genes that control their expression and protect the endothelium strongly on the other, determines whether DXR will occur or not. An EC reaction leading to better resistance to injury has also been reported by Dorling and collegues [52]: immortalized pig ECs challenged for several days with human IgG containing XNA undergo a change in their phenotype. They become more resistant to C mediated lysis and show reduced expression of VCAM and MHC I. Another example pertains to the capacity of ECs to actively build up protection mechanisms. Heme, a hydrophobic iron chelate, aggravates the cytotoxicity engendered by hydrogen peroxide. If ECs are briefly pulsed with heme and then incubated for a prolonged period, they become highly resistant to any further oxidant-mediated injury [38]. This protection has been attributed to the accumulation of ferritin and heme oxygenase, which affords protection from oxidant damage [53].

Genetic manipulations designed to afford protection against HAR work by preventing the release of inflammatory mediators and thrombosis. They are therefore likely to afford some protection against DXR as well. Because elicited IgG is considered in some xenograft models to be an initiating event in DXR, research aimed at defining the xenoantigens eliciting that IgG response will continue to be important. EC activation is regarded as another central event in DXR, as it initiates an amplification loop involving inflammatory and prothrombotic mediators, and also because activated endothelium is the effector 'organ' which mediates the intravascular coagulation process leading to rejection. Consequently, strategies by which the activation of ECs can be prevented have been considered important as topics for research. NF-κB, because it controls the transcription of many inducible genes in ECs, constitutes an ideal target for genetic engineering. Ectopic overexpression of the natural inhibitor IκBα actually blocks NF-κB very effectively *in vitro* [50]. Using a mutated form of IκBα improves the system. In this dominant negative protein, two phosphorylation sites (Ser32/36) have been mutated so that cytoplasmic degradation of IκBα and its release from NF-κB cannot occur and NF-κB is permanantly inactivated [54]. Another strategy consists in the expression of a dominant negative p65 mutant (one of the components of NF-κB) containing the Rel homology domain of the protein which binds to NF-κB sites on DNA but lacks an active transactivation domain [46].

Unlike many other transgenes considered hitherto, those designed to inactivate NF-κB cannot be expressed constitutively in a whole organism: Beg and colleagues [55] have demonstrated that NF-κB (p65/RelA) knockout in mice is lethal. This is essentially due to enhancement of apoptosis in the liver during embryogenesis, leading to hemorrhage on day 16 of gestation. Hematopoietic precursors in these mice, however, were unaffected. The transgenic expression of NF-κB inhibitors in pigs would therefore seem difficult to achieve, unless expression of the transgene could be restricted to the endothelium using EC-specific promoters. Possible promoters would be, for example, those driving the expression of endothelin-1 [56], ICAM-2 [57], vWF [58], tek or tie (receptors tyrosine kinase in EC [59, 60]), flk-1 or flt-1 (VEGF receptors [61, 62]). In addition, improvements in molecular biology have made it possible to express transgenes in a strictly regulated way [63, 64]. In 1996, several authors showed that inactivation of NF-κB (by Rel A/p65 knockout in this case) increases susceptibility to TNFα-induced apoptosis, and that up-regulation of NF-κB gives protection from such injury [65–67]. This observation is surprising because Grimm and colleagues [68] demonstrated that pro-apoptotic genes need NF-κB activation for their expression. It would appear that, at least in some cell types, TNF-α (but not LPS) transmits one signal that elicits cell death and another, dependent on NF-κB, that protects against death by inducing the expression of genes such as A20, Bcl-2 or Bcl-XL. One major concern about NF-κB inactivation is that loss of NF-κB function may be deleterious in xenotransplantation where release of TNF-α has been shown to be associated with DXR [51]. It is possible, however, that partial inhibition of NF-κB would keep ECs quiescent enough to confer protection against DXR, while still allowing cells to escape apoptosis. Alternatively, to avoid cell death it may be necessary to achieve transgenic expression of anti-apoptotic genes in addition to the inhibition of NF-κB. The simultaneous expression of several anti-apoptotic genes could well be necessary, as co-transfection of A20 alone is not sufficient to rescue RelA -/- 3T3 cells from TNF-α induced death. Also very relevant in this regard is the work of C. Ferran, who has shown that the expression of a truncated form of the human p55 TNF-receptor in ECs renders them resistant to human TNFα [69]. The combined expression of NF-κB and such TNF-receptor inhibitors (or other molecules interfering with cell death) may well be one way to inhibit the activation of ECs without increasing their susceptibility to ongoing cell death.

Transgenic pigs expressing CRPs and competitors of α1,3–galactosylation have already been produced and have demonstrated that HAR in primates can be prevented. Anti-coagulant molecules expressed on EC membranes as well as inhibitors of EC activation (together with anti-apoptotic genes) will probably be tried in the near future, giving us an idea of the extent to which it might be possible to achieve further protection against DXR.

Identification for genetic manipulation of target factors involved in cellular rejection

Cell-mediated rejection of vascularized grafts is not as well documented for xenotransplants as it is in allotransplantation. Most of the data are derived from small animal models (guinea pigs or hamsters to rats for instance [51]), whereas almost nothing is known about the cellular response in more relevant pig-to-primate models. Indeed, such is the severity of HAR or of the acute vascular rejection that the expected T cell mediated rejection simply has no opportunity to take place, making it impossible for the cellular response to be studied. In addition, manoeuvres aimed at inhibiting HAR (see above) have always been associated with extremely powerful immunosuppressant treatment, usually with a combination of the three major drugs (steroids/CSA/cyclophosphamide [70]) which further distorts the T cell response. In the hamster-to-rat combination, the use of injected CVF with CSA results in long term survival in the majority of recipients [51]. Macrophages (as in allotransplantation) are the predominant infiltrating cells within the first two weeks [71]. NK cells accumulate later, following the same kinetics as T cells with a peak at about day 15. This NK/macrophage infiltrate occurs to the same extent in nude recipients and is therefore not T cell controlled [72]. It has been claimed that, in a xenograft combination, long term acceptance could depend upon a TH2 dominant T cell response which could promote a non complement fixing isotype of rat Ig (such as IgG2c). The latter could then compete with the more deleterious species usually present in a TH1 context. However, we have recently obtained similar percentages of long survival (S. Brouard et al., submitted) in LEW.1A recipients even though they are unable to mount an IL-4 response when placed in the same protocol, whereas a strong accumulation in the graft of IL-10 and TGFβ mRNA was observed. The possibility that manipulation of the cytokine network will allow the recipient immune response to be redirected is not yet sustained by strong enough evidence. Even in allotransplantation, tissues derived from IL-10 or IL-4 transgeneic recipients were not less vigorously rejected [73]. However, the xenotransplantation context will offer further possibilities of altering the cytokine environment in which presentation of xenoantigens takes place by transgenesis or transduction with an appropriate vector. In vitro experiments have clearly demonstrated that direct xenorecognition of pig MHC molecules does exist in the pig/human or the pig/primate MLR (see for review [3]). Similarly, mature pig dendritic cells elicit a strong response from purified human T cells [3]. Therefore, although a weaker CD4/pig class II interaction could occur, cross reactivity of human TCR for pig MHC molecules is actually taking place [74]. Moreover, second signals also seem to operate normally, such as those for B7/CD28, LF1/ICAM(s) or CD2/LFA3 [3]. However, some decreases in affinity are to be expected, as well as impairment in various species-specific cytokine regulations, such as human IFNγ for pig class I or class II regulation. As in humans, most direct recognition seems to be CD4 mediated, as demonstrated by the inhibiting effect of anti pig class II antibody in cell culture [74]. However pig endothelial cells (which are class II positive) can mount a proliferation of CD8 cells [3]. Therefore, the direct recognition of xenotissues might be expected to mimic what happens in allotransplantation, although less efficiently owing to an altered affinity in receptor/ligand interactions.

One important difference compared to allo interactions lies in the potential role of NK cells. Indeed, human NK cells can be activated and can kill pig endothelial cells in culture in the absence of XNA [75]. This effect could be related to the lack of any negative signal delivered to human NK through KIR by pig class I. However, to what extent, if any, NK cells have a role in xenotransplantation remains unknown. Interestingly, nude animals do not reject xenografts.

The principal difference in the response of human T cells to pig xenografts as compared to allografts may lie in the magnitude of indirect recognition of pig peptides presented in the human APC context. Such presentation, which is thought to be minimal in the early phase of allotransplantation in humans, may have much more relevance in the xeno situation [74]. A considerable degree of indirect presentation would theoretically be expected, owing to the constant presence of XNA – which could direct large numbers of soluble complexes to human APC – and to the great diversity of eligible peptides to be presented after processing and addressing to human class I or II molecules. However, so far there has only been some preliminary documentation of the indirect presentation of pig antigens [3, 74–77]. Interestingly, as would be expected, the responding T cells here are also mostly CD4, and anti-human class II antibodies are potent inhibitors of this pathway. The nature of the xenopeptides presented and how they differ from their counterparts in the allo situation are fundamental questions that will influence our theoretical capacity to intervene on the donor. The importance of peptides processed from MHC molecules in the allogeneic context can be related to the presence of alloantibodies. Despite the possibility that XNA anti HLA antibodies (and the elicited Ig response) could cross react with SLA molecules, it is likely that it is the presence of XNA that modifies the pattern of peptides presented. In addition, while the sequence homologies between human and pig proteins remain to be properly assessed, major variations may be expected, particularly in the extracellular field of membrane glycoproteins [78], rendering possible an extremely aggressive T cell response with a high frequency of anti-xeno epitope clones.

Pig class II antigens, therefore, seem to be the major molecules in the response to xenografts as their role in both direct and indirect presentations appears to be central. Since vascularized grafts from MHC class II KO are not rejected [79], controlling the class II genes in the donor might be a major goal in the xeno context too. Class I gene invalidation may increase the aggressivity of NK cytotoxicity but human class I transgeneic pigs may show an increased direct (and possibly indirect) recognition. Further data are therefore needed for the results of such possible engineering to be worked out. In addition, pig endothelial cell B7 may be just as important [40]. These cells are also class II positive cells *in vivo*, even in their resting configuration [80].

However, several bioreagents can effectively interfere with B7 (or other co-stimulatory molecules such as LFA3 or ICAMs, see review [81]).

Clearly, there will be constraints towards the genetic manipulations that one might like to apply to the pig. The breeding of pigs with a transgenic expression of, or deficiency for, molecules which may lead to an immune deficiency (class II removal for example) may also be difficult to perform, mainly because of the costs of maintaining pigs in germ-free conditions. For this reason, the use of expression systems which restrict transgene expression to defined tissues and which do so in a strictly controlled and inducible way will be a clear step forward for research in xenotransplantation.

References

1. Parker W, Saadi S, Lin SS, Holzknecht ZE, Bustos M, Platt JL. Transplantation of discordant xenografts: a challenge revisited. Immunol. Today 1996; 17(8): 373–378.
2. Bach FH, Winkler H, Ferran C, Hancock WW, Robson SC. Delayed xenograft rejection. Immunol. Today 1996; 17(8): 379–384.
3. Dorling A, Riesbeck K, Lechler RI. The T-cell response to xenografts: molecular interactions and graft-specific immunosuppression. Xeno. 1996; 4(4): 68–76.
4. Bouhours D, Pourcel C, Bouhours JF. Simultaneous expression by porcine aorta endothelial cells of glycolipids bearing the major epitope for human xenoreactive antibodies (Galalpha1–3Gal), blood group H determinant and N-glycolylneuraminic acid. Glycoconjugate J. 1996; 13: 947–953.
5. Parker W, Bruno D, Holzknecht ZE, Platt JL. Characterization and affinity isolation of xenoreactive human natural antibodies. J. Immunol. 1994; 153: 3791–3803.
6. Thibaudeau K, Borche L, Soulillou JP, Blanchard D. Characterization of porcine platelet glycoproteins recognized by human natural 'anti-gal' antibodies. Blood 1996; 87(11): 4636–4642.
7. Mirenda V, LeMauff B, Cassard A, Huvelin JM, Boeffard F, Faivre A, Soulillou JP, Anegon I. Intact pig pancreatic islet function in the presence of human xenonatural antibody binding and comlement activation. Transplantation 1997; in press.
8. Azimzadeh A, Wolf P, Dalmasso A, Odeh M, Beller JP, Fabre M, Charreau B, Thibeaudeau K, Cinqalbre J, Soulillou JP, Anegon I. Assessment of hyperacute rejection in a rat-to-primate cardiac xenograft model. Transplantation 1996; 61: 1305–1313.
9. Saadi S, Platt JL. Transient perturbation of endothelial integrity induced by natural antibodies and complement. J. Exp. Med. 1995; 181: 21–31.
10. Platt JL, Vercellotti GM, Lindman BJ, Oegema TR, Bach FH, Dalmasso AP. Release of heparan sulfate from endothelial cells. Implications for pathogenesis of hyperacute rejection. J. Exp. Med. 1990; 171: 1363–1368.
11. Jurd KM, Gibbs RV, Hunt BJ. Activation of human prothrombin by porcine aortic endothelial cells: a potential barrier to pig to human xenotransplantation. Blood Coagul. Fibrinolysis 1996; 7(3): 336–343.
12. Robson SC, Kaczmarek E, Siegel JB, Candidas D, Koziak K, Millan M, Hancock WW, Bach FH. Loss of ATP diphosphohydrolase activity with endothelial cell activation. J. Exp. Med. 1997; 185(1): 153–163.
13. Dalmasso AP, Vercellotti GM, Platt JL, Bach FH. Inhibition of complement-mediated endothelial cell cytotoxicity by decay-accelerating factor. Transplantation 1991; 52(3): 530–533.
14. Bach FH, Robson SC, Winkler H, Ferran C, Stuhlmeier KM, Wrighton CJ, Hancock WW. Barriers to xenotransplantation. Nature Medicine 1995; 1(9): 869–873.

15. Peerschke EIB, Reid KBM, Ghebrehiwet B. Platelet activation by Clq results in the induction of aIIb/B3 integrins (GPIIb-IIIa) and the expression of P-selection and procoagulant activity. J. Exp. Med. 1993; 178: 579–587.
16. Vanhove B, Martin Rd, Lipp J, Bach FH. Human xenoreactive natural antibodies of the IgM isotype activate pig endothelial cells. Xenotransplantation 1994; 1: 17–23.
17. Sandrin MS, Fodor WL, Mouhtouris E, Osman N, Cohney S, Rollins SA, Guilmette ER, Setter E, Squinto SP, McKenzie IFC. Enzymatic remodelling of the carbohydrate surface of a xenogenic cell substancially reduces human antibody binding and complement-mediated cytolysis. Nature Medicine 1995; 1(12): 1261–1266.
18. Sharma A, Okabe J, Birch P, McCellan SB, Martin MJ, Platt JL, Logan JS. Reduction in the level of Gal(alpha1,3)Gal in transgenic mice and pigs by the expression of an alpha(1,2)fucosyltransferase. Proc. Natl. Acad. Sci. USA 1996; 93: 7190–7195.
19. Hirafuji M, Mencia-Huerta JM, Benveniste J. Regulation of PAF-acether (platelet-activating factor) biosynthesis in cultured human vascular endothelial cells stimulated with thrombin. Biochim. Biophys. Acta 1987; 930: 359–369.
20. Kroshus TJ, Rollins SA, Dalmasso AP, Elliott EA, Matis LA, Squinto SP, R.M. Bolman I. Complement inhibition with an anti-C5 monoclonal antibody prevents acute cardiac tissus injury in an *ex vivo* model of pig-to-human xenotransplantation. Transplantation 1995; 60(11): 1194–1202.
21. Rollins SA, Matis LA, Springhorn JP, Setter E, Wolf DW. Monoclonal antibodies directed against human C5 and C8 block complement-mediated damage of xenogenic cells and organs. Transplantation 1995; 60(11): 1284–1292.
22. Warner SJ, Auger KR, Libby P. Interleukin 1 induces interleukin 1. II. Recombinant human interleukin 1 induces interleukin 1 production by adult human vascular endothelial cells. J. Immunol. 1987; 139(6): 1911–1917.
23. Goodman DJ, vonAlbertini M, Willson A, Millan M, Bach FH. Direct activation of porcine endothelial cells by human natural killer cells. Transplantation 1995; 61(5): 763–771.
24. Kopp CW, Siegel JB, Hancock WW, Anrather J, Winkler H, Geczy CL, Kaczmarek E, Bach FH, Robson SC. Effect of porcine endothelial tissue factor pathway inhibitor on human coagulation factors. Transplantation 1997; 63(5): 749–758.
25. Emeis JJ, Kooistra T. Interleukin 1 and lipopolysaccharide induce an inhibitor of tissue-type plasminogen activator *in vivo* and in cultured endothelial cells. J. Exp. Med. 1986; 163: 1260–1266.
26. Nachman RL, Hajjar KA, Silverstein RL, Dinarello CA. Interleukin 1 induces endothelial cell synthesis of plasminogen activator inhibitor. J. Exp. Med. 1986; 163(6): 1595–1600.
27. Conway EM, Bach R, Rosenberg RD, Koningsberg WH. Tumor necrosis factor enhances expression of tissue factor mRNA in endothelial cells. Throm. Res. 1989; 53(3): 231–241.
28. Ripoche J, Mitchell JA, Erdei A, Madin C, Moffatt B, Mokoena T, Gordon S, Sim RB. Interferon gamma induces synthesis of complement alternative pathway proteins by humlan endothelial cells in culture. J. Exp. Med. 1988; 168(5): 1917–1922.
29. Yoshizumi M, Kurihara H, Morita T, Yamashita T, Oh-hashi Y, Sugiyama T, Takaku F, Yanagisawa M, Masaki T, Yazaki Y. Interleukin 1 increases the production of endothelin-1 by cultured endothelial cells. Biochem. Biophys. Res. Commun. 1990; 166(1): 324–329.
30. Gross SS, Jaffe EA, Levi R, Kilbourn RG. Cytokine-activated endothelial cells express an isotype of nitric oxide synthase which is tetrahydrobiopterin-dependant, calmodulin-independant and inhibited by arginine analogs with a rank-order of potency characteristic of activated macrophages. Biochem. Biophys. Res. Commun. 1991; 178(3): 823–829.
31. Sica A, Matsushima K, VanDamma J, Wang JM, Polentarutti N, Dejena E, Colotta F, Mantovani A. IL-1 transcriptionally activates the neutrophil chemotactic factor/IL-8 gene in endothelial cells. Immunology 1990; 69(4): 548–553.
32. deMartin R, Vanhove B, Cheng Q, Hofer E, Czismadia V, Winkler H, Bach FH. Cytokine-inducible expression in entothelial cells of an IκBa-like gene is regulated by NFκB. EMBO J. 1993; 7: 2773–2779.

33. Rollins BJ, Yoshimura T, Leonard EJ, Pober JS. Cytokine-activated human endothelial cells synthetize and secrete a monocyte chemoattractant, MCP-1/JE. Am. J. Pathol. 1990; 136(6): 1229–1233.
34. Konkle BA, Shapiro SS, Asch AS, Nachman RL. Cytokine-enhanced expression of glycoprotein Ibalpha in human endothelium. J. Biol. Chem. 1990; 265(32): 19833–19838.
35. Bevilacqua MP, Stengelin S, Gimbrone-Jr MA, Seed B. Endothelial leukocyte adhesion molecule 1: an inducible receptor for neutrophils related to complement regulatory proteins and lectins. Science 1989; 243: 1160–1165.
36. Sironi M, Breviario F, Proserpio P, Biondi A, Vecchi A, VanDamme J, Dejana E, Mantovani A. IL-1 stimulates IL-6 production in endothelial cells. J. Immunol. 1989; 142(2): 549–553.
37. Rossi V, Breviario F, Ghezzi P, Dejana E, Mantovani A. Prostacyclin synthesis induced in vascular cells by interleukin-1. Science 1985; 229: 174–176.
38. Balla G, Jacob HS, Balla J, Rosenberg M, Nath K, Apple F, Eaton JW, Vercellotti GM. Ferritin: a cytoprotective antioxydant stratagem of Endothelium. J. Biol. Chem. 1992; 267(25): 18148–18153.
39. Otsuka A, Hanafusa T, Kono N, Tarui S. LPS augments HLA-A,B,C molecule expression but inhibits interferon-gamma-induced HLA-DR molecule expression on cultured human endothelial cells. Immunology 1991; 73: 428–432.
40. Maher SE, Karmann K, Min W, Hughes CC, Pober JS, Bothwell AL. Porcine endothelial CD86 is a major costimulator of xenogeneic human T cells: cloning, sequencing, and functional expression in human endothelial cells. J. Immunol. 1996; 157(9): 3838–3844.
41. Forsyth KD, Chua KY, Talbot V, Thomas WR. Expression of the leukocyte common antigen CD45 by endothelium. J. Immunol. 1993; 150(8): 3471–3477.
42. Seelentag WK, Mermod JJ, Montesano R, Vassali P. Additive effects of IL-1 and TNF alpha on the accumulation of the three granulocyte and macrophage colony-stimulating factor mRNAs in human endothelial cells. EMBO J. 1987; 6(8): 2261–2265.
43. Boutherin-Falson O, Reuse S, Dumont JE, Boeynaems JM. Increased levels of c-fos and c-myc mRNA in ATP-stimulated endothelial cells. Biochem. Biophys. Res. Commun. 1990; 172(1): 306–312.
44. Vanhove B, Hofer-Warbinek R, Kapetanopoulos A, Hofer E, Bach FH, deMartin R. Gem, a GTP-binding protein from mitogen-stimulated T cells, is induced in endothelial cells upon activation by inflammatory cytokines. Endothelium 1997; 5: 51–61.
45. Dixit VM, Green S, Sarma V, Holzman LB, Wolf FW, O'Rourke K, Ward PA, Prochownik EV, Marks RM. TNA alpha induction of novel gene products in human endothelial cells including a macrophage-specific chemotaxin. J. Biol. Chem. 1990; 265(5): 2973–2978.
46. Anrather J, Csizmadia V, Brostjan C, Soares MP, Bach FH, Winkler H. Inhibition of bovine endothelial cell activation *in vitro* by regulated expression of a transdominant inhibitor of NF-κB. J. Clin. Invest. 1997; 99(4): 763–772.
47. Hiscott J, Marois J, Garoufalis J, D'Addario M, Roulston A, Kwan I, Pepin N, Lacoste J, Nguyen H, Bensi G, Fenton M. Characterization of a functional NF-kappa B site in the human interleukin 1 beta promoter: evidence for a positive autoregulatory loop. Mol. Cell. Biol. 1993; 13: 6231–6240.
48. Cheng Q, Cant CA, Moll T, Hofer-Warbinek R, Wagner E, Birnstiel-ML ML, Bach-FH FH, de-Martin R. NK-kappa B subunit-specific regulation of the I kappa B alpha promoter. J. Biol. Chem. 1994; 269(18): 13551–13557.
49. Pan JL, McEver RP. Regulation of the human P-selectin promoter by Bcl-3 and specific homodimer members of the NF-κB/Rel family. J. Biol. Chem. 1995; 270: 23077–23083.
50. Wrighton CJ, Hofer-Warbinek R, Moll T, Eytner R, Bach FH, deMartin R. Inhibition of endothelial cell activation by adenovirus-mediated expression of IκBalpha, an inhibitor of NF-κB. J. Exp. Med. 1996; 183: 1013–1022.
51. Bach FH, Ferran C, Hechenleitner P, Mark W, Koyamada N, Miyatake T, Winkler H, Badrichani A, Candidas D, Hancock WW. Accommodation of vascularize xenografts: expres-

sion of 'protective genes' by donor endothelial cells in a host Th2 cytokine environment. Nature Med. 1997; 3(2): 196–204.
52. Dorling A, Stocker C, Tsao T, Haskard DO, Lechler RI. In vitro accommodation of immortalized porcine endothelial cells. Transplantation 1996; 62: 1127–1136.
53. Abraham NG, Lavrosky Y, Schwartzman ML, Stoltz RA, Levere RD, Gerritsen ME, Shibahara S, Kappas A. Transfection of the human heme oxygenase gene into rabbit coronary microvessel endothelial cells: protective effect against heme and hemoglobin toxicity. Proc. Natl. Acad. Sci. USA 1995; 92: 6798–6802.
54. Brown K, Gestberger S, Carlson L, Franzoso G, Siebenlist U. Control of IκB-a proteolysis by site-specific, signal-induced phosphorylation. Science 1995; 267: 1485–1488.
55. Beg AA, Sha WC, Bronson RT, Ghosh S, Baltimore D. Embryonic lethality and liver degeneration in mice lacking the RelA component of NK-κB. Nature 1995; 376: 167–170.
56. Paul M, Zintz M, Böcker W, Dyer M. Characterization and functional analysis of the rat endothelin promoter. Hypertension 1995; 25(4): 683–687.
57. Cowan PJ, Shinkel TA, Witort EJ, Barlow H, Pearse MJ, D'Apice AJF. Targeting gene expression to endothelial cells in transgenic mice using the human intercellular adhesion molecule 2 promoter. Transplantation 1996; 62(2): 155–160.
58. Aird WC, Jahroudi N, Weiler-Guettler H, Rayburn HB, Rosenberg RD. Human von Willebrand factor gene sequences target expression to a subpopulation of endothelial cells in transgenic mice. Proc. Natl. Acad. Sci. USA 1995; 92: 4567–4571.
59. Dumont DJ, Yamaguchu TP, Conlon RA, Rossant J, Breitman ML. Tek, a novel tyrosine kinase gene located on mouse chromosome 4, is expressed in endothelial cells and their presumptive precursors. Oncogene 1992; 7(8): 1471–1480.
60. Korhonen J, Lahtinen I, Halmekyto M, Alhonen L, Janne J, Dumont D, Alitalo K. Endothelial-specific gene expression directed by the tie gene promoter *in vivo*. Blood 1995; 86: 1828–1835.
61. Morishita K, Johnson DE, Williams LT. A novel promoter for vascular endothelial growth factor receptor (flt-1) that confers endothelial-specific gene expression. J. Biol. Chem. 1995; 270(46): 27948–27953.
62. Patterson C, Perrella MA, Hsieh CM, Yoshizumi M, Lee ME, Haber E. Cloning and functional analysis of the promoter for KDR/flk-1, a receptor for vascular endothelial growth factor. J. Biol. Chem. 1995; 270(39): 23111–23118.
63. Gossen M, Freundlieb S, Bender G, Muller G, Hillen W, Bujard H. Transcriptional activation by tetracyclines in mammalian cells. Science 1995; 268: 1766–1769.
64. Schultze N, Burki Y, Lang Y, Certa U, Bluethmann H. Efficient control of gene expression by single step integration of the tetracycline system in transgenic mice. Nature Biotech. 1996; 14: 499–503.
65. VanAntwerp DJ, Martin SJ, Kafri T, Green DR, Verma IM. Suppression of TNF-alpha-induced apoptosis by NF-κB. Science 1996; 274: 787–789.
66. Wang CY, Mayo MW, Baldwin AS. TNF- and cancer therapy-induced apoptosis: potentiation by inhibition of NF-κB. Science 1996; 274: 784–787.
67. Beg AA, Baltimore D. An essential role for NF-κB in preventing TNF-alpha-induced cell death. Science 1996; 274: 782–784.
68. Grimm S, Bauer MKA, Baeuerle PA, Schulze-Osthoff K. Bcl-2 down-regulates the activity of transcription factor NF-κB induced upon apoptosis. J. Cell. Biol. 1996; 134(1): 13–23.
69. Ferran C, Cooper JT, Brostjan C, Stroka DM, Millan MT, Goodman DJ, Bach FH. Expression of a truncated form of the human p55 TNF-receptor in bovine aortic endothelial cells renders them resistant to human TNF. Transplantation Proc. 1996; 28(2): 618–619.
70. Waterworth PD, Cozzi E, Tolan MJ, Langford G, Braidley P, Chavez G, Dunning J, Wallwork J, White D. Pig-to-primate cardiac xenotransplantation. Transplant. Proc. 1997; 29: 899–900.
71. Josien R, Pannetier C, Douillard P, Cantarovich D, Menoret S, Bugeon L, Kourilsky P, Soulillou JP, Cuturi-MC MC. Graft-infiltrating T helper cells, CD45RC phenotype, and Thl/Th2-related cytokines in donor-specific transfusion-induced tolerance in adult rats. Transplantation 1995; 60(10): 1131–1139.

72. Candinas D, Belliveau S, Koyamada N, Miyatake T, Hechenleitner P, Mark W, Bach FH, Hancock WW. T cell independence of macrophage and natural killer cell infiltration, cytokin production, and endothelial activation during delayed xenograft rejection. Transplantation 1996; 62(12): 1920–1927.
73. Charreau B, Tesson L, Soulillou JP, Pourcel C, Anegon I. Transgenesis in rats: technical aspects and models. Transgenic Res. 1996; 5(4): 223–234.
74. Yamada K, Sachs DH, DerSimonian H. Human anti-porcine xenogeneic T cell response. Evidence for allelic specificity of mixed leukocyte reaction and for both direct and indirect pathways of recognition. J. Immunol. 1995; 155(11): 5249–5256.
75. Kirk AD, Li RA, Kinch MS, Abernethy KA, Doyle C, Bollinger RR. The human antiporcine cellular repertoire. In vitro studies of acquired and innate cellular responsiveness. Transplantation 1993; 55(4): 924–931.
76. Dorling A, Binns R, Lechler RI. Cellular xenoresponses: observation of significant primary indirect human T cell anti-pig xenoresponses using co-stimulator-deficient or SLA class II-negative porcine stimulators. Xenotransplantation 1996; 3: 112–119.
77. Dorling A, Lombardi G, Binns R, Lechler-RI RI. Detection of primary direct and indirect human anti-porcine T cell responses using a porcine dendritic cell population. Eur. J. Immunol. 1996; 26(6): 1378–1387.
78. Murphy PM. Molecular mimicry and the generation of host defense protein diversity. Cell 1993; 72(6): 823–826.
79. Campos L, Naji A, Deli BC, Kern JH, Kim JI, Barker CF, Markmann JF. Survival of MHC-deficient mouse heterotopic cardiac allografts. Transplantation 1995; 59(2): 187–191.
80. Pescovitz MD, Sachs DH, Lunney JK, Hsu SM. Localization of class II MHC antigens on porcine renal vascular endothelium. Transplantation 1984; 37: 627–630.
81. Soulillou JP. Relevant targets for therapy with monoclonal antibodies in allograft transplantation. Kidney Int. 1994; 46(2): 540–553.

PART SIX

Surgical and medical aspects

25. Heart retransplantation: medical and surgical issues

JOHAN VANHAECKE, JOHAN VAN CLEEMPUT,
WALTER DROOGNÉ & WIM DAENEN

Background

In order to look at heart retransplantation in its right perspective, a number of preliminary pieces of information must be kept in mind. First, the actual scope of the problem is limited. From the largest two international heart transplant registries [1, 2] and the organ procurement registries [3], we know that retransplantations currently account for 1.5–2.5% of the 4600–4800 heart transplantations performed annually worldwide, i.e. the total retransplant volume is 70–120 procedures per year. There has been no increase in the proportion of heart retransplantation over the past 10 years (Table 1). Second, the available experience is scattered. A majority of heart transplant centers have at some time performed heart retransplantation, although in any given year only 20–25% of centers report such activity. The number of retransplantations per center is mostly very limited so that worldwide there are probably fewer than 10 centers with a total heart retransplantation experience of >20 patients (Table 2). Third, the global survival rate after retransplantation continues to be inferior to that after a first transplant, even if a slight improvement has been noted over the last years (Table 3). Finally, death rate on the waiting list decreased from 14.5% in 1988 to 12.8% in 1992 and 10.2% in 1996 [1].

Table 1. Heart retransplantation as a percentage of the total transplant volume

	ISHLT[a]	CHTS[b]
1981	5.9	–
1984	–	4.3
1986	2.8	3.2
1991	2.2	2.9
1996	1.5	2.5
Total	2.2	2.5

[a]Registry of the International Society for Heart Transplantation, see Ref. 1.
[b]Registry of the Collaborative Heart Transplant Study, see Ref. 2.

J.L. Touraine et al. (eds.), Retransplantation, 211–216.

Table 2. Center experience in heart retransplantation[a]

	Number of retransplantations	Number of centers (%)
	0	33 (29)
	1–10	67 (60)
	11–20	9 (8)
	>20	3 (3)
Total	467	112 (100)
Median (among centers with $n > 0$)	3	
Mean ± S.D.(among centers with $n > 0$)	5.9 ± 6.7	

[a]Data from the Registry of the Collaborative Heart Transplant Study, see Ref. 2.

Table 3. One year actuarial survival rate after heart transplantation[a]

	1982–1990	1991–1996
First transplant	78.5%	80%
Retransplantation		
Within 9 months	39.6%	42.3%
After >9 months	63.5%	68.7%

[a]Registry of the International Society for Heart Transplantation, see Ref. 1.

Reasons for heart retransplantation

The main causes for retransplantation vary with time after the original surgery. In the initial days to weeks 'primary non-function' of the donor heart can occur as a result of various factors such as poor donor management, brain death related catecholamine toxicity to the myocardium, poor donor heart preservation, elevated pulmonary vascular resistance in the recipient, size mismatch. In the subsequent months 'recalcitrant rejection' may damage the donor heart to the point where retransplantation must be considered. After the first post-transplant year 'graft coronary artery disease' or chronic rejection becomes the leading cause for retransplantation.

Surgical issues

Surgical issues in heart retransplantation are non-specific. They include operating on an immunocompromized patient and experience with (multiple) redo procedures. In urgent retransplantation patients may be on a mechanical support system; besides the requirement for expertise with these systems, the presence of mechanical support prior to retransplantation has been associated with decreased survival [4]. Vascular access can be a problem, especially for the follow-up endomyocardial biopsies and coronary angiography. During the initial hospitalization after repeat transplantation there is an increased incidence of major surgical complications such as mediastinitis, intrathoracic bleeding and acute renal failure requiring dialysis [4].

Medical issues

Patient selection

The cause of graft failure and the potential for rehabilitation are the main issues in selecting patients for heart retransplantation. Early analyses revealed a worse outcome in patients retransplanted because of rejection, as compared to those retransplanted for graft coronary artery disease [4]. This finding was confirmed in more recent single center and multicenter studies [1, 5, 6]. The potential for rehabilitation in retransplant candidates depends on age, motivation, cumulative side effects of medication (renal function, bone disease, obesity, glucose intolerance); acceptable results with combined heart-kidney transplantation, previously known only from anecdotal experience, have recently been reported in somewhat larger numbers of patients [7, 8], intercurrent illnesses (malignancy, infection) and progression of initial disease (cerebrovascular disease, renal and/or peripheral atherosclerosis, diabetic complications).

Immunology

HLA sensitization increases in repeat transplantation patients, with a higher mean PRA, a greater proportion of highly sensitized patients and a higher incidence of positive retrospective donor-specific crossmatches [4]. Because a lower survival has been documented in patients with a positive crossmatch [4], the need for/feasibility of prospective crossmatching must be addressed. Developing a strategy for highly sensitized patients remains a daunting task (regional arrangements between centers, timing of entry on the retransplant waiting list, treatment aimed at lowering HLA-antibody titers). On the other hand uncertainty persists as to the significance of antibodies against B-lymphocytes and the need for/efficacy of augmented immunosuppression after a positive crossmatch. Regardless of the crossmatch results it is unknown if and how the initial and maintenance immunosuppressive regimens should be adapted in repeat transplantation. The significance of repeat HLA mismatches is unknown.

Timing of heart retransplantation

Effect of the duration of the first graft on the outcome of heart retransplantation. In all major registries the outcome of retransplantation is better when the first graft functioned for at least 9–12 months [9–11] and the difference in 1 year survival between 'early' and 'late' retransplantation is quite substantial (Table 3). The reasons for this time effect have not been thoroughly explored, but it is obvious that retransplantation for graft coronary artery disease, which has a better prognosis, will more commonly occur after the first posttransplant year, and conversely retransplantation for acute rejection will be more prevalent early on. Also, 'early' retransplants may be technically more demanding, they are done in a period of more intense immunosuppression and they include a number of urgent retransplantations, which have been shown to yield poor results [12, 13].

According to a recent analysis of ISHLT Registry data [1] this correlation between the duration of function of the first graft and the 1– and 3-year mortality after repeat transplantation would actually be U-shaped, with mortality rising again if the duration of the first transplant exceeds 8 years.

Individual timing of heart retransplantation. When considering a patient for retransplantation, a number of factors have a bearing on the actual time frame for the reintervention. When primary non-function of the graft occurs in the initial days after surgery, its etiology should be well thought over: is it a poor graft or a poor patient, and in either case is there a potential for improvement? A stunned left ventricle may recover if mechanically supported for a period of time, acute right ventricular failure may be overcome with or without a temporary assist device if the pulmonary vascular resistance can be brought down. Alternatively the graft may have been damaged beyond repair or the critical condition of the patient may precipitate multi-organ failure. In this early phase the development of HLA antibodies should be monitored closely in order to avoid hyperacute rejection of the second graft.

Deciding on the time of a 'late' retransplantation for graft coronary artery disease is even more difficult. The rare opportunity for myocardial revascularization (PTCA, coronary stenting, CABG) should of course be excluded. The problem however is with the rate of progression of graft coronary artery disease which is variable and the occurrence of clinical events which is unpredictable in individual patients [14]. If the cardiac function deteriorates to a point where mechanical assistance becomes necessary prior to retransplantation, survival is decreased [4].

Course after heart retransplantation

Most of the increased mortality associated with heart retransplantation occurs during the early posttransplantation period [9–11]. In fact, an analysis of the ISHLT Registry data showed that patients surviving beyond 6 months after repeat transplantation had a long-term survival not significantly different from that in patients surviving 6 months after primary transplantation [4]. Reasons for the excess early mortality include the already mentioned HLA sensitization, frequent requirement for mechanical assistance and more surgical complications. There is also a greater incidence of primary non-function of the second graft which could be due to the acceptance of less ideal donor hearts in these critically ill patients. Available data suggest that in the follow-up of second graft recipients rejection, infection and graft coronary disease do not occur more frequently, while the incidence of malignancy is increased as compared to primary transplant recipients [4].

The Leuven experience in heart retransplantation

Despite all of the above, our current knowledge on when, how and in whom to consider heart retransplantation remains very fragmentary. As an illustration thereof we include in this review the limited experience of our own center.

From a total of 226 heart transplantations performed with a 1 and 5 year actuarial survival rate of 91% and 84% respectively, 10 procedures were second heart transplants (4.4% of the total volume). At the time of retransplantation these 10 patients were 48(15 years old (median 52, range 22–61) and 6 were men; all but one were on a respirator and 6 were on a mechanical assist system. Eight patients were retransplanted 'early' (at 3.9 ± 3.2 days, range 1–11, median 3) because of primary non-function of the first donor heart; one of these died intraoperatively from a hyperacute rejection and one died 3 years later from acute rejection due to non-compliance. Two patients were retransplanted 'late', at 27 and 66 months respectively, for acute rejection with irreversible cardiogenic shock; both are alive and well. The 8 current survivors have a median follow-up of 5.2 years (range 1 month to 7.5 years). For the whole retransplant group 1 and 5 year actuarial survival rate is 90% and 75% respectively. These results are at variance with most of the above mentioned findings from pooled data in that survival after retransplantation is not inferior, urgent retransplantation has acceptable results and retransplantation for rejection seems feasible.

Conclusion

Retransplantation plays but a small part in the cardiac transplantation scene. Although a number of surgical and medical issues have been identified, low numbers and a scattered experience make it difficult to sort out the determinants of a successful outcome. From available data it would appear that the best results are obtained in patients retransplanted after 1–8 years for graft coronary artery disease. Transplant centers differ not only in the extent but also in the nature of their retransplant experience.

Acknowledgements

We gratefully acknowledge the contributions of Prof. Dr. Gerhard Opelz, Heidelberg, Dr. Johan De Meester, Leiden and Leo Roels, Leuven, in generously providing us with some of the registry data referred to in this paper. The first author holds the Michael Ondetti Chair in Cardiology at the University of Leuven, Belgium.

References

1. Griffith BP, Novick RJ. Heart and lung retransplantation: should it be done? Data from the ISHLT and UNOS Registries, presented during a debate at the 17th Annual Meeting and Scientific Sessions of the International Society for Heart and Lung Transplantation, London, England, April 5, 1997.
2. Opelz G. Personal communication of data from the Collaborative Heart Transplant Study, December 1996.
3. Roels L. Personal communication of data from the UNOS and ETCO Registries, December 1996.
4. Ensley RD, Hunt S, Taylor DO et al. Predictors of survival after repeat heart transplantation. J. Heart Lung Transplant. 1992; 11: S142–S158.
5. Smith JA, Ribakove GH, Hunt SA et al. Heart retransplantation: the 25-year experience at a single institution. J. Heart Lung Transplant. 1995; 14: 832–839.
6. Loire R, Boissonnat P. Cardiac retransplantation (42 cases in 38 patients). Indications and outcome. Arch. Mal. Coeur Vaiss 1996; 89: 229–234.
7. Col V, Squifflet JP, Goenen M et al. Combined heart-kidney transplantation: results and indications. Proceedings of the Annual Scientific Meeting of the Belgian Transplantation Society, 1997, March 1, Brussels.
8. Narula J, Bennett LE, DiSalvo T, Hosenpud JD, Semigran MJ, Dec WD. Outcomes in recipients of combined heart–kidney transplantation: multi-organ, same-donor transplant study of the International Society for Heart and Lung Transplantation Society/United Network for Organ Sharing Scientific Registry. Transplantation 1997; 63: 861–867.
9. Opelz G. Data published in Newsletter 2: 1996 of the Collaborative Transplant Study. Heidelberg, April 1, 1996.
10. Hosenpud JD. The Registry of the International Society for Heart and Lung Transplantation: Fourteenth Official Report – 1997. Presented at the 17th Annual Meeting and Scientific Sessions of the International Society for Heart and Lung Transplantation, London, England, April 5, 1997.
11. De Meester J. Personal communication of data from the Eurotransplant Thoracic Database, March 1997.
12. de Boer J, Cohen B, Thorogood J, Zantvoort FA, D'Amaro J, Persijn GG. Results of acute heart retransplantation (letter). Lancet 1991; 337: 1158.
13. Mullins P, Chauhan A, Aravot D et al. Acute heart retransplantation (letter). Lancet 1991; 337: 1552–1553.
14. McGiffin DC, Savunen T, Kirklin JK et al. Cardiac transplant coronary artery disease. A multivariable analysis of pretransplantation risk factors for disease development and morbid events. J. Thorac. Cardiovasc. Surg. 1995; 109: 1081–1089.

26. Intestinal retransplantation

S. SARNACKI & Y. RÉVILLON

Intestinal transplantation is a potential alternative to total parental nutrition (TPN) for the treatment of chronic intestinal failure.

Advancement in surgical technique, perioperative care, and the availability of effective immunosuppressive agents, has made intestinal transplantation a feasible procedure for these patients. Despite improvement in survival, particularly since the use of tacrolimus, the procedure still carries a higher patient and graft loss when compared to other organs.

Retransplantation may theoretically be proposed in such cases of failure of the primary graft. In our previous experience with isolated small bowel transplantation (SB), two patients among seven have been retransplanted. Up to this date, we have performed two additional SB transplantations and six combined liver/small bowel (LSB) grafts and none of these patients have undergone retransplantation. When considering the recent International Intestinal Transplant Registry reported by D. Grant in 1995, this procedure seems actually exceptionally retained: 180 transplantations have been performed in 170 patients and retransplantation, therefore, concerns only 0.05% of this population. These cases are analyzed according to the centre of origin, the cause of primary graft failure, the type of the second graft – liver/small bowel (LSB), isolated small bowel (SB) or multivisceral graft (MV) – the timing and urgency of retransplantation and the outcome of the patient and the graft.

Seven patients died after retransplantation, mainly from sepsis and/or multivisceral failure. Three were reported to be alive but had removal of their grafts mainly because of acute or chronic rejection. Only one case was precisely documented for the immunological status of the recipient and showed a specific reactivity of the patient's serum with endothelial/monocyte antigens, but not with lymphocytes (negative cross-match).

In conclusion, intestinal retransplantation alone or with other abdominal organs is associated with high mortality and morbidity and must be avoided. With this aim in view, the selection of the patients that require intestinal graft must be very rigorous, and perhaps more difficult, the choice of the type of the graft carefully discussed in a multidisciplinary approach. Finally, the development of new immunosuppressive treatments based on the molecular analysis of alloreactivity and tolerance seems to be essential, particularly in the case of intestinal transplantation to improve the survival of patients and grafts.

J.L. Touraine et al. (eds.), Retransplantation, 217.

PART SEVEN

Ethical and operational issues

27. Should we retransplant lung?

JAMES H. DAUBER

Introduction

Transplantation of the lung has become an accepted form of therapy for a variety of endstage lung diseases. Despite recent improvements in surgical techniques and immunosuppression, graft failure, particularly in the late post transplant period from chronic rejection, continues to extract an unacceptable toll leading to a strong desire on the part of both the afflicted patient and physician for retransplantation. Given the growing disparity between the size of donor and recipient pools, however, the practice of retransplanting lung is controversial. Information on the survival post retransplantation is limited due to the relatively few numbers that have been performed world wide. Most recent figures indicate that overall survival is only half the rate seen for a first transplant. In selected centers it is better but still not as good as after a first transplant. Leading causes of death after retransplantation are infection and respiratory failure from chronic rejection. Factors associated with a favorable outcome after retransplantation include ambulatory status of the recipient, interval between first and second transplants and retransplantation for conditions other than chronic rejection. Survival also seems to be higher if retransplantation is performed at centers which have done more than five procedures. Functional status following retransplantation may achieve virtually normal levels, but in recipients retransplanted for chronic rejection, recurrence of this complication occurs in nearly two thirds leading to significant declines in both their functional status and survival. Given these results the rationale for continuing to perform retransplantation may be questioned. None-the-less it is the opinion of the author that retransplantation should be performed at selected centers but only with rigid selection of recipients, close monitoring of results and a willingness to share this information with the transplant community.

Present status of lung transplantation

Candidate and donor pools

The number of first time lung transplants has grown steadily since 1981 when the modern era of lung transplantation began. Recent figures from the United Network for Organ Sharing (UNOS) registry document steady growth in the number of procedures being done in the United States [1]. There is a suggestion

J.L. Touraine et al. (eds.), Retransplantation, 221–228.

from the registry published by the International Society for Heart and Lung Transplantation (ISHLT), however, that by 1995 the volume of lung transplants worldwide has plateaued to around 1000 cases annually [2]. In order to accommodate for this growth the donor pool had to greatly enlarged. This was done to some degree by including older donors. Consequently the average age of donors has increased from around 20 to more than 28 years [2]. Registration of candidates on the United Network for Organ Sharing (UNOS) waiting list has grown to 1706, an increase of over ten fold in the last 8 years [1]. Since growth of the donor pool has not kept pace with registrations, the average waiting time has doubled in the last 5 years to 548 days. Waiting times often exceed 2 years for double lung transplantation at The University of Pittsburgh Medical Center and other active transplant centers in the United States (J. Dauber, Unpublished Data).

Outcomes

Operative mortality remains around 10% overall but varies considerably for different indications [1]. One, 3 and 5 year survivals in the UNOS registry are 72, 57 and 41%, respectively. These survival rates, although much improved over those in the early and mid 1980's still are lower than those for liver and heart where 5 year survivals approach 70% [1]. After a successful lung transplant there is unequivocal improvement in functional status and quality of life [3] and the vast majority of recipients do not regret undergoing the procedure, even when the outcome is not optimal.

Major causes of mortality

In the perioperative period the major causes of death are primary graft failure and infection. Both of these conditions are not uncommonly associated with multiorgan failure. Bacteria account for the vast majority of infectious deaths, but fungi definitely contribute to mortality and morbidity in this period [4]. Acute rejection is rarely fatal at this time unless it is severe and occurs along with the other major complications described above.

In the first two years after hospital discharge, infection continues to be the major cause of mortality and is often related to augmentation of immune suppression that it needed to treat recurrent episodes of acute cellular rejection which are a frequent event for most recipients. Airway complications also contribute to mortality in this period but are becoming much less common causes of death as management techniques improve [5].

In long term survivors the leading cause of mortality is chronic rejection. Chronic lung rejection is characterized chiefly by inflammation and scarring of the small airways. The histological hallmark is obliterative bronchiolitis (OB). Over 50% of long term survivors will experience this complication which causes obstruction to airflow and predisposes to infection, particularly with

Table 1. Grading of bronchiolitis obliterans syndrome

Grade of BOS	Decline in FEV_1[a]
0	<20%
1	20 to 35%
2	35 to 50%
3	>50%

[a] Decline is measured by substracting new value for FEV_1 from best baseline value determined by averaging at least two sets of consecutive measurements made 4–6 weeks apart [7].

Pseudomonas aeruginosa. The major risk factor appears to be the severity of acute rejection in the early postransplant period [6]. Optimally the diagnosis is confirmed by detecting OB in the allograft, but transbronchial lung biopsy is often insensitive [3]. For this reason a clinical diagnosis may be made if there is reduction in airflow that cannot be attributed to any other condition. The latter is referred to as the bronchiolitis obliterans syndrome which is graded in severity (Grades 0–3) base on the degree in reduction of flow rates [7] (Table 1). Treatment with augmented immune suppression improves lung function in less than one-third of afflicted recipients. Typically it will stabilize lung function at a lower level for a variable period of time before there is a relapse. Up to one third of recipients will essentially fail to respond and develop severe respiratory insufficiency over a three to six month period. Even when not fatal, chronic rejection diminishes the functional status and quality of life of recipients and greatly increases medical costs. It is the major cause of death in the late transplant period and represents a major barrier to the wide-spread acceptance of lung transplantation as a treatment for end stage lung and pulmonary vascular disease [3].

Recent experience with retransplantation of the lung

Indications for and frequency of retransplantation

Allograft failure in both the early and late transplant periods has driven transplant centers and recipients to pursue retransplantation. The principal indications for retransplantation along with the median time to retransplantation are listed in Table 2 [8]. In keeping with the discussion above, bronchiolitis obliterans syndrome is the leading cause for retransplantation today, whereas in the early and mid 1980's it was primary graft failure and airway complications.

In comparison to the total number of first time transplants, the number of retransplants is quite small, never accounting for more than 3–4% of all transplants on a yearly basis since 1991 [1]. Several centers which have

Table 2. Indications and timing for retransplantation of the lung. Source: Pulmonary Retransplantation Registry [8]

Indication	Percentage of cases	Days after first transplant (median)
Chronic rejection (BOS)	58	624
Primary graft failure	25	13
Airway complications	9	119
Severe acute rejection	5	23
Miscellaneous	3	206

Table 3. Causes of death following retransplantation of the lung. Source: Pulmonary Retransplantation Registry [8]

Cause of death	Percentage of deaths
Infection	42
Failure of second organ system	26
Chronic rejection (BOS)	26
Airway complications	3

performed more than 15 retransplant procedures have recently published their experience [9, 10, 11, 12] but the most extensive analysis of outcomes has been derived from the Pulmonary Retransplantation Registry which is maintained in London, Ontario [8].

Mortality after retransplantation

Survival at all times following retransplantation is significantly lower than for a first time transplant. Results from both the Retransplantation Registry and UNOS are similar and indicate that one year survival is around 45% [1, 8]. By 4 years survival has dropped to about 30%. Survival after retransplantation for heart and liver is also lower than for first time transplants, but four year survival is about 50% for both, rate 60% higher than for the lung [1]. The major causes of death after retransplantation are infection, second organ system failure and chronic rejection [8]. Airway complications extract only a very minor toll (Table 3). It should be noted, though, that two year survival after retransplantation of the lung is about fifty percent in centers which have done more than five procedures [11, 12], a rate that is 2.5 times better than in centers which have done fewer than five procedures [8]. Nonetheless, the rate for 2-year survival in experienced centers is still less than what is seen for first time transplants (approximately 65%) [1].

Several factors associated with the recipient of a second lung transplant appear to affect mortality. The most prominent is the ambulatory status at the time of retransplant. When a retransplant is performed on an ambulatory recipient, the survival rate at three months is nearly three times that for a non-ambulatory recipient [8]. Improved survival after 2 years is also seen for ambulatory recipients compared to non-ambulatory recipients, but the advantage may also reflect the experience of the transplant center in addition to the status of the recipient [8]. None-the-less the message from the Retransplant Registry seems to be clear that non-ambulatory recipients have a very poor survival rate. Experience at centers with above average experience with retransplantation support this finding [10].

A second factor which may influence outcome is the duration of time between the first and second procedures [10]. Results from several individual centers including the University of Pittsburgh suggest that the longer the interval, the better the survival. The most recent analysis from the Retransplant Registry, however, does not demonstrate a survival advantage for this factor [8].

A third factor which may confer survival advantage is the indication for retransplantation. If done for chronic rejection, long term survival may be lower than for recipients done for other conditions due to the relatively high rate of obliterative bronchiolitis in the group done for OB. Within 3 years after retransplantation 69% of recipients done for OB will have recurrent OB whereas only 17% of recipients done for other conditions will develop this complication [8]. In addition, the severity of OB in recipients retransplanted for this condition was much greater than that in recipients who developed OB after being retransplanted for other conditions. Approximately 80% of recipients with Grade III BOS three years after retransplantation were done for graft failure from chronic rejection [8].

Functional status after retransplantation

According to the Retransplant Registry 53% of recipients who were retransplanted and survived for a median of 780 days achieved a New York Heart Association functional status of Class I. Of the remaining, 34% were Class II, 10% Class III and only 3% Class IV. Eight of 59 subjects in this analysis group were on chronic oxygen therapy, though. One of the major causes for a poor functional status is probably the decline in pulmonary function that occurs in recipients who were retransplanted for OB. On average this group experienced a progressive decline in flow rates over three years (Table 4). Flow rates in the group transplanted for other conditions did not decline over the same period and were significantly higher than those in the former group at years two and three [8].

The retransplantation controversy

Proponents of retransplantation cite the following facts to support the procedure. First, survival after retransplantation is steadily improving and approaching rates for first time transplants in selected patients done at experi-

Table 4. FEV_1 for patients retransplanted for BOS and for other conditions. Source: Pulmonary Retransplantation Registry [8]

Month after retransplant	Retransplanted for BOS	Retransplanted for other conditions
3	1.8 ± 0.2	2.0 ± 0.2
12	1.7 ± 0.3	2.2 ± 0.3
24	1.3 ± 0.3^{a}	2.0 ± 0.3
36	$1.1 \pm 0.2^{a,b}$	1.9 ± 0.3

$^{a}p < 0.05$, 3 months vs 36 months.
$^{b}p < 0.05$, BOS vs other conditions.

enced centers. With more experience and better selection, rates should continue to improve. Second, valuable experience will be gained with new immunosuppressive regimens devised to prevent recurrence of OB in recipients retransplanted for this condition. Attempting to use new regimens with potentially more toxicity in this group is justifiable given the great propensity for these recipients to develop chronic rejection. These newer techniques for immune suppression can then be applied to first time transplant recipients as needed. Third, survival after heart-lung transplantation is not much better than that for retransplantation at experienced centers and yet heart-lung transplants are not categorically denied due to poor survival. Finally, survival rates after retransplantation of liver and heart are not as good as rates after first transplants and yet retransplantation of these organs is widely practiced. From the standpoint of the physician–patient relationship, the possibility of retransplantation also offers hope for recipients with a failing graph and their families, and may allow them to adapt better to a declining functional status imposed by chronic rejection.

Adversaries of retransplantation cite the growing disparity between the size of donor and recipient pools and the suboptimal survival and functional status following retransplantation as the overriding reasons for not offering retransplantation. They argue that scarce donor lungs should be used only for first time transplants to insure that the greatest good is being done for the largest number of patients with endstage lung and pulmonary vascular diseases. Using increasing proportion of organs for retransplantation will deny a chance for a life saving operation for first time recipients without a comparable outcome. Other reasons for limiting or eliminating retransplantation are the following. First, in an era where health care costs are coming under close scrutiny and major efforts are being made to limit the growth of expenditures, retransplantation is less attractive due to the potential to impose high costs on transplant programs. Second, the expectation that outcomes following retransplantation will equal those after a first transplant may never be realized and provide a false hope to those recipients contemplating undergoing a second transplant and their families. Experiencing a rapid decline in graft function soon after a second transplant could devastate recipients and their families. These are compelling arguments when applied in an analytical manner. In the presence of a dying recipient who is seeking salvation, though, they tend to lose some of their impact and make the transplant team seem impersonal and unconcerned about the individual's plight.

Recommendations regarding retransplantation

It is the opinion of this author that retransplantation of the lung should not be halted summarily, but that it should be performed only at centers with a high level of experience and a good record of success with retransplantation. Such centers should not be expected to accept recipients from other programs who have developed graft failure and would potentially benefit from a retransplant. Having to accept such outside recipients would unduly penalize retransplantation centers and the candidates waiting for a first transplant in these programs.

In order to optimize outcomes after retransplantation, designated centers must exercise the same criteria for selection as they do for first time transplants. Recipients for retransplantation should be ambulatory and have no evidence of insufficiency of other major organ systems that would jeopardize their chance of a successful outcome. About half of the recipients with severe chronic graft failure at the University of Pittsburgh today would not meet these criteria and, therefore, be denied candidacy (J. Dauber, unpublished results).

Retransplant centers should form a consortium to devise optimal patient selection and treatment strategies. Careful monitoring of outcomes and rapid dissemination of results are essential, and after a designated period of 3–5 years, if outcomes are not meeting expectations, consideration should be given to further limiting or even abandoning the procedure.

In coming to this conclusion, I have tried to balance the interests and needs of society as a whole and of the patient as an individual. This is not an easy task and given the same considerations another physician could easily come to the opposite conclusion. As long as transplant centers are given some autonomy in the selection of recipients, it is likely that retransplantation will continue to be done. For this reason I appeal to those centers performing retransplantation to work together to address the issues discussed above.

References

1. 1996 Annual Report of the U.S. Scientific Registry of Transplant Recipients and the Organ Procurement and Transplantation Network. UNOS and the Division of Transplantation, Bureau of heath Resources Develoment, Heath Resources and Services Administration, U.S Department of Health and Human Services, 1997.
2. Hosenspud JD, Novick RJ, Bennett LD, Keck BM, Fiol B, Daily OP. The Registry of the International Society for heart and lung transplantation: Thirteenth Official Report – 1996. J. Heart Lung Transplant. 1996; 15: 655–674.

3. Trulock EP. State of the art: lung transplantation. Am. J. Resp. Crit. Care Med. 1997; 155: 789–818.
4. Dauber, JH, Paradis IL, Dummer JS. Infectious complications in pulmonary allograft recipients. Clin. Chest Med. 1990; 11: 291–308.
5. Higgins R, McNeil K, Dennis C et al. Airway stenoses after lung transplantation: management with expanding stents. J. Heart Lung Transplant. 1994; 13: 774–778.
6. Paradis IL, Yousem SA, Griffith BP. Airway obstruction and bronchiolitis obliterans after lung transplantation. Clin. Chest Med. 1993; 14: 751–763.
7. Cooper JD, Billingham M, Egan T et al. A working formulation for the standardization of nomenclature and for clinical staging of chronic dysfunction in lung allografts. J. Heart Lung Transplant. 1993; 12: 713–16.
8. Novick RJ, Stitt L, Schafers H-J et al. Pulmonary retransplantation: does the indication for operation influence postoperative lung function? J. Thorac. Cardiovasc. Surg. 1996; 112: 1504–1514.
9. Haverich A, Hirt SW, Wahlers T, Schafers H-J, Zink C, Borst H-G. Functional results after lung retransplantation. J. Heart Lung Transplant. 1994; 13: 48–55.
10. Wekerle T, Kelpetko W, Wisser W et al. Lung retransplantation: institutional report on a series of twenty patients. J. Heart Lung Transplant. 1996; 15: 182–189.
11. Novick RJ, Schafers H-J, Stitt L et al. Seventy-two pulmonary retransplantations for obliterative bronchiolitis: predictors of survival. Ann. Thorac. Surg. 1995; 60: 111–116.
12. Al Kattan K, Tadjkarimi S, Banner N, Khaghani N, Yacoub M. Pattern of survival and functional results of single lung transplantation for obliterative bronchiolitis (abstract). J. Heart Lung Transplant. 1996; 15: S69.

28. A single center experience with heart retransplantation: the 29 year experience at a single institution

SHARON A. HUNT, ROBERT C. ROBBINS, EDWARD B. STINSON, PHILLIP E. DYER, NORMAN E. SHUMWAY & BRUCE A. REITZ

The subject of organ retransplantation has generated a great deal of debate and discussion as physicians, ethicists and health care payers as well as patients address such intrinsically conflicting principles as distributive justice and the drive to maximize individual patient survival. As is the case with other organ allografts, it is inevitable that a certain number of cardiac allograft recipients will redevelop some form of end-stage heart disease and become potential candidates for retransplantation. While there may be no strictly right or wrong answer to the question of whether heart retransplantation should ever be performed, we felt that examining the experience at a single relatively high-volume institution which has performed retransplantation over a several decade period could be instructive both in terms of assessing what the best result to be obtained might be as well as identifying subsets of retransplant candidates with predictable better outcome than others. Thus, we present a retrospective analysis of our institutions 29 year experience with cardiac retransplantation.

Methods

In the period between Stanford's first heart transplant in January 1968, and March 1997, a total of 841 heart transplant procedures have been performed at Stanford University Medical Center. Of these, 67 procedures (8%) were retransplant procedures (64 first time and 3 second time) in 64 patients. Figure 1 shows the annual numbers of primary and repeat heart transplant procedures at Stanford and demonstrates a variable number per year, but only one re-transplant procedure since 1993. Nineteen of these 67 retransplant procedures were performed before the introduction of cyclosporine as the mainstay of immunosuppressive therapy in 1981; the remaining 48 have received cyclosporine therapy. Fifty-three of the patients were male (reflecting the overall male preponderance of our patient population) and they ranged in age from 3 to 62 years (with a mean of 41 years) at the time of retransplantation. Indications for retransplantation included constrictive diseases in 3, primary allograft failure in 9, acute allograft rejection in 17, and graft vasculopathy in 38 patients.

J.L. Touraine et al. (eds.), Retransplantation, 229–236.

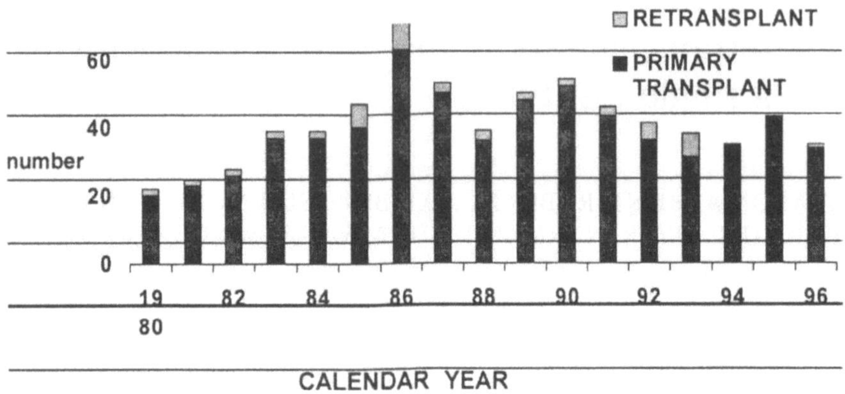

Fig. 1. Graph of annual numbers of retransplant and primary transplant procedures in Stanford program.

Of note, the patients undergoing retransplantation for primary allograft failure or acute allograft rejection were, in general, quite hemodynamically unstable and all were in the intensive care unit setting, most requiring inotropic support. Six of these additionally required the use of mechanical circulatory support (five an intra-aortic balloon pump and one a left ventricular assist device) until a suitable donor heart could be obtain for retransplantation. On the other hand, patients who underwent retransplantation because of advanced graft vasculopathy tended to be more hemodynamically stable. Although most had already sustained ischemic events and had left ventricular dysfunction, the majority waited either at home or in a non-intensive care unit setting for a suitable donor heart to become available.

Principles applied in selection of retransplant recipients were generally the same as those applied in selecting primary transplant recipients, although (in contrast to loosening or less stringent criteria for primary transplant recipients over time) they have evolved and become increasingly restrictive. Our selection committee takes into account not only such obvious contraindications as active sepsis and severe hepatic or pulmonary dysfunction, but also such less quantifiable factors as limitations on quality of life due to intercurrent medical problems such as osteoporosis, neurologic events or infections. Of note, three patients underwent primary kidney transplantation at the time of heart retransplantation, all because of end-stage renal disease due primarily to cyclosporine nephrotoxicity. All three were one year survivors after retransplantation.

Immunosuppressive regimens, including rejection surveillance and therapy were identical in retransplantation and primary transplant recipients at any given point in time. These regimens included azathioprine and corticosteroids in patients undergoing procedures prior to 1981 and triple drug immunosuppression with cyclosporine, azathioprine and corticosteroids as well as induction therapy with antithymocyte globulin or OKT3 in patients since 1981. For example, a pre-cyclosporine patient who underwent retransplantation after 1981 would be started on what was then considered to be state-of-the-art cyclosporine-based immunosuppression.

Follow up for all patients is complete through March, 1997. Actuarial rates of survival and freedom from infection and rejection were calculated for all patients and for the subset who underwent retransplantation since 1981. Cutler–Ederer calculations were used to derive Kaplan–Meier actuarial rates [1] and the Gehan test [2] was used for statistical analysis comparing actuarial curves.

Results

Hospital mortality

Of the 67 retransplantation procedures there were 17 in-hospital deaths (25%). Causes of in-hospital death included infection in 8 patients, acute allograft rejection in 3, multiple organ failure in 3, pulmonary hypertension in 2, and a cerebrovascular accident in one. Of the 9 patients who underwent retransplantation for primary allograft dysfunction, 5 died in the perioperative period. In the subgroup of 48 patients who underwent retransplantation since 1981 there were 11 perioperative deaths and 8 of these occurred in patients who underwent retransplantation less than 6 months after their primary transplant procedure.

Long term survival

Actuarial survival rates for the group of all 64 patients undergoing retransplantation between 1968 and 1997 (55%, 33%, and 22% at 1, 5, and 10 years, respectively) were significantly worse than those for patients undergoing primary transplantation (81%, 62%, 44%, at 1, 5, and 10 years, respectively; Figure 2). This inferior survival was also found in the group of 47 who underwent retransplantation since 1981 (54% and 33% at 1 and 5 years, respectively). Survival was worst in the group of patients undergoing retransplantation prior to 1981 (Figure 3) with only a 35% one year survival rate in these 19 patients.

Of note, most deaths occurred in the perioperative period and the actuarial curves tend to parallel each other after 12 months. The 1 year actuarial survival of patients who underwent retransplantation for acute allograft rejection or primary graft failure since 1981 (42%) was significantly worse ($p < 0.05$) than those who underwent retransplantation during the same time period because of graft vasculopathy (Figure 4).

Rejection

All patients who underwent retransplantation for acute rejection had at least one episode of rejection in their retransplanted heart during the first 6 postoperative months and 3 died of acute rejection. This is in contrast to the group

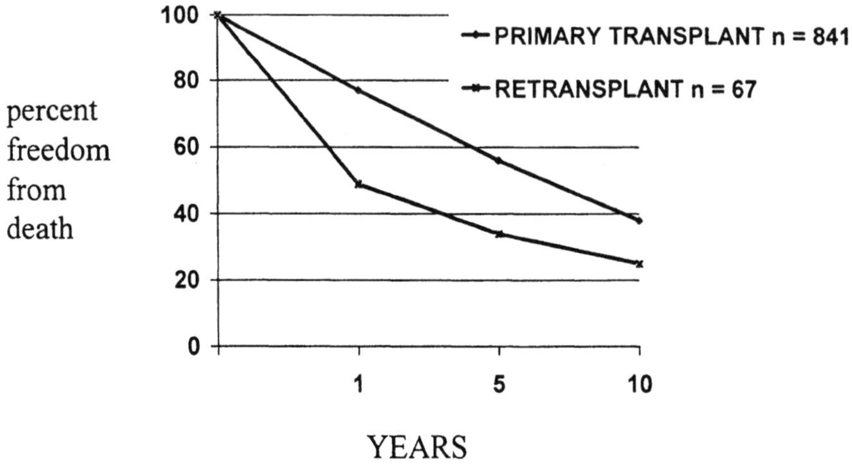

Fig. 2. Actuarial survival curves comparing group of primary transplant recipients with group of retransplant recipients between 1968 and 1997 in Stanford program.

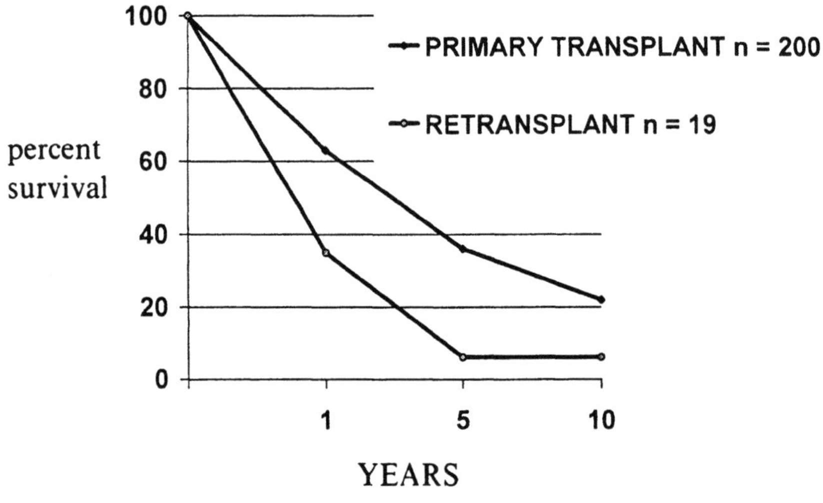

Fig. 3. Actuarial survival curve for cohort of retransplant recipients operated prior to 1981.

who underwent retransplantation for graft vasculopathy, 33% of whom were free of any rejection at 6 months.

Graft atherosclerosis

The actuarial freedom from angiographically visible atherosclerosis in the entire heart retransplantation population at 5 years was 89% and was 91% for the subgroup who underwent retransplantation because of graft vasculopathy.

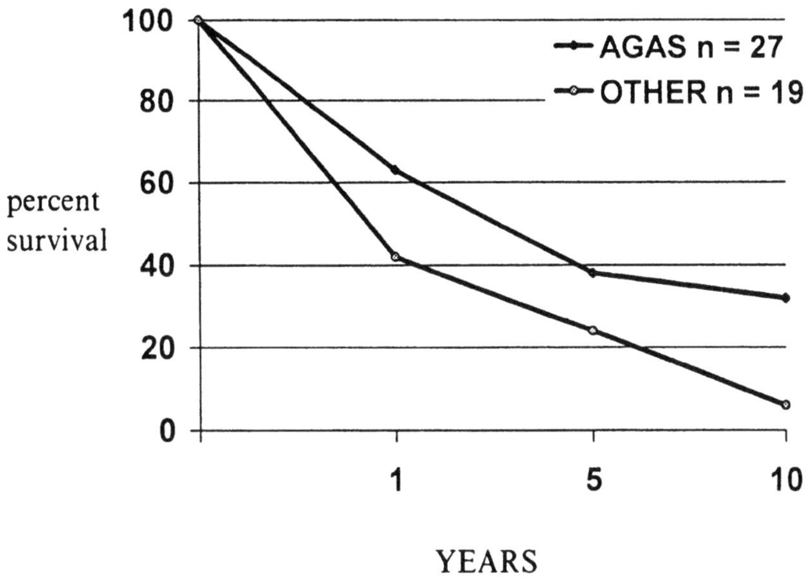

Fig. 4. Actuarial survival curve comparing group of patients undergoing retransplantation for acute rejection or primary graft failure with those undergoing retransplant for graft vasculopathy since 1981.

Functional class

Of the 47 patients who left the hospital after their retransplant procedure, 37 (79%) returned to functional class I and independent, productive lives. The longest-term retransplant patient is currently 13 years post-transplant (23 years since his primary transplant) and is a professor and chief of a department at a local university.

Costs

The mean hospital charge (±SE) for the 15 patients undergoing heart retransplantation since 1990 was \$386 000 ± 133 000. This charge was significantly greater ($p < 0.05$) than that in 100 of the 162 patients undergoing primary heart transplant during the same time period for whom accurate financial data was available (\$162 000 ± 10 000). These charges do not include any intensive care unit charges incurred by patients in United Network for Organ Sharing status 1 during the waiting period prior to transplant. These costs are normalized to 1992 dollars.

Discussion

Heart transplantation has for some time been widely accepted as standard therapy for selected patients with truly end-stage heart disease and markedly improves the prognosis for long-term survival in individual patients [3]. Truly widespread use of the procedure is, (and most likely always will be) limited, however, by the availability of donor organs, at a plateau of about 2500 hearts per year worldwide since the late 1980s [4]. This plateau is contrasted with estimates of up to 16000 patients per year worldwide who potentially could benefit from heart transplantation [5]. Many predict that the gap will ultimately be filled with the use of animal organs as breakthroughs in genetic engineering and control of immune responses permit the introduction of xenotransplantation [6]. Competing technology may also include the introduction of permanent non-biological replacement of the heart in the form of completely implantable left ventricular assist devices [7]. In the time until either or both of these advances comes to pass, however, it behooves the medical profession and society as a whole to make the best possible use of the scarce resource of donor hearts. In this context we have sought to examine the success rates seen with retransplantation of the heart in an effort to determine how the cardiac allograft recipient who re-develops end-stage heart disease in his new heart should be evaluated in the allocation scheme for scarce donor hearts.

In order to evaluate sensibly the efficacy of such a radical form of therapy as retransplantation we first need to examine what is known about the prognosis of patients who develop some condition that could lead to retransplantation. The available data do indeed suggest a grim prognosis for patients developing severe disease in a cardiac allograft. There are three main categories or conditions that lead to retransplantation. The first of these is primary graft failure, probably a condition with a variety of causes including poor graft preservation, hyperacute rejection, and probably others. There are no published data, but most would agree that the mortality of this condition (without retransplantation) approaches 100%. The second potential indication to pursue retransplantation is acute allograft rejection. For patients who develop hemodynamically compromising rejection there are some data available [8] which show very high mortality rates (in the range of 60% at 18 months) after hemodynamically compromising rejection.

The majority of patients being considered for retransplantation in recent years have developed ischemic dysfunction as a result of advanced allograft vasculopathy. Data on the prognosis of such patients in the absence of retransplantation were analyzed by our our group several years ago [9]. In this study of 54 patients with angiographically at least moderate graft coronary disease, survival was directly related to disease severity, with the poorest outcome in patients with a 70% or higher grade obstruction or with three-vessel involvement. Survival with 2-vessel disease was only 41% at 2 years and with 3 vessel disease 13% at 2 years. Survival after onset of any symptoms due to ischemia was approximately 30% at one year.

Given the very poor prognosis for any individual patient who develops either primary graft failure, acute allograft rejection, or severe graft vasculopathy, one must next ask what improvement in that prognosis may be expected with retransplantation. Several sources of such data are published. Perhaps the most widely quoted is the annual update of the Registry of the International Society for Heart and Lung Transplantation. According to the most recent published update [4], 653 retransplantation procedures have been performed worldwide with an overall 52% one year actuarial survival. One notable subset of patients with better survival in the Registry data includes patients undergoing retransplantation more than 6 months after primary transplant (almost all for graft vasculopathy), who have a 63% one year survival after retransplantation.

Several years ago 13 major United States heart transplant centers pooled their data on retransplantation on the theory that high volume centers would have better results than those from an international registry which included results from all programs regardless of their volume or success rates [10]. The pooled data included information on 125 repeat transplant recipients from the 13 centers and did, in fact, show higher one year survival rates than those for the 499 retransplantation recipients then reported to the ISHLT Registry – 60% vs 48%. These results were still quite inferior to the 79% one year survival for primary transplant recipients in the Registry database. As is the case with the Registry data as well as our own data reported here, subsets of patients undergoing retransplantation more than 6 months after primary transplant or for the indication of graft vasculopathy or after 1985 enjoyed better survival rates than the rest. However, even the ideal candidate defined by these predictive variables had a 1 year survival probability in the 13 centers data base of only 64%.

Our own data, derived from a single institution with a long and consistent base of experience, clearly confirm the experience of others. Based on what is known about the prognosis of retransplant candidates, it is clear that the individual patient's prognosis is considerably improved by retransplantation. However, the retransplantation procedure is costly (over double the cost of a primary procedure in our institution) and the graft survival rates are not as good as if the graft were used in a primary transplant procedure.

These facts lead to the ethical conflict between the position of patient advocacy which tries to maximize every patients chance of survival and not abandon patients and the position of distributive justice in which the difference in efficacy between primary transplantation and retransplantation makes the latter untenable [11]. This is a conflict which those in our field face on a daily basis and there seems to be a consensus evolving that, although there can be few dogmatic policies, retransplantation should be reserved for occasional very highly selected patients if it is done at all. Our own centers record of having performed only one retransplant in the past four years is a testimony to our own evolving philosophy as well as to the fact that we have not completely abandoned the procedure.

References

1. Cutler SJ, Ederer F. Maximum utilization of the life table method in analyzing survival. J. Chronic Dis. 1958; 8: 699–712.

2. Gehan A. Generalized Wilcoxon test for comparing arbitrary single-censored samples. Biometrika 1965; 52: 203–222.
3. Mudge GH, Goldstein S, Addonizio LJ, Caplan A, Mancini D, Levine TB et al. Task force 3: recipient guidelines/prioritization. J. Amer. Coll. Cardiol. 1993; 22: 21–31.
4. Hosenpid JD, Novick RJ, Bennet LE, Keck BM, Fiol B, Daily OP. The Registry of the International Society for Heart Lung Transplantation: thirteenth official report – 1996. J. Heart Lung Transplant. 1996; 15: 655–674.
5. O'Connell JB, Gunnar RM, Evans RW, Fricker J, Hunt SA, Kirklin JK. Task Force 1: organization of heart transplantation in the U.S. In: 24th Bethesda Conference. J. Am. Coll. Cardiol. 1993; 22: 8–14.
6. Skolnick AA. Transplantion pioneer predicts successful xenotransplant soon. JAMA 1993; 269: 2951–2958.
7. Oz MC, Argenziano M, Catanese KA, Gardocki MT, Goldstein DJ, Ashton RC et al. Bridge experience with long-term implantable left ventricular assist devices: are they an alternative to transplantation? Circulation 1997; 95: 1844–1852.
8. Mills RM, Naftel DC, Kirklin JK, Van Bakel A, Jaski B, Massin E. Cardiac transplant rejection with hemodynamic compromise: a multi-institutional study of the role of endomyocardial cellular infiltrate. J. Heart Lung Transplant. (in press).
9. Keogh AM, Valantine HA, Hunt SA, Schroeder JS, McIntosh N, Oyer PE, Stinson EB. Impact of proximal or midvessel discrete coronary artery stenoses on survival after heart transplantation. J. Heart Transplant. 1992; 11: 892–901.
10. Ensley RD, Hunt S, Taylor DO, Renlund DG, Menlove RL, Karwande SV et al. J. Heart Lung Transplant. 1992; 11: S 142–158.
11. Ubel PA, Arnold RM, Caplan AL. Rationing failure: the ethical lessons of the retransplantation of scarce vital organs. JAMA 1993; 270: 2469–2474.

29. Should we retransplant liver?

CHRISTIAN DUCERF

This is a difficult question which involves medical, ethical, economic and social considerations. The pool of available liver grafts is limited so liver grafts have to be used with the best efficiency. Unfortunately results for liver retransplantation are not as good as for first liver transplantation [1]. The number of first transplantations in Europe and in the United States is from 3000 to 5000 and the frequency of retransplantation is from 11% to 20% [2]. The rate of retransplantation decreases with the teams experience and it can be noted the results of transplantation are improved. Retransplantation is more frequent in emergency [3]. The main causes of retransplantation in emergency [4] are, first: primary non function of the graft, second: hepatic artery thrombosis of the graft, third: refractory acute rejection episodes and chronic rejection diseases leading to graft loss.

The main reasons to retransplant patients are directly due to the graft itself or to the technique of transplantation. In such case, it is very difficult to refuse the efficient treatment alone in order to save the patient suffering from an hepatic insufficiency disease leading rather quickly to death. In fact, there is no artificial procedure to bridge the critical period as in renal or hemodynamic insufficiency syndrome. It is the beginning of a vicious circle, needing one liver transplantation whatever the graft poor or not because there is emergency conditions. Sometimes this leads to a second liver transplantation or third and so on and so forth. On another hand, using 2, 3 or more grafts for one patient is an ethical dilemma all the more so there is a shortage of available liver grafts.

The results of retransplantation are worse as the number of retransplantation increases especialy after more than 3 liver transplantations for the same patient [5].

The first way to avoid retransplantation is to avoid primary nonfunction (PNF), hepatic artery thrombosis (HAT), and rejection episodes (RE). To prevent PNF it is important to use good grafts. It is not a good way or a good deal to use all grafts available even in the case of major steatosis or after ischemic damage [6]. Of course the potential pool of liver grafts is increasing but in this case the risk of retransplantation is increasing too. Hence 2 or more liver grafts have to be used. So it seems better to refuse poor graft rather than risking to use 2 livers. It is well known the rate of PNF increases as the degree of steatosis of the liver graft does. In the same way, modern preservation solution such as UW is more efficient to reduce preservation lesions within liver grafts.

J.L. Touraine et al. (eds.), Retransplantation, 237–240.

The second way to reduce retransplantation is technical. The procedure to make arterial anastomosis must be perfect to avoid arterial thrombosis. Making arterial anastomosis is probably more hazardous when liver reduction technique or split liver technique is used. Of course problems with arterial anastomosis are more frequent in pediatric surgery because of the size of the vessels. It is advisable to use a microscope if the vessels diameter are less than 5 mm. Stenoses develop at the site of anastomosis. It is possible to detect arterial narrowing with echodoppling and thus to treat arterial stenosis using radiological technique of angioplasty in order to prevent arterial thrombosis of the graft which is the next step leading moreoften to retransplantation [7]. Explaining of development of stenosis is not obvious even if the procedure is perfect other factors such as immunological reaction can be interfering. Molecules expression of the major complex of histocompatibility could be activated by physical process such as traumatism when making anastomosis.

The third way to reduce retransplantation rate is to prevent rejection episodes more accurately. Monoclonal antibodies such as OKT3 efficiently decrease refractory acute cellular rejection episodes and thus reduce the retransplantation rate. Nowadays new immunosuppressive drugs are available. The use of FK506 (Prograf®) in liver transplantation is very efficient in reducing the rate of corticosteroid resistant episodes [8].

Some indications for liver transplantation lead to a higher retransplantation rate such as acute BuddChiari syndrome and primary sclerosis cholangitis. Retransplantations are probably due to thrombosis complications in BuddChiari syndrome and perhaps to recurrence of the disease or immunological problems in primary sclerosis cholangitis.

Let us move now to the results of liver transplantation. It is important to try to avoid retransplantation because the results are not so good as in the case of a first transplantation. How do we explain these bad results? some risk factors leading to death after retransplantation are known. Variables such as donor age, female donor, recipient age, preoperative ventilation assistance, creatinine level, bilirubine level, and immunosuppressive drugs choice (cyclosporine or FK506) induce a higher risk [1]. Time between first and second liver transplantation matters as risk factor: urgent retransplantation is worse than elective one because it's impossible to choose a good graft and look for it in an emergency situation, it's necessary to accept any liver graft even an uncompatible one. The results of retransplantation depend on the number of organs failing. In case of more than four organs showing acute failure, the post operative rate of mortality is over than 90%. It is not uncommon to observe such deficiency as renal, pulmonary, cardiac and of course hepatic failure in emergency conditions or after two, three, or more liver retransplantations. In such case, liver retransplantation indications should be considered with caution.

The other circumstance requiring liver retransplantation is disease recurrence in the graft. Retransplantation is made later after the first graft. The commonest disease in such case is viral hepatitis. There are no many papers on this subjects in literature. Once again recurrence has to be prevented. Unfortunately, not many treatments are available. In case of cirrhosis due to virus B, immunopassive prophylacxis with specific antibodies is efficient [9]. In case of recurrence of hepatitis B on the graft, after prophylacty failure or no prophylacty use, the results of retransplantation are very poor with less than 10% survival rate one year after retransplantation. There is a little hope with new efficient drugs against virus B, may be these new therapeutics such as Lamivudine [10] and Famciclovir will be a help in the treatment of recurrence after retransplantation. In case of posthepatitic cirrhosis due to virus C, there is no efficient prophylacty against recurrence after liver transplantation. Unfortunately recurence is very common, observed in more than 70% of cases, but recurrence evolution is more progressive than it is with hepatitis B. Moreover frequency of cirrhosis C is important and that is at present the main indication for liver graft. Therefore it is easy to imagine a high rate of recurrences in the future. Antiviral treatments such as interferon and Ribavirine are studied [11] to reduce the evolution of recurence and to slow down inflammation and fibrosis in the liver graft. Indications for this treatment in such a case remain to be discussed.

The last point to deal with is economics. The retransplantation cost is two times higher than the first transplantation one [12]. The main reason for this over cost is intensive care unit stay and this is moreoften due to organ failure. Hence all the previously described factors are linked together. Of course the cost of retransplantation is an economic problem at what's more a social problem even, I would go as far as saying a choice by society.

Conclusion

Retransplantation remains an ethical problem because there are not enough liver grafts available but there are no other way to treat acute liver failure, so it is extremely important to avoid this complication after the first transplantation. The risk factor of mortality should be evaluated in function of anamnesis before taking a decision. Late retransplantations could be a more acute problem in the future because of the recurrence rate of liver diseases in specific indications of liver transplantation mainly viral cirrhosis. For ending economic problem is still opened to discussion.

References

1. Doyle HR, Morelli F, McMichael J, Doria C, Aldrighetti L, Starzl TE, Marino IR. Hepatic retransplantation – an analysis of risk factors associated with outcome. Transplantation 1996; 10: 1499–1505.
2. European Liver Transplant Registry. Registry of the European liver Transplant Association. Hôpital Paul Brousse, Villejuif.
3. Anthuber M, Pratschke E, Jauch KW, Zuelke C, Groh J, Welte M, Forst H. Liver retransplantation – indications, frequency, results. Transplant. Proc. 1992; 24: 1965–1966.
4. Fangmann J, Ringe B, Hauss J, Pichlmayr R. Hepatic retransplantation: the Hannover experience of two decades. Transplant. Proc. 1993; 25: 1077–1078.

5. Mora NP, Klintmalm GB, Cofer JB, Poplawski SS, Goldstein RM, Gonwa TA, Husberg BS. Results after liver retransplantation (Retx): a comparative study between elective vs nonelective Retx. Transplant. Proc. 1990; 22: 1509–1511.
6. Ploeg RJ, D'Alessandro AM, Knechtle SJ et al. Risk factors for primary dysfunction after liver transplantation – a multivariate analysis. Transplantation 1993; 55: 807–813.
7. Abbasoglu O, Levy MF, Vodapally MS, Goldstein RM, Husberg BS, Gonwa TA, Klintmalm. Hepatic artery stenosis after liver transplantation – incidence, presentation, treatment, and long term outcome. Transplantation 1997; 63: 250–255.
8. Williams R, Neuhaus P, Bismuth H, McMaster P et al. Two year data from the European Multicentre Tacrolimus (FK506) Liver Study. Transpl. Int. 1996; 9: 1–7.
9. Burbach GJ, Bienzle U, Neuhaus R, Hopf U, Metzger WG, Pratschke J, Neuhaus P. Intravenous or intramuscular anti-HBs immunoglobulin for the prevention of hepatitis B reinfection after orthotopic liver transplantation. Transplantation 1997; 63: 478–480.
10. Ben-Ari Z, Shmueli D, Mor E, Shapira Z, Tur-Kaspa R. Beneficial effect of lamivudine in recurrent hepatitis B after liver transplantation. Transplantation 1997; 63: 393–397.
11. Bizollon T, Palazzo U, Ducerf C, Chevallier M, Elliot M, Baulieux J, Trepo C. Pilot study of a combination of alpha interferon and ribavirin as therapy of recurrent hepatitis C after liver transplantation. Hepatology 1997; in press.
12. D'Alessandro AM, Ploeg RJ, Knechtle ST et al. Retransplantation of the liver – a seven-year experience. Transplantation 1993; 55: 1083–1087.

30. Should we retransplant pancreas?

BÉATRICE CUZIN, NAOUFEL BENRAIS, NICOLE LEFRANÇOIS, MARWAN DAWAHRA, XAVIER MARTIN & JEAN MICHEL DUBERNARD

Introduction

The success rate and the frequency of pancreas transplants have increased in recent years. Pancreas transplantation establishes a neuglycemic, insulin-independant state, and the potential to favorably influence the evolution of secondary complications of diabetes involving the eyes, nerves, and kidneys has been shown. Failure of a pancreas transplant is not an immediate life threatening problem, nevertheless the original course of diabetes is resumed. Thus justifications of pancreas retransplantation will be herein discussed in examining three steps: efficacy justification, economical justification, ethical justification.

Data have been collected from an extensive review of literature (MEDLINE data base from 1986 through 1997): less than 10 articles have been published about the subject.

Efficacy of pancreas retransplant

Overall results of pancreas retransplant

Few experiences have been published about pancreas retransplantation: University of Minnesota Hospital (Minneapolis) experience [1–5], University of Nebraska Medical Center and Clarkson Hospital (Omaha) experience [6] and E. Herriot Hospital of Lyon (France) experience [7].

The University of Minnesota has performed 327 pancreas transplants from 1978 through 1989 including 68 retransplants (21%). The mean age of patients was 33 ± 7 years. Forty seven percent of pancreas retransplant were pancreas alone, 35% were pancreas after kidney retransplants, 18% were simultaneous pancreas and kidney retransplants. Overall patient actuarial survival rates at 1 year were similar after retransplantation and primary transplant (89% versus 91%: non significant (NS)). Overall graft functional actuarial rate at 1 year were also similar after retransplantion and primary transplant (43% versus 46%: NS). Causes of graft losses at one month were similar for retransplants and primary transplants (technical failures 16% versus 18%: NS; rejection 3% versus 6%: NS)

The University of Nebraska Medical Center and Clarkson Hospital have performed 175 pancreas transplants from April 1989 to May 1995 including

J.L. Touraine et al. (eds.), Retransplantation, 241–244.

12 retransplants (7%). Mean age of patients was 37 years; mean duration of diabetes was 25 years and mean follow up was 21 months. Four retransplants were pancreas alone, 7 pancreas after kidney retransplants and 1 simultaneous pancreas and kidney. Mean waiting time for pancreas retransplant was 3.4 months. Overall patient actuarial survival rate at 2 year was 91% and overall graft functional actuarial survival rate at 2 years was 73%. Rejections and major infections were reported in 58% of the patients and operative complications in 12%.

We have performed 220 pancreas transplants from 1986 through 1996 including 17 retransplants (8%). Mean age of the patients was 38 years (range 26–46 years), mean follow up has been 68 months (range 15–123 months). Eleven retransplants were pancreas alone and 6 simultaneous pancreas and kidney. Overall patient survival rate at 1 year and 2 years were 94% and 82% respectively. Overall pancreas graft functional rate at 1 year and 2 years were 64% and 41%; overall kidney graft functional rate at 1 year and 2 years were 94% and 70%. Complications have concerned 52% of the patients: 2 infections (local), 4 early vessels thrombosis, 1 bladder fistula, 1 important bleeding, 1 lymphorrhea.

Risk factors of pancreas retransplant related to patients

Experience from the University of Minnesota Hospital [1–3] has focused on different subpopulations of patients who could represent high risk patients for pancreas retransplantation. Forty-eight second transplants have been performed, 18 third transplants and 4 fourth transplants. There were no significant difference in graft function rates for second versus third and fourth transplants at 1 year: 40% versus 49%: NS; 40% versus 50%: NS. Thus, number of retransplants does not seem to be a risk factor of retransplantation. Eight cases of immediate retransplants after thrombosis of pancreas graft have been performed [3]. Survival rates for patient, pancreas and kidney were similar to other pancreas retransplants. Immediate retransplants does not seem to be a risk factor of retransplantation, but follow up has been limited at 6 months. Of the retransplantations, 13% were performed after a previous pancreas graft had been lost because of an intra-abdominal infection [2]. Ninety two percent were again complicated by intra-abdominal infection, mainly caused by the same microbial species that had caused failure of the previous graft 1 to 5 years earlier. In 83% of infected retransplants, a graft pancreatectomy was necessary to control the infection, in 17% the infection resolved with persistent graft function. Thus, pancreas graft loss caused by intra-abdominal infection is a contraindication to retransplantation.

Risk factors of pancreas retransplant related to technique

Graft function rates according to drainage technique were not significantly different in the experience of University of Minnesota [1], data are not available for the two other centers (small series): with duct occluded technique, graft function rate at 1 year was 10% for retransplants versus 18% for primary transplants: (NS); with intestinal drainage technique, graft function rate at 1 year was 39% for retransplants versus 42% for primary transplants: (NS); with intestinal bladder technique, graft function rate at 1 year was 53% for retransplants versus 60% for primary transplants: (NS).

Graft function rates according to grafted organs for the University of Minnesota Hospital experience [1]: within the pancreas transplant alone and kidney categories, there were no significant differences in graft function rates for retransplants versus primary transplants: at 1 year 48% versus 41% (NS) for all pancreas alone, 40% versus 35% (NS) for all pancreas after kidney, 68% versus 54% (NS) for bladder drained pancreas alone, and 50% versus 53% (NS) for bladder drained pancreas after kidney transplants. However, for simultaneous pancreas and kidney (all bladder drained), the results with retransplants were significantly different than with primary transplants, with 1 year pancreas graft function rates of 32% versus 68% ($p = 0.05$). Within the pancreas transplants alone, four in eleven retransplants were functional at 1 year and five in six within the simultaneous pancreas and kidney transplants. There was no penalty for placing a pancreas retransplant in the same side as a previous transplant [1].

Discussion

Efficacy of pancreas retransplantation seems to be similar to primary transplantation but few data are avalaible, experience is limited, studies are retrospective and non comparative. Conclusion about best retransplantion technique is difficult and results are preliminary. Actually, the best functional results would be obtained with intestinal drainage technique. Even if no data with retransplants have been published with the technique, for the moment, it could be relevant to use it.

Economic justification of pancreas retransplantion

No economic data are available for or against the pancreas retransplantation policy. Economic data are relevant in medicine, only if they provide costs correlated with outcome results (and quality of life): cost-utility, cost-effectiveness studies. Preliminary results from personal sources to be published, have established that the most cost-effective strategy is simultaneous pancreas kidney transplantation compared with other treatment options for type I diabetics with end stage renal disease (dialysis, kidney alone transplant from a cadaver or living donor), but have not focused on pancreas retransplantation.

Ethical justification of pancreas retransplantation

Even in a period of organ shortage, pancreas retransplantation seems to be acceptable. Retransplantation is rare in our experience and in University of

Nebraska Medical Center experience [6]: less than 10% of pancreas transplants. Nevertheless in University of Minnesota experience [1, 2], it represents 20% of overall pancreas transplants. In the centers, mainly pancreas alone retransplants are performed so that it does not appear as harmful to other organ transplants or to primary pancreas transplants (simultaneous pancreas kidney transplants). Waiting time for pancreas alone retransplant is low: it could contribute towards limit the wainting stress of the patient. Indications of simultaneous pancreas kidneys retransplants ought to be discussed since mean waiting time is increased these last years and since primary pancreas transplants are concerned by the decision.

Conclusion

In the pancreas retransplantation policy, efficacy justification seems to be acceptable so that ethical justification. Economical justification is not yet available. Thus, for the moment, pancreas retransplantation appears as a reasonable alternative to be proposed to diabetic patients with pancreas graft loss except for those caused by intra-abdominal infection.

References

1. Morel P, Schlumpf R, Dunn DL, Moudry-Munns K, Najarian JS, Sutherland DER. Pancreas retransplants compared with primary transplants. Transplantation 1991; 51: 825–833.
2. Benedetti E, Troppmann C, Gruessner AC, Sutherlan DER. Pancreas graft loss caused by intra-abdominal infection. A risk factor for a subsequent pancreas retransplantation. Arch. Surg. 1996; 131: 1054–1060.
3. Boudreaux JP, Corry RJ, Sutherland DER. Combined experience with immediate pancreas retransplantation. Transplant. Proc. 1991; 23: 1628–1629.
4. Schlumpf R, Morel P, Moudry-Munns K, Dunn DL, Sutherland DER. An analysis of pancreas retransplants with bladder drainage. Transplant. Proc. 1990; 22: 1602.
5. Morel P, Schlumpf K, Moudry-Munns K, Dunn DL, Sutherland DER. Pancreatic retransplants: an analysis of the outcome. Transplant. Proc. 1990; 22: 620–621.
6. Stratta RJ, Taylor RJ, Sudan D, Sindhi R, Castaldo P. Experience with pancreas retransplantation. Transplant. Proc. 1995; 27: 3020–3021.
7. Sanseverino R, Dubernard JM, Melandri M, Camozzi L, Martin X, Faure Jl, Lefrançois N, Gelet A. Pancreas and kidney retransplantation in insulin-dependant diabetic patients. Diabetes 1989; 38: 238–239.

31. Problems related to retransplantation in pediatric patients

CHRISTER HOLMBERG & JARMO LAINE

During the last 10 years results of kidney, liver and heart transplantation in childhood have steadily improved and are at least equal to those in adults. After renal transplantation five year patient and graft survivals of over 90 and 80%, respectively, can be achieved with FK 506, induction or triple therapy, and in all age groups [1, 2]. The most common causes of graft loss are chronic rejection, acute rejection, recurrence of the basic disease, and technical problems [3].

After liver transplantation 70% of recipients survive more than five years and during the last three years, with increasing use of living related donors, over 80% survival rates have been reported [4]. Causes of graft loss include technical problems, especially hepatic artery trombosis, which is common in small children, rejection and primary non-function.

After heart transplantation 70% survive for 5 years and the results are better for patients with cardiomyopathy compared with children with a congenital defect [5]. Although some patients are lost because of acute rejection, chronic rejection or transplant cardiovascular disease is the most common cause of graft loss also in children [6].

Thus, 20–30% of all children receiving a new kidney, liver or heart lose their new organ and can avoid chronic dialysis or death (in liver and heart recipients) only by successful retransplantation. We will shortly discuss special problems related to, and the results of, retransplantation in childhood.

Recurrence of the original disease

Oxalosis is a metabolic disease in which the main defect is in the liver, but the metabolic disturbance secondarily leads to terminal renal failure. Results of kidney transplantation in these children are poor [7]. Combined liver and kidney transplantation should today be performed, or only liver transplantation early enough to avoid renal pathology. Recurrence of the primary renal disease is seen after glomerulonephritis, amyloidosis and hemolytic-uremic syndrome, but the most problematic diseases in childhood are focal segmental glomerulosclerosis (FSGS), mesangiocapillary glomerulonephritis type I and congenital nephrosis of the Finnish type (CNF). In FSGS recurrence rates of 20% in the first, and up to 70% in the second graft have been reported [8]. Cochat et al.

J.L. Touraine et al. (eds.), Retransplantation, 245–249.

[8] has recently reported success with early treatment of nephrotic syndrome after transplantation with plasmapheresis and cyclophosphamide in three FSGS patients. The recurrence rate of mesangiocapillary glomerulonephritis type I is 13% [9] and we have seen a 17% recurrence rate of severe nephrotic syndrome in CNF children after renal transplantation. Seven out of 39 CNF patients transplanted at our institution developed a nephrotic syndrome after transplantation: two went into permanent remission with early institution of cyclophosphamide instead of azathioprine. Three patients developed nephrosis in the second graft and two of these went into remission with cyclophosphamide. The only common denominator was that all children with a nephrotic syndrome had one DR mismatch and most patients a preceeding CMV or EBV infection [10].

Immunological factors

As discussed in preceeding articles about adult patients, the results after a second renal transplant depend on HLA match. Patients who not share previous mismatches, not have any DR mismatches, and receive a living related donor graft do better after retransplantation also in childhood. Early loss of the first graft and PRA > 20 have led to a less favourable prognosis after retransplantation. Also, early retransplantation, during the first 6 to 12 months after graft loss is followed by a worse outcome [11].

Surgical factors

Although renal retransplantation may be technically more complicated, the main technical problems are encountered in small children with a previous liver transplantation. Reconstruction of vascular anastomosis and biliary flow is much more time consuming and difficult, and extensive blood loss and perforation of the bovel during the operation are more common.

Side effects of immunosuppression

Organ transplantation to a 2–5-year-old child can be considered successful only if normal growth and development are achieved, and a life expectancy of 30–40 years can be assured. Normal growth and development depend on graft function, nutritional and endocrinological status and absence of complications. Even with normal graft function some renal transplant recipients and many liver transplanted children show suboptimal growth [12]. Steroid medication is the main factor causing this growth retardation. Thus, many attempts have been made to stop steroids. However, up to 50% of all renal graft recipients develop late acute rejections and long-term graft function may be reduced after steroid withdrawal [13]. Selected liver transplanted patients can be weaned off steroids without short-time side effects. However, we do not know about their long term graft function, and if steroid withdrawal leads to higher cyclosporine or FK 506 doses the end result may be renal failure in the long run.

Candidates for retransplantation have had several attempts to save their first graft: higher steroid dosing, rescue treatment with FK 506, monoclonal or polyclonal antilymphocyte globulins or mycophenolate mofetil. This period is often accompanied by suboptimal or zero growth. If more aggressive immunosuppression is considered after retransplantation growth inhibition may be severe.

The current immunosuppressants not only have growth inhibiting side effects. The nephrotoxicity of cyclosporine and FK 506 is well known. When we switched our liver transplant patients 1:1 from conventional cyclosporine to the new microemulsion formulation glomerular filtration rate (GFR) decreased more than 15% in one-third of our patients. This change was reversible in most patients with a reduction of their dose [14]. Similarly McDiarmid et al. reported a decrease in GFR from 97 to 51 ml/min/1.73 m^2 when their liver transplanted patients were switched from cyclosporine to FK 506 in a rescue study [15].

High doses and a combination of several immunosuppressants may also increase the risk for future malignancies. Most standard protocols report a 5% risk of developing lymphoproliferative disease, but according to Millis et al. [16] the use of OKT3 or FK 506 as rescue treatment increased this risk to 10%, and a combination of OKT3 and FK 506 to 28%.

Noncompliance

Noncompliance occurs in 25–50% of all pediatric patients and is especially common in adolescents [17]. If a graft is lost due to noncompliance it can be questioned if a second transplantation is justified considering the shortage of grafts. Troppman et al. [18] reported retransplantation in noncompliant patients after thorough interdisciplinary evaluation with excellent results. Our own experience with adolescent patients support their experience. With interdiciplinary support, and after getting through their pubertal crisis, outcome is mostly good.

Results of retransplantation

After renal retransplantation the long term results in children are similar to those in adults. There is no significant difference in survival between first and second living related transplant [19]. Retransplantation with a cadaver graft has a significantly worse outcome than the first cadaver graft. The NAPRTCS data show a 5 year graft survival of 65 and 48%, respectively. Additional risk factors are the previously mentioned ones: suboptimal matching, high PRA, early first graft loss and young or old donors.

Results of liver retransplantation are not encouraging and considering the shortage of organs it can be questioned. However, the timing of the second transplantation has a big influence on outcome. If retransplantation is performed 20–60 days after the first operation failure probability is 70–80%. Early and late retransplantation has a more favourable prognosis [20]. This is explained by the fact that patients with early graft loss due to rejection or more commonly hepatic artery trombosis or primary non function, who not get a new liver within the first days, go into severe liver failure, develop infections, often with multiorgan failure and reduced general condition. Retransplantation in this clinical condition is mostly unsuccesful. On the other hand, children who immediately obtain a new liver or early retransplantation for chronic rejection have an excellent long-term outcome.

There are very few reports of cardiac retransplantation in childhood. Michler et al. [6] reported retransplantation in 17 children with a three year survival of 47%. All four patients retransplanted within 2 months after the first operation died. Eleven patients were retransplanted because of transplant cardiovascular disease and three developed it again in the second graft. All three subsequently died.

Conclusion

Retransplantation with a living related kidney graft has a similar prognosis as in primary transplantation. When retransplantation with a cadaver kidney is considered this should not be performed within the first 6–12 months after the first transplantation. One should avoid similar and DR mismatches, donors less than 16 and more than 40 year old and transplanting patients with high PRA. Retransplantation in children with FSGS is a problem and aggressive treatment of nephrotic syndrome should probably be instituted early [8]. In CNF children it is possible that a prerequisite for transplantation should be zero mismatches in DR. Thus, nephrosis in the first graft with recurrence in the second might be avoided.

After liver transplantation retransplantation should probably only be performed within the first weeks after transplantation if the child still is in good general condition and no infection is present. Another good candidate is a child with chronic rejection without major complications.

Retransplantation after heart transplantation is questionable. Exceptions may be children, who develop transplant coronary artery disease late after transplantation and whose general condition is still good. Recurrence will probably be seen in many patients.

In all children with allografts one has to consider growth, development, renal function and quality of life for the child and the family. We must bear in mind that aggressive immunosuppression, massive rescue therapy and stronger immunosuppression after retransplantation may lead to reduced growth, renal failure, early malignancy and reduced quality of life. Thus treatment has to be individualized and must aim at normal growth and development in addition to a functioning allograft.

References

1. Shapiro R, Scantlebury VP, Jordan ML et al. FK 506 in pediatric kidney transplantation – primary and rescue experience. Pediatr. Nephrol. 1995; 9: S43–S48.
2. Holmberg C, Laine J, Rönnholm K, Ala-Houhala M, Jalanko H. Congenital nephrotic syndrome. Kidney Int. 1996; 49 (Suppl. 53): S51–S56.
3. Chavers B, Kim E-M, Matas AJ, Gillingham KJ, Najarian JS, Mauer SM. Causes of single allograft loss in a large pediatric population at a single center. Pediatr. Nephrol. 1994; 8: 57–61.
4. Salt A, Noble-Jamieson G, Barnes ND et al. Liver transplantation in 100 children: Cambridge and King's College Hospital series. BMJ 1992; 304: 416–421.
5. Koerner MM, Tenderich G, Mannebach H et al. Heart transplantation at the Heart Center North Rhine-Westphalia in Bad Oeyenhausen – 1995 report. In: Cecka JM, Terasaki PI (eds.), Clinical Transplantation 1995. Los Angeles, UCLA Tissue Typing Laboratory, 1996; 137–144.
6. Michler RE, Edwards NM, Hsu D et al. Pediatric retransplantation. J. Heart Lung Transplant. 1993; 12: S319–S327.
7. Broyer M, Brunner FP, Brynger H et al. Kidney transplantation in primary oxalosis: Data from the EDTA registry. Nephrol. Dial. Transplant. 1990; 5: 332–336.
8. Cochat P, Kassir A, Colon S et al. Recurrent nephrotic syndrome after transplantation: early treatment with plasmapheresis and cyclophosphamide. Pediatr. Nephrol. 1993; 7: 50–54.
9. Habib R, Gagnadoux M, Broyer M. Recurrent glomerulonephritis in transplanted children. Contrib. Nephrol. 1987; 55: 123–135.
10. Laine J, Jalanko H, Holthöfer H et al. Posttransplantation nephrosis in patients with congenital nephrotic syndrome of the Finnish type. Kidney Int. 1993; 44: 867–874.
11. Almond PS, Matas AJ, Gillingham K et al. Risk factors for second renal allografts immunosuppressed with cyclosporine. Transplantation 1991; 52: 253–258.
12. Sarna S. Mechanisms and treatment of growth retardation in children with liver transplants (dissertation). Helsinki (Finland): Univ. of Helsinki, 1997.
13. Reisman L, Lieberman KV, Burrows L, Schanzer H. Follow-up of cyclosporine-treated pediatric renal allograft recipients after cessation of prednisone. Transplantation 1990; 49: 76–80.
14. Laine J, Hoppu K, Jalanko H, Rönnholm K, Holmberg C. Kidney function after 1:1 conversion to the cyclosporine microemulsion formulation in children with liver allografts. Transplantation 1997 (in press).
15. McDiarmid SV, Wallace P, Vargas J, Ament ME, Busuttil RW. The treatment of intractable rejection with tacrolimus (FK506) in pediatric liver transplant recipients. J Pediatr. Gastroent. Nutr. 1995; 20: 291–299.
16. Millis JM, Alonso EM, Piper JB et al. Liver transplantation at the University of Chicago. In: Cecka JM, Terasaki PI (ed.), Clinical Transplantation 1995. Los Angeles: UCLA Tissue Typing Laboratory, 1996: 187–197.
17. Meyers K, Weiland H, Thomson P. Pediatric renal transplantation non-compliance. Pediatr. Nephrol. 1995; 9: 189–192.
18. Troppman C, Benedetti E, Gruessner RWG et al. Retransplantation after renal allograft loss due to noncompliance. Transplantation 1995; 59: 467–471.
19. Tejani A, Sullivan EK. Factors that impact on the outcome of second renal transplantation in children. Transplantation 1996; 62: 606–611.
20. Doyle HR, Morelli F, McMichael J et al. Hepatic retransplantation – an analysis of risk factors associated with outcome. Transplantation 1996; 61: 1499–1505.

32. Living donors in kidney retransplantation

DAVID E. R. SUTHERLAND, KRISTIN GILLINGHAM, MICHAEL CECKA, JOHN S. NAJARIAN, WILLIAM D. PAYNE, RAINER W. G. GRUESSNER & ARTHUR J. MATAS

Introduction

Living donors have been used for a large number of kidney retransplants, but so rarely for extra-renal organs that an analysis is not possible. Hence, the data and discussion presented here on living donors is restricted to the kidney.

Much of the debate on retransplants evolves around the use of a scarce resource – suitable cadaver organs. If one argues that organs should be given to individuals with the highest probability of successful outcome, there are some candidates for retransplants who have a higher probability of success than some candidates from primary transplants. If one argues that the organ should go to those whose treatment alternatives are the worst, then again there are retransplant candidates who should have priority for a cadaver organ.

The arguments regarding allocation of cadaver organs go on endlessly, but the debate is completely stilled by use of living donors. Here the debate is only on the risk to the donor and the right to take a risk to do good for someone else, someone else usually being a loved one.

It is, of course, of interest to compare the results of retransplants to those of primary transplants, and within both categories the results with living versus cadaver donors. In this paper the data from two analyses are presented, one from a registry and one from a single center. The first set of data is for transplants done in the USA as reported to the UNOS/UCLA Registry during the period 1988–95. The second is for transplants done at the University of Minnesota between 1980 and 1986 in cyclosporine-treated recipients.

UNOS USA kidney graft analyses

Within the UNOS data base two analyses were done. The first simply compared overall results for living donors versus cadaver donor retransplants in recipients in which the first transplant was done either before or after 1997 (Table 1 and Figure 1). The second UNOS analysis compared the results of retransplants in which both the first and second transplant were done since 1987 in one or the other of the following sequences (1st/2nd): cadaver/cadaver, living/living, cadaver/living, living/cadaver (Figure 2).

In regard to the overall UNOS analysis for primary versus retransplant (Table 1) in both the living donor and cadaver donor categories, the results of

J.L. Touraine et al. (eds.), Retransplantation, 251–259.

Table 1. UNOS kidney transplant 1 and 3 year graft survival rates for all cases, 1988–1995

	Primary (*N*) 1 year	Retransplant (*N*) 3 year	Primary (*N*) 3 year	Retransplant (*N*) 3 year
LRD	92% (19 591)	90% (1631)	84% (19 591)	82% (1631)
CAD	83% (48 597)	78% (8702)	74% (48 597)	67% (8702)

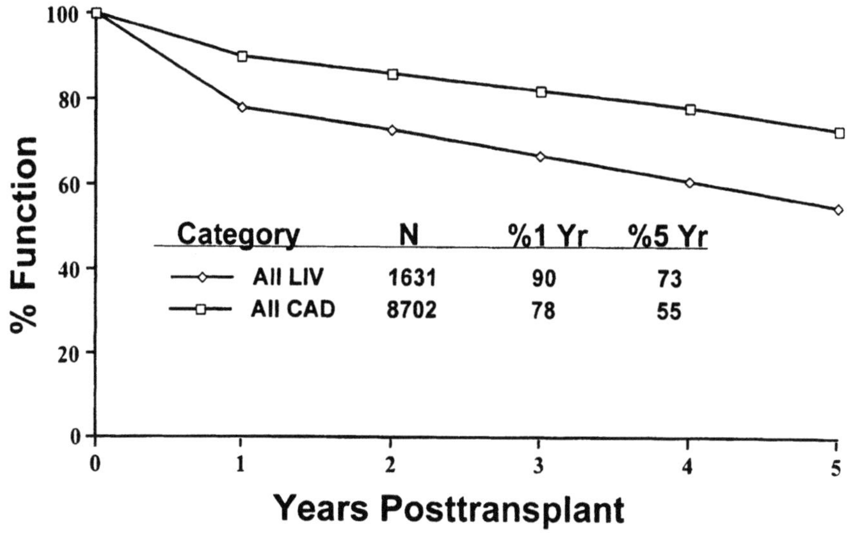

Fig. 1. UNOS USA retransplant graft survival rates by 2nd donor type (1st transplant pre- or post-1987), 1988–1996.

retransplants were only slightly less good that for primary transplants. Living donor results were also considerably better than cadaver donor results including in the retransplant categories (Figure 1). Indeed, living donor retransplant results were better than primary cadaver results (Table 1).

In regard to outcome with living donor and cadaver retransplants according to source of the first transplant (living or cadaver) in the UNOS data base, the only factor that mattered was the source of the second transplant (Figure 2). Kidney graft survival rates (non-death censored) were similar for living donor retransplants done after failure of a cadaver or living donor graft. Likewise, cadaver donor kidney retransplant survival rates were similar for those done after failure of a cadaver or living donor graft. The important point is that living donor retransplants have higher graft survival rates than cadaver donor retransplants no matter what the source of the first transplant (Figure 2).

It should be noted that in the UNOS data, retransplants done after 1987 in patients transplanted before 1987 have higher graft survival rates that those done in patients whose first transplant was post-1987. The difference may be

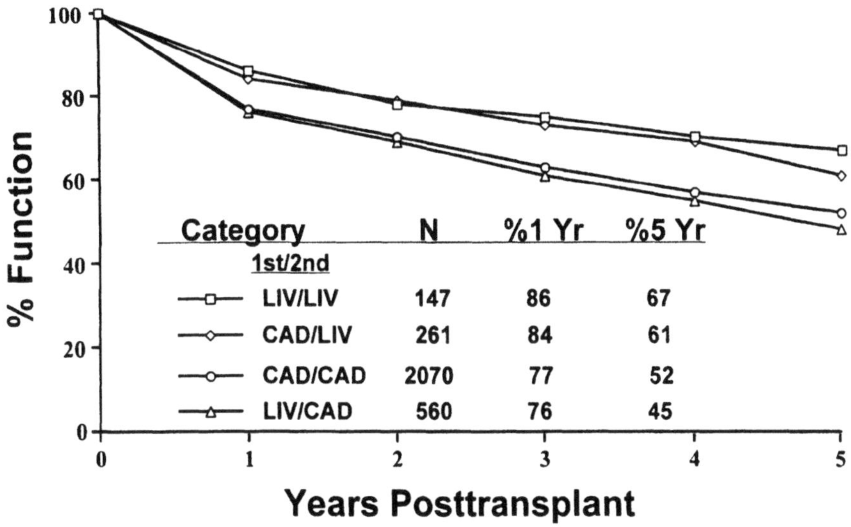

Fig. 2. UNOS USA retransplant graft survival rates by 1st/2nd donor type (both transplants post-1987), 1988–1996.

because many pre-1987 first transplant recipients receive less potent immunosuppression (no cyclosporine or FK506 available), but were able to receive these drugs for retransplants, while the first transplant recipients done post-1987 rejected while on cyclosporine or FK506 and there is nothing more potent to offer (true high responders).

University of Minnesota analysis

The Minnesota data is mostly concordant with the UNOS data, although the retransplant graft survival rates tend to be higher in the various categories. In the analysis of kidney retransplant graft survival rates (non-death censored) for living donor versus cadaver donor transplants according to the source of the first transplant (living or cadaver), again an important factor is the source of the retransplant, living donor retransplants doing equally well after failure of the first transplant from either a cadaver or living donor and better than cadaver retransplants done after failure of either a cadaver or living donor first transplant (Figure 3).

Patient survival rates did not differ for living versus cadaver donor retransplant recipients regardless of donor source of the first transplant (Figure 4). Interestingly, in the death censored analysis, there was really little difference in retransplant graft survival rates according to donor source (Figure 5). Indeed, in this analysis, the graft survival rates were highest when the donor category of the retransplant was the same as the first transplant. It

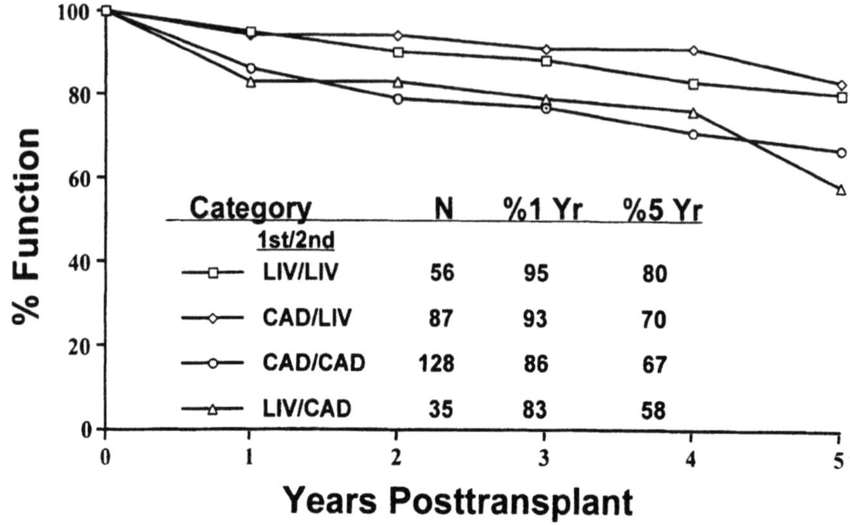

Fig. 3. Minnesota kidney retransplant graft function in CSA Rx patients by 1st/2nd donor type, 1980–1996.

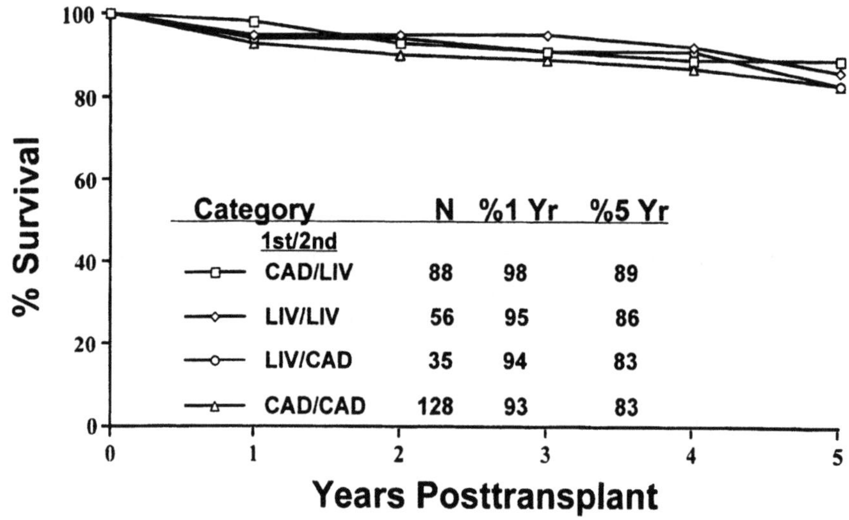

Fig. 4. Minnesota kidney retransplant recipient survival in CSA Rx patients by 1st/2nd donor type, 1980–1996.

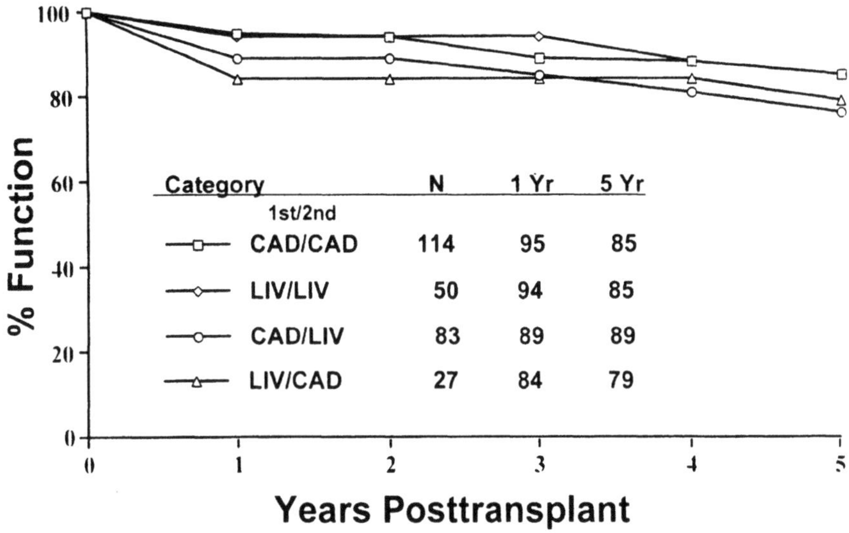

Fig. 5. Minnesota death censored kidney retransplant graft survival by 1st/2nd donor type, 1984–1997.

Table 2. One year graft function rate for kidney retransplants

1st	2nd	2nd
	CAD/CAD (*N*)	**LIV/CAD (*N*)**
Technical failure	83% (12)	100% (2)
Immunological loss	90% (103)	79% (25)
	CAD/LIV (*N*)	**LIV/LIV (*N*)**
Technical failure	89% (9)	100% (3)
Immunological loss	88% (74)	89% (47)

also means death with a functioning retransplant was more likely to occur in a cadaver/cadaver sequence than with the other sequences. With this caveat, again it is apparent that it is preferable to retransplant from a living donor.

We also analyzed Minnesota transplant results according to whether the first transplant was lost for technical or immunological reasons (Table 2). There were very few first transplant losses for technical reasons ($N = 26$) and following retransplantation only three second kidney were lost for any reason. Thus, retransplants after technical loss of the first graft were highly successful. On the other had, retransplants after immunological losses are equally high, particularly when the second kidney comes from a living donor.

In regard to a comparison of Minnesota primary versus retransplant results within the cadaver donor category there is no difference in graft (non-death censored) (Figure 6) or patient survival (Figure 7) rates, regardless of the donor

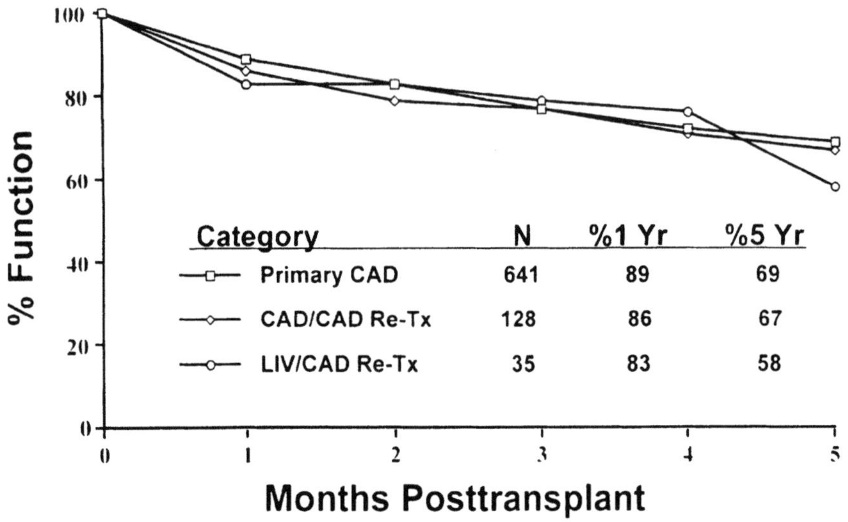

Fig. 6. Minnesota cadaver kidney graft function for primary vs retransplant CSA Rx patients 1980–1996.

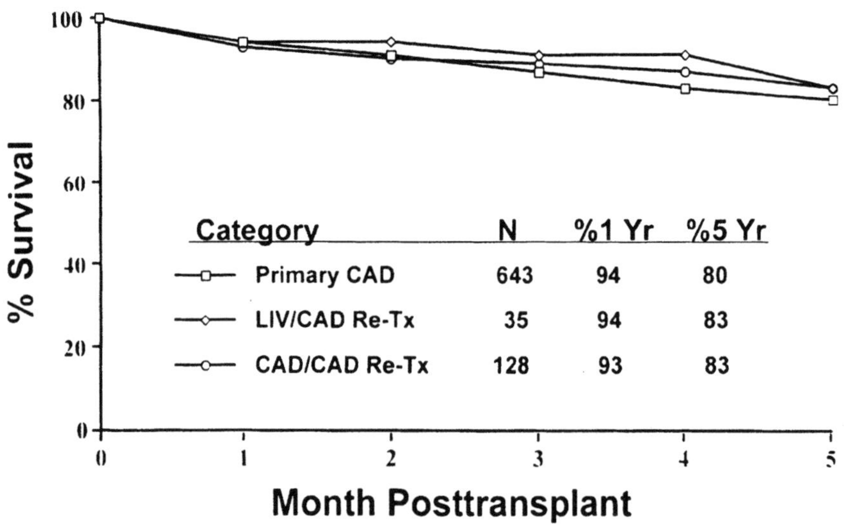

Fig. 7. Minnesota cadaver donor kidney recipient survival for primary vs retransplant CSA Rx patients, 1980–1996.

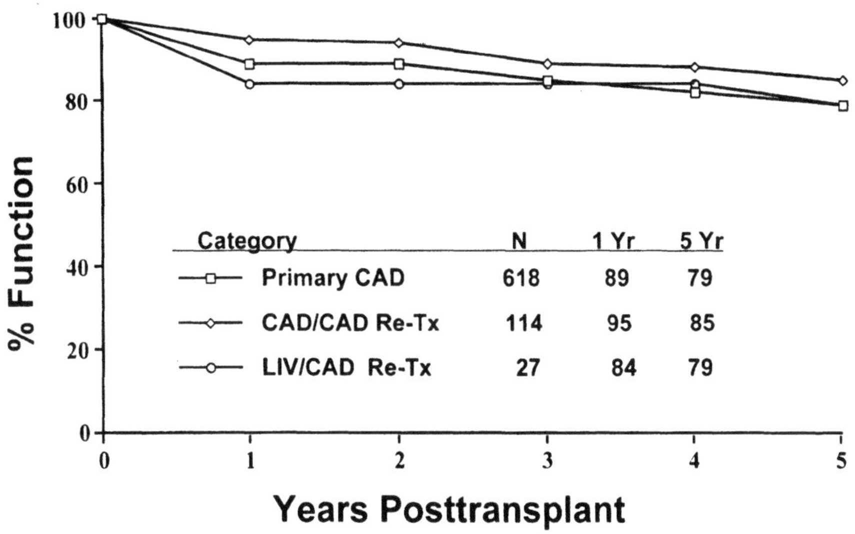

Fig. 8. Minnesota death censored kidney graft function for cadaver primary vs retransplants, 1984–1997.

source of the first transplant. The death censored analysis also showed that the results of primary and retransplants from cadaver donors were similar (Figure 8). There is, however, a greater tendency for recipients of sequential cadaver donor transplants to die with a functioning retransplant.

In the living donor category the graft survival rates (non-death censored) for primary and retransplants were similar of the source of the first transplant (Figure 9). After one year, living donor retransplant graft survival rates were slightly less good for those in whom the first transplant was from a cadaver donor.

Patient survival rates were identical for recipients of primary or retransplants from living donors regardless of the source of the patients kidney (Figure 10). Graft survival rate within the death censored analysis were similar for primary and living donor retransplants when the first transplant was also from a living donor (Figure 11). For living donor retransplants in recipients whose first graft was from a cadaver, second graft survival rates were slightly less high than for primary transplants.

Summary and conclusion

Living donor kidney retransplants survival rates are similar (living/living) or nearly similar (cadaver/living) to those with primary living donor transplants. A living donor is always preferable for a retransplant because waiting time is eliminated and graft survival rates are higher than those of cadaver donor

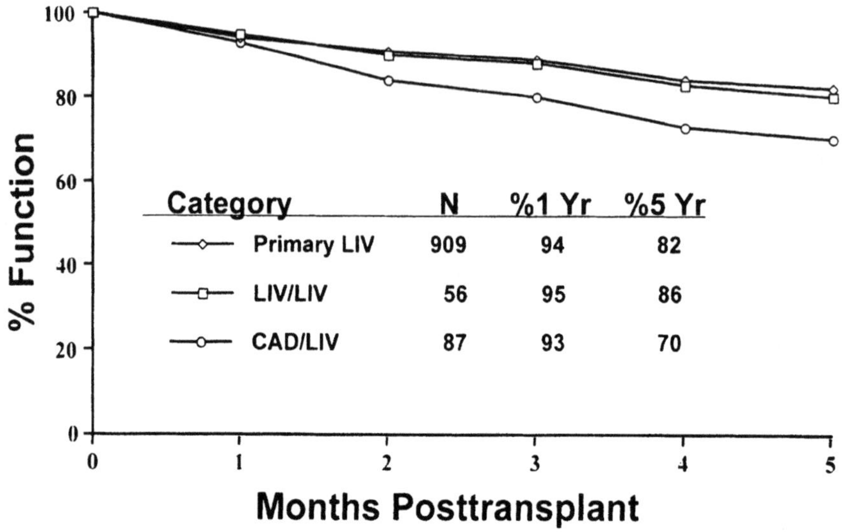

Fig. 9. Minnesota living donor kidney graft function for primary vs retransplant CSA Rx patients, 1980–1996.

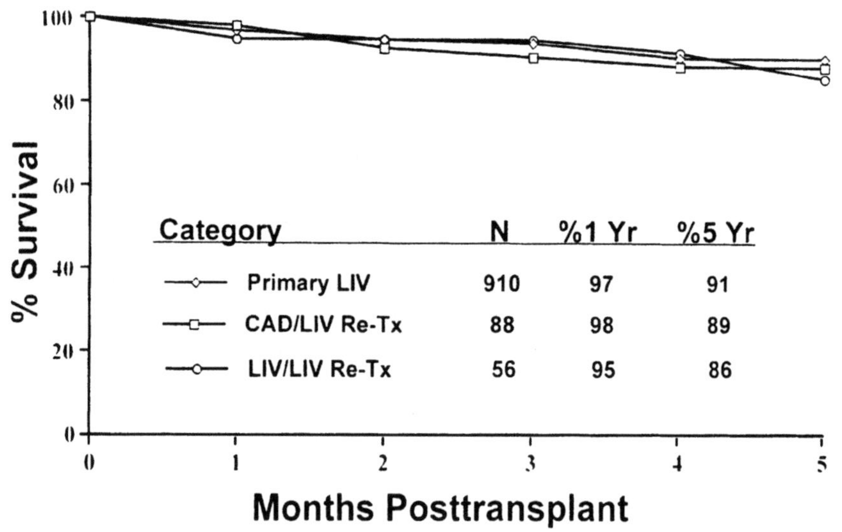

Fig. 10. Minnesota living donor recipient survival for primary vs retransplant CSA Rx patients, 1980–1996.

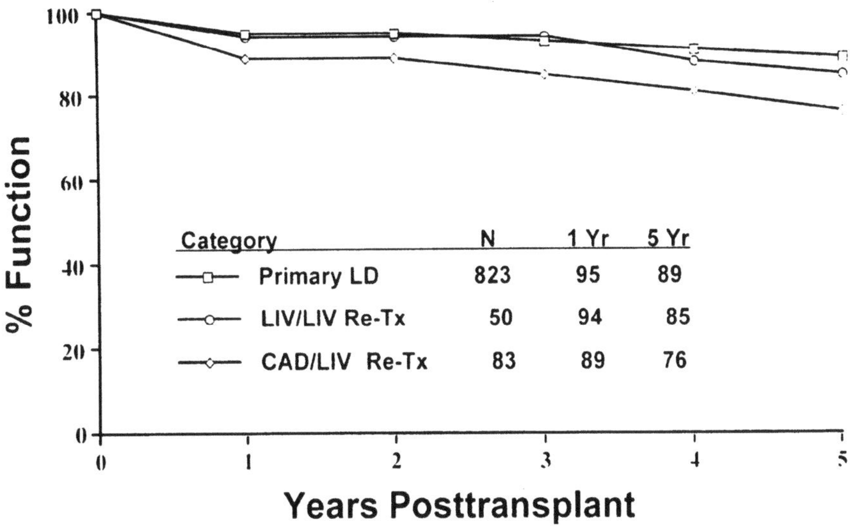

Fig. 11. Minnesota death censored kidney graft function for living primary vs retransplants.

retransplants. Indeed, living donor retransplant results are better than cadaver donor primary transplants. Even thought the results of cadaver kidney transplants were also good, some individuals suggest that retransplant candidates should have a lower priority than primary transplant candidates for access to a scarce resource. Living donor retransplants completely obviates this argument, and also gives the highest probability of success.

33. Retransplantation: is the trouble worth the effort?

ROGER W. EVANS & DANIEL J. KITZMANN

The merits of retransplantation have often been debated [1–15]. Opponents are of the opinion that patients who have not had a previous transplant should be given a fair opportunity to receive one. Proponents of retransplantation argue that organs should be allocated based on medical urgency. They believe that patients awaiting their first graft stand a reasonable chance of receiving a donor organ at a later date. A retransplant candidate often has a diminished probability of survival.

Fairness is an abstract concept that is relative to circumstances. Although informative, philosophical debate on this topic rarely serves as the basis for unequivocal public policy. People with opposing views usually offer plausible arguments on metaphysical issues. Data are not always available to inform decisions and, when they exist, their validity is frequently disputed.

Costs and outcomes, as well as risks and benefits, are no longer pedestrian issues in transplantation [16–23]. They are often at the forefront of any discussion concerning the allocation of public and private resources.

By any standard, transplantation constitutes expensive medical technology [24, 25]. As shown in Figure 1, the total first year cost of all transplants exceeds \$100 000, with liver transplants costing over three times as much [24, 25]. Five-year charges are even more impressive (Figure 2). Based on these data, it

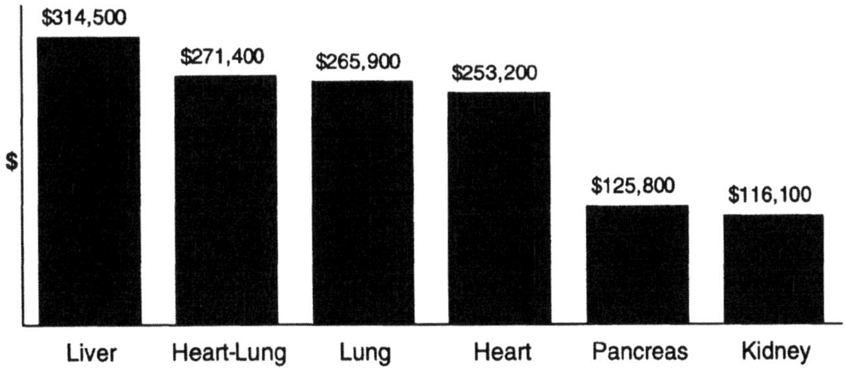

Fig. 1. Estimated total first-year transplantation charges, 1996. Source: Ref. 25.

J.L. Touraine et al. (eds.), Retransplantation, 261–273.

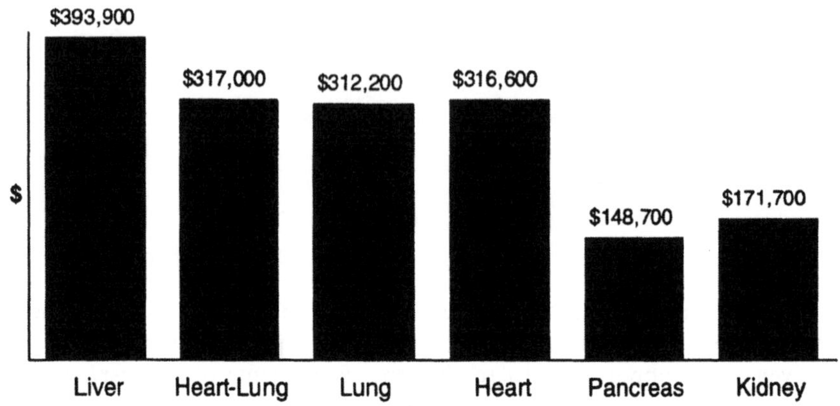

Fig. 2. Estimated total five-year transplantation charges, 1996. Source: Ref. 25.

is clear why public policy makers remain concerned as to the economic implications of organ transplantation.

Outcomes have also become a major issue in public debate concerning health care reform [26–35]. Providers are expected to compete on the basis of both outcomes as well as costs. Those organizations that are able to provide cost-effective transplant services in an economically efficient manner are in the best position to maintain a favorable market share [23].

The prudent management of risk is a major challenge for viable transplant programs [23]. Conservative patient selection is essential if costs are to be contained and outcomes are to be enhanced. Programs that insist on transplanting high-risk patients will jeopardize their future. Their services are likely to be excessively expensive and of poor quality in comparison with the competition. Moreover, as has been suggested, there is a clear public mandate for cost-effective health care. In turn, this constitutes a utilitarian philosophical orientation to health care [36].

Given these data, thoughts, and expectations, we will attempt to put retransplantation into perspective. We will not rely on abstract philosophical arguments that are often as dubious as the persons who express them. From a sociological perspective, we must interpret the pervasive currents that now dominate contemporary thinking concerning health care policy.

Data

Two primary data sources have been used for this analysis. The first of these is the United Network for Organ Sharing (UNOS) Scientific Registry for Organ Transplantation [37]. The second is the National Cooperative Transplantation Study (NCTS) [38, 39].

UNOS Scientific Registry

The UNOS Scientific Registry contains data that facilitates the continuous evaluation of the clinical and scientific status of transplantation in the Untied States. The specific goals of the Registry are (1) to collect, in a computer system, data on all transplant patients and all transplant programs in the USA, (2) to provide a database enabling periodic reporting of transplantation effectiveness, nationwide, and (3) to provide a national database for basic and clinical research on organ transplantation. The Scientific Registry collects data about recipient status at the time of transplant and at time of post-transplant hospital discharge. The Registry also collects follow-up data on transplant recipients until 2 years following graft failure or until the patient dies, regardless of cause of death. Each year, summary results of the Scientific Registry are published by UNOS in an annual report. Less frequently, a separate report is published on 'center-specific' graft and patient survival [40].

National Cooperative Transplantation Study

In August 1989, all kidney, heart, liver, heart-lung, and pancreas transplant programs in the United States were invited to participate in the National Cooperative Transplantation Study (NCTS) [38, 39]. The NCTS is the only national study ever conducted to examine the financial aspects of all transplant procedures. It is unlikely that a study such as the NCTS will ever be conducted again. Not only was the study expensive, but the competitive pressures of managed care make it unlikely that transplant centers will share financial data. In doing so, their competitive advantage may be compromized.

For purposes of the NCTS, financial data were to be provided on up to 25 patients for each type of transplant each transplant center performed. This restriction was imposed because of the considerable effort required to retrieve detailed billing data from each transplant hospital. The data were also restricted to transplants performed in 1988. Patients were randomly selected from a national sampling frame maintained by UNOS. Each patient within each transplant center had an equal probability of selection.

A hospital cost summary form was completed by a hospital financial representative for each patient. This form included an itemized list of transplant procedure charges, as well as information regarding length of hospital stay, sources of payment, and the amount reimbursed by third-party payers. The itemized charges included (1) medical, surgical, and central supplies, (2) operating room and anesthesia, (3) pharmacy, (4) laboratory and diagnostic tests, (5) radiology and nuclear medicine, (6) blood administration, (7) oxygen and gas mixtures, (8) room and board, (9) histocompatability testing, (10) dialysis, (1 1) other, (12) professional fees, including surgeons and others, and (13) donor organ acquisition.

Results

Table 1 summarizes data pertaining to the UNOS waiting list and the number of transplants performed for 1988 and 1995 [37]. As shown, in 1988, the year-end waiting list consisted of 16 026 patients, compared with 42 744 in 1995. In 1988, extrarenal transplant candidates represented 13% of the patients on the list, compared with 17.1% in 1995. The number of transplants performed increased by 57% between 1988 and 1995. In 1988, 43.5% of all transplants were extrarenal, compared with 57.1% in 1995 [37].

Table 2 provides summary data on the distribution of retransplant candidates on the year-end UNOS waiting list for 1988 and 1995 [37]. A separate percentage is shown for organ-specific transplant candidates, as well as all transplant candidates. In 1988, cadaveric donor kidney transplant candidates constituted 24.6% of the waiting list. This percentage decreased to 16.5% in 1995. Overall, of those persons awaiting a transplant at year end in 1988, 26% were retransplant candidates, compared with 18% in 1995.

As indicated in Table 2, the actual number of patients awaiting retransplant at year end has increased considerably – from 70 in 1988 to 613 in 1995 [37]. In 1988, 98% of all retransplant candidates were awaiting a kidney, compared with 91% in 1995. In 1995, liver transplant patients constituted 5% of all retransplant candidates.

Table 3 provides summary data on retransplant recipients for 1988 and 1995 [37]. As indicated, in 1988, patients receiving a regraft constituted 13% of all transplant recipients, compared with 9% in 1995. The actual number of retransplant recipients increased by about 16% (from 1596 to 1846). In 1988, patients who received kidney retransplants constituted 71% of all repeat procedures, compared with 59% in 1995.

As these data indicate, the number of persons on the waiting list in need of a retransplant has continued to increase, as has the number of persons who actually receive a retransplant procedure.

Survival data

Primary and regraft transplant recipient survival data are summarized in Table 4 [37]. As shown, the data for cadaveric kidney transplant recipients is similar, whether the patient receives a primary or a regraft procedure. Living donor kidney retransplant results diminished with time in comparison with primary grafts. Most importantly, however, patient survival for liver, pancreas, and kidney transplant regraft recipients is much poorer than that of patients who have received only one transplant. At 5 years, the differences are 22.9%, 13.1%, and 29.5%, respectively.

Table 5 summarizes data similar to the above for graft survival [37]. As shown, at 5 years, there are substantial differences between regraft and primary

Table 1. Distribution of all patients on the UNOS waiting list at year end, including transplant recipients

	Waiting list				Transplants			
Transplant	1988		1995		1988		1995	
Cadaveric kidney	13943	(87.0%)	31 149	(72.9%)	7230	(56.5%)	8598	(42.9%)
Living donor kidney	–	–	–	–	1811	(14.2%)	3212	(16.0%)
Liver	616	(3.8%)	5701	(13.3%)	1713	(13.4%)	3926	(19.0%)
Pancreas	163	(1.0%)	286	(0.7%)	249	(1.9%)	1028	(5.1%)
Heart	1030	(6.4%)	3468	(8.1%)	1676	(13.1%)	2360	(11.8%)
Lung	69	(0.4%)	1932	(4.5%)	33	(0.3%)	871	(4.3%)
Heart-lung	205	(1.3%)	208	(0.5%)	74	(0.6%)	69	(0.3%)
Totals	16026	(99.9%)	42744	(100.0%)	12786	(100.0%)	20064	(100.0%)

Source: Ref. 37.

Table 2. Distribution of retransplant candidates on the year-end UNOS waiting list

Transplant	1988			1995		
	No.	As % of organ-specific transplant candidates	As % of all transplant candidates	No.	As % of organ-specific transplant candidates	As % of all transplant candidates
Cadaveric kidney	3937	28.2	25.57	7043	22.6	16.48
Living donor kidney	–	–	–	–	–	–
Liver	39	6.3	0.24	354	6.2	0.83
Pancreas	4	2.5	0.02	85	29.7	0.20
Heart	26	2.5	0.16	90	2.6	0.21
Lung	1	1.4	0.00	78	4.0	0.18
Heart-lung	0	0.0	0.00	6	2.9	0.01
Totals	4007	–	25.99	7656	–	17.91

Table 3. Distribution of retransplant recipients based on year-end UNOS data

Transplant	1988			1995		
	No.	As % of organ-specific transplant recipients	As % of all transplant recipients	No.	As % of organ-specific transplant recipients	As % of all transplant recipients
Cadaveric kidney	1130	15.7	8.84	1083	13.4	5.40
Living donor kidney	152	8.4	1.19	266	8.8	1.33
Liver	247	14.4	1.93	388	9.9	1.93
Pancreas	18	7.2	0.14	31	3.0	0.15
Heart	45	2.7	0.35	64	3.5	0.32
Lung	2	6.1	0.12	13	2.0	0.06
Heart-lung	2	2.7	0.12	1	1.9	0.00
Totals	1596	–	12.69	1846	–	9.19

Source: Ref. 37.

graft survival rates for all transplant procedures. Once again, however, the differences are greatest for liver, pancreas, and heart transplantation.

Clearly, as these data show, the results of retransplantation are inferior to those associated with primary procedures. In fact, as shown in Table 6, since 1988 there has been virtually no change in the results for heart transplantation [11]. Meanwhile, both the primary and regraft survival rates for liver transplantation have improved remarkably, although the margin of difference between primary and regraft procedures is now greater than it was previously (18.6% versus 24.9%).

Table 4. Primary and regraft transplant recipient survival rates

Transplant	One year (%)			Three year (%)			Five year (%)		
	Primary	Regraft	Difference	Primary	Regraft	Difference	Primary	Regraft	Difference
Cadaveric kidney	93.4	93.3	−0.1	87.5	88.0	+0.5	80.5	81.5	+1.0
Living donor kidney	97.4	96.4	−1.0	94.4	92.1	−2.3	90.6	87.1	−3.5
Liver	83.2	58.3	−24.9	76.6	52.7	−23.9	71.7	48.8	−22.9
Pancreas	90.7	87.5	−3.2	84.5	73.0	−11.5	79.7	66.6	−13.1
Heart	83.4	58.6	−24.8	75.7	48.9	−26.8	68.5	39.0	−29.5
Lung	73.5	43.0	−30.5	57.8	32.7	−25.1	n.d.	n.d.	n.d.
Heart-lung	62.9	n.d.	n.d.	50.1	n.d.	n.d.	39.7	n.d.	n.d.

n.d. = no data.
Source: Ref. 37.

Table 5. Primary and retransplant recipient graft survival rates

Transplant	One year (%)			Three year (%)			Five year (%)		
	Primary	Regraft	Difference	Primary	Regraft	Difference	Primary	Regraft	Difference
Cadaveric kidney	82.0	76.0	−6.0	70.6	64.9	−5.7	60.2	54.1	−6.1
Living donor kidney	91.7	88.8	−2.9	84.4	81.0	−3.4	75.9	71.3	−4.6
Liver	73.1	50.3	−22.8	65.3	42.5	−22.8	59.8	37.8	−22.0
Pancreas	74.7	50.9	−23.8	65.2	25.1	−40.1	53.3	23.7	−29.6
Heart	82.4	57.3	−25.1	74.1	46.6	−27.5	66.5	36.6	−29.9
Lung	71.9	41.1	−30.8	54.6	31.3	−23.3	40.1	n.d.	n.d.
Heart-lung	62.9	n.d.	n.d.	50.1	n.d.	n.d.	39.7	n.d.	n.d.

n.d. = no data.
Source: Ref. 37.

Table 6. Comparative 1-year patient survival rates for primary grafts and retransplantation in 1988 and 1995

Transplant	Year 1988	Year 1995
Heart		
Primary	83.3%	83.4%
Regraft	60.9	58.6
Liver		
Primary	68.7	83.2
Regraft	50.1	58.3

Source: Ref. 11.

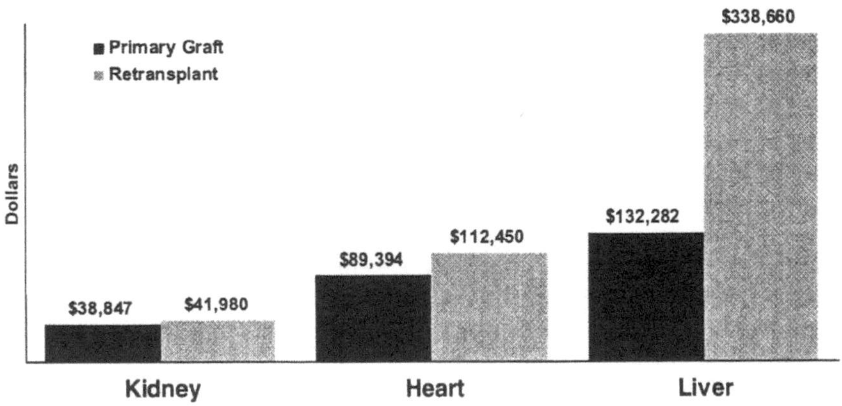

Fig. 3. Comparative charges for primary grafts and retransplantation. Source: Ref. 11.

Cost data

Figure 3 summarizes the relevant financial data for primary grafts and retransplant procedures [11]. As shown, for kidney, heart, and liver transplantation, the charges for retransplantation exceed those for primary grafts. However, the differences are most striking for heart and liver transplantation, but relatively small for kidney transplantation. Thus, taken together, these data suggest that kidney retransplantation is about as cost-effective as a primary procedure.

Discussion

In absolute numbers, the demand for retransplantation continues to increase. Unfortunately, with the exception of kidney retransplantation, regrafts are typically inferior to primary grafts with respect to both outcomes and costs.

As a result, retransplantation compromises the overall cost-effectiveness of transplantation at the very same time health care policymakers are vigorously debating the appropriate allocation of increasingly limited health care dollars [41–58]. In this regard, clinicians must recognize that each donor organ is a resource from which society must extract maximum utility. For every retransplant performed, another patient is potentially denied an opportunity to ever benefit from a donor organ. However, in the event that no other suitable candidate is awaiting a transplant, a donor organ may be appropriately allocated to a retransplant candidate. However, even under this circumstance, cost-effectiveness should remain a consideration.

The clinical mentality is rarely consistent with public health goals yet, today, policymakers are asking physicians to think in what must be regarded as a foreign language. Managed care is little more than a system that requires implicit rationing at the local level [59–67]. Thus, as policymakers promote public health, they expect managed care to be the mechanism whereby their principles are put into action [68–70]. As a result, few clinicians understand the insidious nature of the relationship between managed care and the rationing of health care resources. Historically, rationing has been thought of in terms of explicit criteria applied at the societal level. Clearly, this approach has been obviated by policymakers. Physicians are now responsible for making the very decisions they have preferred to avoid.

Managing care means limiting resource utilization consistent with an available budget. In the case of transplantation, there are two different resources that must be managed – donor organs and costs. In many respects, retransplantation represents a gross mismanagement of both these resources. As such, the trouble is not worth the effort.

References

1. Stratta RJ, Oh CS, Sollinger HW, Pirsch JD, Kalayoglu M, Belzer FO. Kidney retransplantation in the cyclosporine era. Transplantation 1988; 45: 40–45.
2. Dein JR, Oyer PE, Stinson EB, Starnes VA, Shumway NE. Cardiac retransplantation in the cyclosporine era. Ann. Thorac. Surg. 1989; 48: 350–355.
3. Salmela K, Kyllonen L, Eklund B, Isoniemi H, Hockerstedt K, Ahonen J. The value of repeated renal transplantation. Transplantation 1990; 50: 984–986.
4. Gordon RD, Hartner CM, Casavilla A et al. The liver transplant waiting list – a single-center analysis. Transplantation 1991; 51: 128–134.
5. Mora NP, Klintmalm GB, Cofer JB et al. Results after liver retransplantation in a group of 50 regrafted patients: two different concepts of elective versus emergency retransplantation. Transplant. Int. 1991; 4: 231–234.
6. Candinas D, Keusch G, Conrad B, Schlumpf R, Decurtins M, Largiader F. A 20-year follow-up of cadaveric kidney allotransplantation. Transplant Proc. 1992; 24: 2711–2713.
7. Ensley RD, Hunt S, Taylor DO et al. Predictors of survival after repeat heart transplantation. The Registry of the International Society for Heart and Lung Transplantation, and Contributing Investigators. J. Heart Lung Transplant. 1992; 11: S142–S158.
8. Karwande SV, Ensley RD, Renlund DG et al. Cardiac retransplantation: a viable option? The Registry of the International Society for Heart and Lung Transplantation. Ann. Thorac. Surg. 1992; 54: 840–844.

9. Retransplantation termed unfair, cost-ineffective. UNOS Update 1992; 8: 4.
10. Evans RW. A cost-outcome analysis of retransplantation: the need for accountability. Transplant. Rev. 1993; 7: 163–175.
11. Evans RW. Is retransplantation cost-effective? Transplant. Proc. 1993; 25: 1694–1696.
12. Michler RE, Edwards NM, Hsu D et al. Pediatric retransplantation. J. Heart Lung Transplant. 1993; 12: S319–S327.
13. Michler RE, McLaughlin MJ, Chen JM et al. Clinical experience with cardiac retransplantation. J. Thorac. Cardiovasc. Surg. 1993; 106: 622–631.
14. Mentzer SJ, Reilly JJ, Caplan AL, Sugarbaker DJ. Ethical considerations in lung retransplantation. J. Heart Lung Transplant. 1994; 13: 56–58.
15. Smith JR, Ribakove GH, Hunt SA et al. Heart retransplantation: the 25-year experience at a single institution. J. Heart Lung Transplant. 1995; 14: 832–839.
16. Evans RW, Manninen DL, Dong FB. An economic analysis of liver transplantation: costs, insurance coverage, and reimbursement. Gastroenterol Clin. North Am. 1993; 22: 451–473.
17. Evans RW. Organ transplantation and the inevitable debate as to what constitutes a basic health care benefit. In: Terasaki PI, Cecka JM (eds.), Clinical Transplants, 1993. Los Angeles, CA: UCLA Tissue Typing Laboratory, 1994: 359–391.
18. Evans RW. Liver transplantation in a managed care environment. Liver Transplant. Surg. 1995; 1: 61–75.
19. Evans RW. Organ transplantation in an era of economic constraint: liver transplantation as a case study. Semin. Anesthesiol. 1995; 14: 127–135.
20. Evans RW. Socioeconomic aspects of heart transplantation. Curr. Opin. Cardiol. 1995; 10: 169–179.
21. Evans RW. Effect of liver transplantation on local, regional, and national health care. In: Busuttil RW, Klintmalm GB (eds.), Transplantation of the Liver. Philadelphia, PA: W.B. Saunders, 1996: 869–879.
22. Evans RW, Kitzmann DJ. Contracting for services: liver transplantation in the era of mismanaged care. Clinics in Liver Disease 1997; 1: (in press).
23. Evans RW, Kitzmann D. The 'arithmetic' of donor liver allocation. In: Terasaki PI, Cecka JM (eds.), Clinical Transplants, 1996. Los Angeles, CA: UCLA Tissue Typing Laboratory, 1997.
24. Hauboldt RH. Cost Implications of Human Organ Transplantations, An Update: 1993. Brookfield, WI: Milliman and Robertson, Inc., 1993.
25. Hauboldt RH. Cost Implications of Human Organ and Tissue Transplantation, An Update: 1996. Brookfield, WI: Milliman & Robertson, 1996.
26. Relman AS. Assessment and accountability; the third revolution in medical care. N. Engl. J. Med. 1988; 319: 1220–1222.
27. Lohr KN. Outcome measurement; concepts and questions. Inquiry 1988; 25: 37–50.
28. Epstein AM. The outcomes movement – will it get us where we want to go? N. Engl. J. Med. 1990; 323: 266–270.
29. Geigle R, Jones SB. Outcomes measurement: a report from the front. Inquiry 1990; 27: 7–13.
30. Hopkins A, Costain D. Measuring the Outcomes of Medical Care. London, England: Royal College of Physicians of London, 1990.
31. Clinton JJ. Outcomes research – a way to improve medical practice. JAMA 1991; 266: 2057.
32. Delamothe T. Outcomes into Clinical Practice. London: BMJ Publishing, 1994.
33. Guadagnoli E, McNeil BJ. Outcomes research: hope for the future or the latest rage? Inquiry 1994; 31: 14–24.
34. Dauphinee WD. Assessing clinical performance: where do we stand and what might we expect? JAMA 1995; 274: 741–743.
35. Hayward J. Promoting clinical effectiveness. Br. Med. J. 1996; 312: 1491–1492.
36. Evans RW. A critical perspective on the tools to support clinical decision making (editorial). Transfusion 1996; 36: 671–673.
37. Annual Report of the U.S. Scientific Registry for Transplant Recipients and the Organ Procurement and Transplantation Network – Transplant Data. Richmond, VA: UNOS and the U.S. Department of Health and Human Services, 1996.

38. Evans RW, Manninen DL, Dong FB. The National Cooperative Transplantation Study: Final Report. Seattle, WA: Battelle-Seattle Research Center, 1991.
39. Evans RW. Executive Summary: The National Cooperative Transplantation Study. Report BHARC-100-91-020. Seattle, WA: Battelle-Seattle Research Center, 1991.
40. Division of Organ Transplantation, United Network for Organ Sharing. 1994 Report of Center-Specific Graft and Patient Survival Rates: Liver Data. Rockville, MD: Health Resources and Services Administration, 1994.
41. Evans RW. Health care technology and the inevitability of resource allocation and rationing decisions, Part I. JAMA 1983; 249: 2047–2053.
42. Evans RW. Health care technology and the inevitability of resource allocation and rationing decisions, Part II. JAMA 1983; 249: 2208–2219.
43. Evans RW. Advanced medical technology and elderly people. In: Binstock RH, Post SG (eds.), Too Old for Health Care? Controversies in Medicine, Law, Economics, and Ethics. Baltimore, MD: The Johns Hopkins University Press, 1991: 44–74.
44. Evans RW. Rationale for rationing. Health Management Quarterly 1992; 14: 14–17.
45. Smith R. Rationing in Action. London: BMJ Publishing Group, 1993:
46. Bowling A, Jacobson B, Southgate L. Health service priorities: exploration in consultation of the public and health professionals on priority setting in an inner London health district. Soc. Sci. Med. 1993; 37: 851–857.
47. Heginbotham C. Health care priority setting: a survey of doctors, managers, and the general public. In: Smith R (ed.), Rationing In Action. London: BMJ Publishing Group, 1993: 141–156.
48. Ham C. Health care rationing. Br. Med. J. 1995; 310: 1483–1484.
49. Smith R. Being creative about rationing. Br. Med. J. 1996; 312: 391–392.
50. Bowling A. Health care rationing: the public's debate. Br. Med. J. 1996; 312: 670–674.
51. Maynard A. Rationing health care. Br. Med. J. 1996; 313: 1499.
52. Klein R. Defining a package of healthcare services the NHS is responsible for: the case against. Br. Med. J. 1997; 314: 506–509.
53. New B. Defining a package of healthcare services the NHS is responsible for: the case for. Br. Med. J. 1997; 314: 503–505.
54. Kmietowciz Z. Rationing is now accepted as inevitable by all sides. Br. Med. J. 1997; 314: 461.
55. Harrison S. Central government should have a greater role in rationing decisions: the case against. Br. Med. J. 1997; 314: 970–973.
56. Lenaghan J. Central government should have a greater role in rationing decisions: the case for. Br. Med. J. 1997; 314: 967–970.
57. Doyal L. Rationing within the NHS should be explicit: the case for. Br. Med. J. 1997; 314: 1114–1118.
58. Coast J. Rationing within the NHS should be explicit: the case against. Br. Med. J. 1997; 314: 1118–1122.
59. Iglehart JK. The American health care system: managed care. N. Engl. J. Med. 1992; 327: 742–747.
60. Iglehart JK. Physicians and the growth of managed care. N. Engl. J. Med. 1994; 331: 1167–1171.
61. Iglehart JK. The struggle between managed care and fee-for-service practice. N. Engl. J. Med. 1994; 331: 63–67.
62. Jolt H, Leibovici MM. Managed Care: Principles and Practice. Philadelphia, PA: Hanley & Belfus, 1995.
63. Kassirer JP. Is managed care here to stay? N. Engl. J. Med. 1997; 336: 1013–1014.
64. Jensen GA, Morrisey MA, Gaffney S, Liston DK. The new dominance of managed care: insurance trends in the 1990s. Health Aff. 1997; 16: 125–136.
65. Chernew M, Fendrick AM, Hirth RA. Managed care and medical technology: implications for cost growth. Health Aff. 1997; 16: 196–206.
66. Herzlinger RE. Market-driven health care: who wins, who loses in the transformation of America's largest service industry. Reading: Addison-Wesley, 1997.

67. Wilkerson JD, Devers KJ, Given R. Competitive Managed Care: The Emerging Health Care System. San Francisco: Jossey-Boss, 1997:
68. Reiser SJ. Medicine and public health: pursuing a common destiny. JAMA 1996; 276: 1429–1430.
69. Hearn W. Time for medicine, public health to join forces. Am. Med. News. 1996; 39: 3.
70. Stapleton S. Linking medicine, public health. Am. Med. News 1997; 40: 3.

34. Ethics of retransplantation in a context of organ shortage

R. M. ARNOLD

Objective

To critically analyze the ethical arguments for and against the retransplantation of solid organs.

Data sources

Literature review of both biomedical and ethical sources, and informal discussions with transplant surgeons, organ procurement staff, and philosophers. A previously published article, Ubel PA, Arnold RM, Caplan AL. Rationing failure: the ethical lessons of the retransplantation of scare, vital organs. *JAMA* 1993; 20(270): 2469–2474, was relied on heavily.

Data extraction

Cognitive analysis of the various arguments and counter-arguments found in the literature.

Data synthesis

The most common arguments for retransplant found in the literature are that: (1) transplant surgeons have a special responsibility to patients they have transplanted and (2) that if retransplantations are discouraged, surgeons will be less likely to utilize 'marginal donors' increasing mortality. Arguments against retransplantation concentrate on: (3) the argument that retransplant candidates should not get a 'second chance' until everyone gets a first chance. Argument (1), (2) or (3) are not defensible.

The decision on retransplantation should depend on whether there is a significant difference in efficacy between primary transplantation and retransplantation. Answering this question raises a number of other issues: (a) balancing a transplantation's efficacy and the urgency of a patient's need; (b) determining what constitutes a significant difference in mortality; (c) determining what constitutes sufficient evidence of a difference in mortality; and (d) determining how to handle retransplantation in light of insufficient data.

Conclusion

Neither the most common arguments for or against transplantation hold up to critical analysis. The only defensible argument concerning the defensibility of retransplantation depends on its efficacy compared to primary transplantation. Further work to reach agreement regarding what constitutes valid data and what constitutes a significant difference in mortality needs to be done.

J.L. Touraine et al. (eds.), Retransplantation, 275.

35. Improving long-term graft survival as a means to reduce retransplantation

LEENDERT C. PAUL

Introduction

Long-term follow-up studies of renal transplant patients have shown that chronic rejection is the single most prevalent cause of graft failure after the first post-transplant year [1]. It is not known how many of these patients will undergo retransplantation but data from our own institution suggest that 60–70% of retransplants lost a previous graft due to chronic rejection. There are no large registry data available to directly confirm this impression but of the more than 14 000 second cadaver kidney transplants reported to the Collaborative Transplant Study Registry, 57% had a previous graft that had lasted for more than 6 months and 49% had a previous graft that had lasted for more than 1 year. As chronic rejection is the single most important cause of graft failure in this time frame, it would seem that avoidance of chronic rejection will reduce the need for retransplantation. The aim of the current review is to evaluate the risk factors of chronic rejection and to suggest strategies to decrease its prevalence.

Chronic rejection

Chronic rejection is a slowly progressive form of graft dysfunction that usually becomes clinically apparent after the first 6 post-transplant months, does not respond to currently used immunosuppressive drugs and is characterized by irreversible lesions in the vessels, the glomerular and peritubular capillaries and the tubulointerstitial compartment [2]. The most characteristic lesion is graft atherosclerosis, a picture consisting of concentric intimal thickening accompanied by infiltration of the vessel wall with mononuclear cells and reduction in the luminal area available for blood flow as a result of adventitial fibrosis [3]. The vascular lesions are usually accompanied by variable glomerular and peritubular capillary lesions, tubular atrophy and interstitial fibrosis [4–6]. The latter lesion is most sensitive but least specific for chronic rejection [7]. While its exact pathogenesis remains to be determined, recent clinical and experimental studies have pointed out that both immune and non-immune mechanisms are involved that all seem to converge in a growth factor cascade that results in excessive formation of scar tissue and irreversible organ damage.

J.L. Touraine et al. (eds.), Retransplantation, 277–287.

Risk factors

Transplant registries and single centre studies have identified various risk factors of chronic rejection including prolonged ischemic exposure, delayed graft function, acute rejection episodes, impaired graft function at 6 months and perhaps viral infections, hyperlipidemia and hypertension.

Acute rejection episodes. The most consistently identified risk factor of chronic rejection of kidney transplants is the occurrence of acute rejection episodes, an observation at variance with the findings in heart transplant patients in whom acute rejection episodes have only a small impact on the long-term prognosis [8]. As most acute rejection episodes in renal transplant patients do not result in chronic rejection, it is not entirely clear which acute rejection episodes impact on the long-term outcome. It has been suggested that the number of acute rejection episodes [9–12], their timing of occurrence [10–13], their severity [12], their histopathologic expression pattern [14] or the residual graft function following anti-rejection treatment [8] are important determinants. Whereas the overall number of acute rejection episodes is an independent risk factor in many studies [9–12], the timing of their occurrence seems also important as rejection episodes within the first 3 months do not impact on the late outcome; rejections after the first or second year, on the other hand, are strongly associated with chronic rejection [10–12]. Severe rejection episodes, defined by 50% or more decline in graft function, are also associated with an increased likelihood of chronic rejection [11]. Experimental studies have shown that the rejection frequency, severity and duration combined correlate strongly with histopathological features of chronic rejection later on [15].

A cohort study of cadaveric renal transplants followed for up to 10 years after transplantation showed that early vascular rejection, occurring within 3 months after transplantation is the most important predictor of both early and late graft loss [14]. During the first 3 months, 16% of patients developed vascular rejection and 24% developed interstitial rejection. One-year graft survival of patients without rejection, with interstitial rejection, and with vascular rejection was 88%, 87% and 49% respectively; the five-year survival was 74%, 71% and 34% respectively [14].

Finally, recent data from the Collaborative Transplant Group show that the long-term graft survival in patients who attained a 1-year serum creatinine value of <130 μmol/l after a rejection treatment was only slightly lower compared to patients who experienced no rejection episodes during the first year while the long-term prognosis was inferior in patients with a history of one or more acute rejection episodes who had an impaired graft function at 1 year [8]. Of interest is the finding that an impaired graft function at 1 year in patients without an acute rejection episode is also associated with an inferior prognosis compared with patients with an acute rejection episode but an excellent graft function at 1 year [8]. A similar effect of graft function at

6 months and long-term prognosis has been reported from single centre studies [16, 17].

Ischemia-reperfusion damage. Several studies have demonstrated the impact of ischemia-reperfusion damage on both short – and long-term graft outcome [18–20]. Analysis of the UNOS data file has shown a significant negative effect of delayed graft function on the graft attrition rate after the first transplant year [19].

The Munich transplant group conducted several years ago a randomized controlled trial in which the free radical scavenger superoxide dismutase was administered to renal transplant patients at the time of surgery to mitigate post-ischemic injury and demonstrated that the drug decreased the incidence of late graft loss [21, 22]. Further support for a role of ischemia-reperfusion damage in the development of chronic graft rejection comes from experimental studies that have shown that prolonged ischemia enhances immune-dependent lesions in kidney grafts with chronic rejection [23].

Cytomegalovirus infection. Viral infections, specifically cytomegalovirus (CMV) infections, have been implicated in the pathophysiology of chronic rejection in various animal models, including kidney models of chronic rejection [24–26]. Sero-epidemiologic studies in heart transplant patients have furthermore shown a correlation between post-transplant CMV infection and graft atherosclerosis [27]. Although CMV infections in renal transplant patients have been associated with a specific glomerular lesion postulated to evolve into transplant glomerulopathy, later studies have failed to confirm this relationship [28]. Several more recent studies have shown a lack of correlation between CMV infection and chronic kidney graft rejection [12, 29].

Hyperlipidemia. Abnormalities in circulating lipoproteins are common after renal transplantation and include elevations in total and LDL cholesterol and increases in VLDL and triglycerides. Although it is tempting to speculate that risk factors for systemic atherosclerosis could also contribute to the pathogenesis of chronic rejection, the evidence is indirect. The vascular lesions of chronic rejection may contain foam cells and lipoprotein deposits [30] and experimental studies of cardiac and aortic transplants have shown that hypercholesterolemia [31] alone or in combination with hypertriglyceridemia [32] acts synergistically with allogeneic immune reactions in the pathogenesis of graft atherosclerosis. Many clinical studies reported associations between pre- or post- transplant cholesterol and chronic rejection [33–37] while others studies found no correlation [36, 38]. A multivariate analysis of multiple post-transplant risk factors has shown that only hypertriglyceridemia is a risk factor for chronic rejection, independent of many risk factors known to raise triglycerides, such as diabetes mellitus [12].

Treatment of heart transplant patients with the HMG-CoA reductase inhibitor pravastatin decreases the incidence of clinically severe acute rejection episodes, resulting in an improvement in one year survival and a decrease in both the incidence and progression of graft vascular disease [39]. In kidney transplant patients, pravastatin also decreased the incidence of acute rejection episodes [40] but it is unclear whether this beneficial effect is related to the lipid-lowering properties of the drug or whether it results from drug-related increased immunosuppression. It is furthermore unknown whether these drugs will protect against the development of chronic rejection.

Hypertension. The presence of hypertension in the post-transplant period portends a poorer outcome for the renal transplant, with a faster decline in creatinine clearance and a greater likelihood of return to dialysis or death [36, 41, 42]. Univariate analysis showed that hypertension is a risk factor for chronic rejection but this effect is not independent of other risk factors [12]. Interestingly, it was recently reported that hypertension was an important predictor of chronic rejection in African–Americans but not in Caucasians [43]. There is insufficient clinical data available that show that lowering of the blood pressure improves graft prognosis [42, 44].

Immunosuppression

Standard immunosuppression prior to 1982 consisted of the combination of corticosteroids, azathioprine and, in a few selected centres, the prophylactic use of anti-T cell antisera or antibodies. The addition of cyclosporine A in the 1980s resulted in a decrease in the incidence of acute rejection episodes and an improved 1-year graft survival rate but it has not affected the rate of graft attrition after the first post-transplant year [45]. This raises the question whether its beneficial immunosuppressive effect is counterbalanced by its nephrotoxic side effects [46] or whether inadequate drug doses have been utilized in the late post-transplant period because of concerns of nephrotoxicity [13, 47]. However, immunosuppressive drug regimens in which cyclosporine was administered for only a limited time period shortly after transplantation have shown no differences in long-term graft survival, at least in centres with mostly well-matched grafts [48]. Moreover, non-controlled comparison of less well matched patients treated with or without cyclosporine has failed to show any beneficial effect of cyclosporine on graft loss from chronic rejection in either univariate or multivariate analysis [12].

A single centre study of the effect of immunosuppressive regimens on the incidence of chronic rejection has suggested that powerful treatment regimens, including the prophylactic use of anti-T cell antibodies may prevent the development of chronic rejection [49]. However, analysis of a large group of patients reported to the Collaborative Transplant Study showed no significant influence of prophylactic treatment with polyclonal or monoclonal antibodies on long-term outcome [8]. When analyzing patients whose rejections had been treated either with steroid pulses or with polyclonal or monoclonal antibodies, the long-term outcome in patients with a 1-year creatinine level of $<130\ \mu$mol/l was similar, suggesting that even severe rejections have no marked deleterious effect on long-term outcome, provided they are completely reversible [8]. One could argue, however, that anti-rejection treatments with biological products is a priori more likely to result in more complete reversal of a rejection episode and therefore a better graft function at one year.

There has been a recent surge of new immunosuppressive drugs and approaches that have all shown to be effective to prevent chronic rejection in animal models. Experimental immune-tolerance inducing strategies using blockade of T cell co-stimulatory pathways can prevent chronic rejection [50, 51]. Rapamycine [52–54], deoxyspergualin [55], leflunamine [56–58] and mycophenolic mofetil [59, 60] have all been shown to inhibit chronic rejection to a variable degree in various models but their clinical efficacy to prevent or treat chronic rejection remains to be tested.

Several of these drugs have recently been introduced for clinical use, including FK506 (tacrolimus) and CellCept® (mycophenolate mofetil), while other drugs like rapamycin (sirolimus) are currently undergoing phase III clinical testing. A recently published multicentre study compared the efficacy of FK506 with cyclosporine gel capsules and found a significant reduction in the incidence of biopsy-confirmed acute rejection episodes in the FK506 group [61]. Comparison of long-term graft survival in a small group of FK506-treated patients with more than 35 000 cyclosporine-treated patients reported to the UNOS Kidney Transplant Registry showed a significantly longer projected half-life in FK506-treated patients [62], suggesting that FK506 may be more effective to prevent chronic rejection but caution is warranted since the data were not obtained from a randomized trial, the FK506 follow-up data were scarce and centre-restricted, and important data regarding dosing levels, rejection therapies and protocols were not analyzed.

The efficacy of mycophenolate mofetil to prevent acute rejection has recently been tested in three multicentre clinical trials. Each of these trials showed that the drug reduced the incidence of acute rejection episodes by about 40% [63–66] but it remains to be seen whether this is associated with a decrease in chronic rejection as the drug seems to be effective to prevent early rejection episodes and it is unknown whether it affects vascular rejection episodes, the type of acute rejection that is associated with late graft loss [14].

Growth factor cascade

The stereotypic tissue response following injury consists of cell migration and proliferation, matrix remodelling and programmed cell death, processes controlled by a myriad of enzymes, cytokines and growth factors released in response to injury. Growth factors are produced by a variety of cells in response to a range of stimuli and exert their action by binding to their respective receptors on cell surfaces, followed by activation of intracellular signal transduction pathways and nuclear transcription factors. The same peptide ligand can have both stimulatory or inhibitory activities in a single cell in-vitro, depending on the differentiation state of the cell and the presence of other growth factors [67]. Therefore, the combination of growth factors and cytokines, rather than the presence of one particular growth factor is the most important determinant for a given biological response.

Experimental studies have shown increased expression of various macrophage-derived cytokine mRNAs and proteins in rat renal transplants with chronic rejection, including RANTES and monocyte chemoattractant protein-1 [68], platelet-derived growth factor and the corresponding receptor [69], transforming growth factor β and fibroblast growth factor-1 while the levels of epidermal growth factor are decreased [70]. As many more growth regulatory molecules may be involved, it remains to be determined which of these molecules is rate limiting in the tissue remodelling process and amenable to therapeutic interventions.

Interventions

As alluded to, experimental studies have shown that immune tolerance in experimental animals can prevent chronic rejection [50, 51] but there is no evidence to date that a similar approach in humans is feasible. Moreover, most of the newer immunosuppressive drugs, especially those that also inhibit proliferation of smooth muscle cells or myofibroblasts, prevent chronic rejection when given prophylactically in such animal models [54, 60] but there is currently no maintenance immunosuppressive regimen that has unequivocally shown to decrease chronic rejection in humans. Uncontrolled comparisons of different drug regimens have suggested that FK506-based immunosuppression is associated with a reduced rate of graft attrition after the first year but there are no formal studies to test this hypothesis [62]. Mycophenolate mofetil and rapamycine are currently tested in clinical trials [66] but their efficacy to prevent chronic rejection remains to be demonstrated.

Several non-immunosuppressive drugs have been tested in experimental models, including eicosanoid and PAF-antagonists (reviewed in [71]), heparinoids [72], somatostatin analogs [73], insulin-like growth factor antagonists [74], angiotensin-converting enzyme inhibitors, and angiotensin receptor blockers [75, 76]. Although anecdotal clinical studies support the hypothesis that angiotensin receptor blockers are beneficial in chronic rejection [77], controlled clinical trials are needed to provide formal proof. However, any intervention aimed to reduce graft loss from chronic rejection will require large numbers of patients that will need several years of follow-up [78, 79].

While none of the recommendations proposed to avoid chronic rejection have been tested formally, it would seem prudent to recommend the following strategies. First, avoid graft damage as a result of ischemia-reperfusion injury. While superoxide dismutase given at the time of surgery seems effective to prevent chronic rejection [21], the drug does not universally prevent changes [80] and the availability of the drug is questionable. For now, the only practical way to minimize ischemia-reperfusion damage is to keep cold and warm ischemia as short as possible. It is conceivable that monoclonal antibodies that prevent the influx of neutrophils in damaged tissues will soon be used in clinical practise. Secondly, acute rejection episodes should be treated aggressively to ensure complete reversal of graft function [8]. Surveillance biopsies are perhaps needed to diagnose vascular lesions which should be treated promptly [14]. It is unknown more aggressive treatment of late acute rejection episodes will decrease the incidence of chronic rejection. The impact of anti-viral therapy on chronic rejection is unknown at this stage and there is no clinical data to show that lipid or blood pressure lowering will decrease graft loss from chronic rejection. The lack of data is no justification to ignore the post-transplant hypertension and hyperlipidemia as they will very likely impact on patient cardiovascular morbidity and mortality. Based on animal data, the use of antihypertensive drugs, especially angiotensin-converting enzyme inhibitors or angiotensin receptor blockers prolongs graft survival in chronic rejection [75] but careful monitoring of graft function and electrolytes is necessary.

Strategies to treat post-transplant hyperlipidemia have recently been reviewed [81, 82]. With the current financial pressures on health care systems there is a tendency to transfer long-term follow up of renal transplant patients to primary health care physicians but careful long-term follow up with appropriate counselling on medication and monitoring of drug adherence [83] should remain a high priority in all transplant centres.

References

1. Schweitzer EJ, Matas AJ, Gillingham KJ et al. Causes of renal allograft loss. Progress in the 1980s, challenges for the 1990s. Ann. Surg. 1991; 214: 679–688.
2. Paul LC, Häyry P, Foegh M et al. Diagnostic criteria for chronic rejection/accelerated graft atherosclerosis in heart and kidney transplants: joint proposal from the Fourth Alexis Carrel Conference on Chronic Rejection and Accelerated Arteriosclerosis in Transplanted Organs. Transplant. Proc. 1993; 25: 2022–2023.
3. Luo H, Nishioka T, Eigler NL et al. Coronary artery restenosis after balloon angioplasty in humans is associated with circumferential coronary constriction. Arterioscler. Thromb. Vasc. Biol. 1996; 16: 1393–1398.
4. Barrientos A, Portoles J, Herrero JA et al. Glomerular hyperfiltration as a nonimmunologic mechanism of progression of chronic renal rejection. Transplantation 1994; 57: 753–756.
5. Cheigh JS, Mouradian J, Soliman M et al. Focal segmental glomerulosclerosis in renal transplants. Am. J. Kidney Dis. 1983; 2: 449–455.
6. Hamburger J, Crosnier J, Dormont JA. Observations in patients with a well tolerated homotransplanted kidney. Ann. NY Acad. Sci. 1964; 120: 558–577.
7. Solez K, Axelsen RA, Benediktsson H et al. International standardization of criteria for the histologic diagnosis of renal allograft rejection: The Banff working classification of kidney transplant pathology. Kidney Int. 1993; 44: 411–422.

8. Opelz G. Critical evaluation of the association of acute with chronic graft rejection in kidney and heart transplant recipients. Transplant. Proc. 1997; 29: 73–76.
9. Ferguson R. Acute rejection episodes-best predictor of long-term primary cadaveric renal transplant survival. Clin. Transplant. 1994; 8: 328–331.
10. Matas AJ, Gillingham KJ, Payne WD, Najarian JS. The impact of an acute rejection episode on long-term renal allograft survival (*t*1/2). Transplantation 1994; 57: 857–859.
11. Massy ZA, Guijarro C, Kasiske BL. Clinical predictors of chronic renal allograft rejection. Kidney Int. 1995; 48 (Suppl. 52): S85–S88.
12. Massy ZA, Guijarro C, Wiederkehr MR, Ma JZ, Kasiske BL. Chronic renal allograft rejection: immunologic and nonimmunologic risk factors. Kidney Int. 1996; 49: 518–524.
13. Almond PS, Matas A, Gillingham KJ et al. Risk factors for chronic rejection in renal allograft recipients. Transplantation 1993; 55: 752–757.
14. Van Saase JLCM, Van der Woude FJ, Thorogood J et al. The relation between acute vascular and interstitial renal allograft rejection and subsequent chronic rejection. Transplantation 1995; 59: 1280–1285.
15. Yilmaz S, Yilmaz A, Häyry P. Chronic renal allograft rejection can be predicted by area under the serum creatinine versus time curve (AUC_{Cr}). Kidney Int. 1995; 48: 251–258.
16. Cole E, Naimark D, Aprile M et al. An analysis of predictors of long term cadaveric renal allograft survival. Clin. Transplant. 1995; 9: 282–288.
17. Ferguson RM. Aspects of allograft rejection. II: risk factors in renal allograft rejection. Transplant. Rev. 1995; 9: 121–126.
18. Sanfilippo F, Vaughn WK, Spees EK, Lucas BA. The detrimental effects of delayed graft function in cadaver donor renal transplantation. Transplantation 1984; 38: 643–648.
19. Cecka JM, Terasaki PI. The UNOS scientific renal transplant registry. In: Terasaki PI, Cecka JM (eds.), Clinical Transplants 1994. Los Angeles: UCLA Tissue Typing Laboratory, 1995: 1.
20. Ojo AO, Wolfe RA, Held PJ, Port FK, Schmouder RL. Delayed graft function: risk factors and implications for renal allograft survival. Transplantation 1997; 63: 968–974.
21. Land W. The potential impact of the reperfusion injury on acute and chronic rejection events following organ transplantation. Transplant. Proc. 1994; 26: 3169–3171.
22. Schneeberger H, Aydemir S, Illner WD, Land W. Nonspecific primary ischemia/reperfusion injury in combination with secondary specific acute rejection-mediated injury of human kidney allografts contributes mainly to development of chronic transplant failure. Transplant. Proc. 1997; 29: 948–949.
23. Yilmaz S, Paavonen T, Häyry P. Chronic rejection of rat renal allografts. II. The impact of prolonged ischemia time on transplant histology. Transplantation 1992; 53: 823–827.
24. Li F, Grauls G, Yin M, Bruggeman CA. Initial endothelial injury and cytomegalovirus infection accelerate the development of allograft arteriosclerosis. Transplant. Proc. 1995; 27: 3552–3554.
25. Yilmaz S, Koskinen PK, Kallio E, Bruggeman CA, Häyry PJ, Lemström KB. Cytomegalovirus infection-enhanced chronic kidney allograft rejection is linked with intercellular adhesion molecule-1 expression. Kidney Int. 1996; 50: 526–537.
26. Lautenschlager I, Soots A, Krogerus L et al. CMV increases inflammation and accelerates chronic rejection in rat kidney allografts. Transplant. Proc. 1997; 29: 802–803.
27. Grattan MT, Moreno-Cabral CE, Starnes VA, Oyer PE, Stinson EB, Shumway NE. Cytomegalovirus infection is associated with cardiac allograft rejection and atherosclerosis. JAMA 1989; 261: 3561–3566.
28. Herrera GA, Alexander RW, Cooley CF et al. Cytomegalovirus glomerulopathy: a controversial lesion. Kidney Int. 1986; 29: 725–733.
29. Nadasdy T, Smith J, Laszik Z, Waner JL, Johnson LD, Silva FG. Absence of association between cytomegalovirus infection and obliterative transplant arteriopathy in renal allograft rejection. Mod. Pathol. 1994; 7: 289–294.
30. Vollmer E, Bosse A, Bogeholz J et al. Apolipoproteins and immunohistological differentiation of cells in the arterial wall of kidneys in transplant arteriopathy. Morphological parallels with atherosclerosis. Pathol. Res. Pract. 1991; 187: 957–962.

31. Fellström B, Dimény E, Larsson E, Claesson K, Tufveson G. Rapidly proliferating arteriopathy in cyclosporin-induced permanently surviving rat cardiac allografts simulating chronic vascular rejection. Clin. Exp. Immunol. 1990; 80: 288–292.
32. Räisänen-Sokolowski A, Tilly-Kiesi M, Ustinov J et al. Hyperlipidemia accelerates allograft arteriosclerosis (chronic rejection) in the rat. Arterioscler. Thromb. 1994; 14: 2032–2042.
33. Dimény E, Fellström B, Larsson E, Tufveson G, Lithell H. Chronic vascular rejection and hyperlipoproteinemia in renal transplant patients. Clin. Transplant. 1993; 7: 482–487.
34. Dimény E, Tufveson G, Lithell H, Larsson E, Siegbahn A, Fellström B. The influence of pretransplant lipoprotein abnormalities on the early results of renal transplantation. Eur. J. Clin. Invest. 1993; 23: 572–579.
35. Isoniemi H, Taskinen E, Häyry P. Histological chronic allograft damage index accurately predicts chronic renal allograft rejection. Transplantation 1994; 58: 1195–1198.
36. Brazy PC, Pirsch JD, Belzer FO. Factors affecting renal allograft function in long-term recipients. Am. J. Kidney Dis. 1992; 19: 558–566.
37. Markell MS, Sumrani N, Dibenedetto A, Friedman EA. Effect of early hyperlipidemia on graft and patient survival in cyclosporine-treated renal transplant patients. Am. J. Kidney Dis. 1993; 22: 233–239.
38. Knight RJ, Kerman RH, Welsh M et al. Chronic rejection in primary renal allograft recipients under cyclosporine prednisone immunosuppressive therapy. Transplantation 1991; 51: 355–359.
39. Kobashigawa JA, Katznelson S, Laks H et al. Effect of pravastatin on outcomes after cardiac transplantation. N. Engl. J. Med. 1995; 333: 621–627.
40. Katznelson S, Wilkinson AH, Kobashigawa JA et al. The effect of pravastatin on acute rejection after kidney transplantation – a pilot study. Transplantation 1996; 61: 1469–1474.
41. Modena FM, Hostetter TH, Salahudeen AK, Najarian JS, Matas AJ, Rosenberg ME. Progression of kidney disease in chronic renal transplant rejection. Transplantation 1991; 52: 239–244.
42. Cheigh JS, Haschemeyer RH, Wang JCL et al. Hypertension in kidney transplant recipients. Effect on long-term renal allograft survival. Am. J. Hypertens. 1989; 2: 341–348.
43. Cosio FG, Falkenhain ME, Pesavento TE et al. Relationships between arterial hypertension and renal allograft survival in African-American patients. Am. J. Kidney Dis. 1997; 29: 419–427.
44. Barenbrock M, Colmorgen U, Firschka E et al. A multicenter, randomized, double-blind, placebo-controlled, two-year trial to study the effect of nitrendipine on chronic renal transplant function. Clin. Nephrol. 1995; 43: 388–391.
45. Terasaki PI, Cecka JM, Gjertson DW, Cho Y, Takemoto S, Cohn M. A ten year prediction for kidney transplant survival. In: Terasaki PI, Cecka JM (eds.), Clinical Transplants 1992. Los Angeles: UCLA Tissue Typing Laboratory, 1992: 501.
46. Myers BD, Ross J, Newton L, Leutscher J, Perlroth M. Cyclosporine-associated chronic nephropathy. N. Engl. J. Med. 1984; 311: 699–705.
47. Burke JF, Pirsch JD, Ramos EL et al. Long-term efficacy and safety of cyclosporine in renal-transplant patients. N. Engl. J. Med. 1994; 331: 358–363.
48. Hollander AAMJ, Van Saase JLCM, Kootte AMM et al. Beneficial effects of conversion from cyclosporin to azathioprine after kidney transplantation. Lancet 1995; 345: 610–614.
49. Isoniemi H, Nurminen M, Tikkanen MJ et al. Risk factors predicting chronic rejection of renal allografts. Transplantation 1994; 57: 68–72.
50. Larsen CP, Elwood ET, Alexander DZ et al. Long-term acceptance of skin and cardiac allografts after blocking CD40 and CD28 pathways. Nature 1996; 381: 434–438.
51. Azuma H, Chandraker A, Nadeau K et al. Blockade of T-cell costimulation prevents development of experimental chronic renal allograft rejection. Proc. Natl. Acad. Sci. USA 1996; 93: 12439–12444.
52. Geerling RA, Bruin RWF de, Scheringa M et al. Suppression of acute rejection prevents graft atherosclerosis after allogeneic aorta transplantation in the rat. Transplantation 1994; 58: 1258–1263.

53. Gregory CR, Huang X, Pratt RE et al. Treatment with rapamycin and mycophenolic acid reduces arterial intimal thickening produced by mechanical injury and allows endothelial replacement. Transplantation 1995; 59: 655–661.
54. Schmid C, Heemann U, Azuma H, Tilney NL. Rapamycin inhibits transplant vasculopathy in long-surviving rat heart allografts. Transplantation 1995; 60: 729–733.
55. Räisänen-Sokolowski A, Yilmaz S, Tufveson G, Häyry P. Partial inhibition of allograft arteriosclerosis (chronic rejection) by 15–deoxyspergualin. Transplantation 1994; 57: 1772–1777.
56. MacDonald AS, Sabr K, MacAuley MA, McAllister VC, Bitter-Suermann H, Lee L. Effects of leflunomide and cyclosporine on aortic allograft chronic rejection in the rat. Transplant. Proc. 1994; 26: 3244–3245.
57. Morris RE, Huang X, Gregory CR et al. Studies in experimental models of chronic rejection: use of rapamycin (sirolimus) and isoxazole derivatives (leflunomide and its analogue) for the suppression of graft vascular disease and obliterative bronchiolitis. Transplant. Proc. 1995; 27: 2068–2069.
58. Swan SK, Crary GS, Guijarro C, O'Donnell MP, Keane WF, Kasiske BL. Immunosuppressive effects of leflunomide in experimental chronic vascular rejection. Transplantation 1995; 60: 887–890.
59. Räisänen-Sokolowski A, Aho P, Myllärniemi M, Kallio E, Häyry P. Inhibition of early chronic rejection in rat aortic allografts by mycophenolate mofetil (RS61443). Transplant. Proc. 1995; 27: 435.
60. Azuma H, Binder J, Heemann U, Tullius SG, Tilney NL. Effect of RS61443 on chronic rejection of rat kidney allografts. Transplant. Proc. 1995; 27: 436–437.
61. Pirsch JD, Miller J, Deierhoi MH, Vincenti F, Filo RS, for the FK506 kidney transplant study group. A comparison of tacrolimus (FK506) and cyclosporine for immunosuppression after cadaveric renal transplantation. Transplantation 1997; 63: 977–983.
62. Gjertson DW, Cecka JM, Terasaki PI. The relative effects of FK506 and cyclosporine on short- and long-term kidney graft survival. Transplantation 1995; 60: 1384–1388.
63. Sollinger HW. Mycophenolate mofetil for the prevention of acute rejection in primary cadaveric renal allograft recipients. Transplantation 1995; 60: 225–232.
64. The European Mycophenolate Mofetil Cooperative Study Group. Placebo controlled study of mycophenolate mofetil combined with cyclosporin and corticosteroids for prevention of acute rejection. Lancet 1995; 345: 1321–1326.
65. Keown P, Häyry P, Mathew T et al. A blinded, randomized clinical trial of mycophenolate mofetil for the prevention of acute rejection in cadaveric renal transplantation. Transplantation 1996; 61: 1029–1037.
66. Halloran P, Mathew T, Tomlanovich S, Groth C, Hooftman L, Barker C. Mycophenolate mofetil in renal allograft recipients – a pooled efficacy analysis of three randomized, double-blind, clinical studies in prevention of rejection. Transplantation 1997; 63: 39–47.
67. Sporn MB, Roberts AB. Peptide growth factors are multifunctional. Nature 1988; 332: 217–219.
68. Nadeau KC, Azuma H, Tilney NL. Sequential cytokine dynamics in chronic rejection of rat renal allografts: Roles for cytokines RANTES and MCP-1. Proc. Natl. Acad. Sci. USA 1995; 92: 8729–8733.
69. Akyürek LM, Paul LC, Funa K, Larsson E, Fellström BC. Smooth muscle cell migration into intima and adventitia during development of transplant vasculopathy. Transplantation 1996; 62: 1526–1529.
70. Stein-Oakley AN, Tzanidis A, Fuller PJ, Jablonski P, Thomson NM. Expression and distribution of epidermal growth factor in acute and chronic renal allograft rejection. Kidney Int. 1994; 46: 1207–1215.
71. Häyry P, Isoniemi H, Yilmaz S et al. Chronic allograft rejection. Immunol. Rev. 1993; 134: 33–81.
72. Aziz S, Tada Y, Gordon D, McDonald TO, Fareed J, Verrier ED. A reduction in accelerated graft coronary disease and an improvement in cardiac allograft survival using low molecular weight heparin in combination with cyclosporine. J. Heart Lung Transplant. 1993; 12: 634–643.

73. Häyry P, Räisänen A, Ustinov J, Mennander A, Paavonen T. Somatostatin analog Lanreotide inhibits myocyte replication and several growth factors in allograft arteriosclerosis. FASEB J. 1993; 7: 1055–1060.
74. Häyry P, Myllärniemi M, Aavik E et al. Stable D-peptide analogue of insulin-like growth factor-1 inhibits smooth muscle proliferation after carotid ballooning injury in the rat. FASEB J. 1995; 9: 1336–1344.
75. Benediktsson H, Chea R, Davidoff A, Paul LC. Antihypertensive drug treatment in chronic renal allograft rejection in the rat. Effect on structure and function. Transplantation 1996; 62: 1634–1642.
76. Furukawa Y, Matsumori A, Hirozane T, Sasayama S. Angiotensin II receptor antagonist TCV-116 reduces graft coronary artery disease and preserves graft status in a murine model – a comparative study with captopril. Circulation 1996; 93: 333–339.
77. Barnas U, Schmidt A, Haas M, Oberbauer R, Mayer G. The effects of prolonged angiotensin-converting enzyme inhibition on excretory kidney function and proteinuria in renal allograft recipients with chronic progressive transplant failure. Nephrol. Dial Transplant. 1996; 11: 1822–1824.
78. Hunsicker LG, Bennett LE. Design of trials of methods to reduce late renal allograft loss: the price of success. Kidney Int. 1995; 48 (Suppl. 52): S120–S123.
79. Kasiske BL, Massy ZA, Guijarro C, Ma JZ. Chronic renal allograft rejection and clinical trial design. Kidney Int. 1995; 48 (Suppl. 52): S116–S119.
80. Myllärniemi M, Räisänen-Sokolowski A, Vuoristo P, Kallio E, Land W, Häyry P. Lack of effect of recombinant human superoxide dismutase on cold ischemia-induced arteriosclerosis in syngeneic rat aortic transplants. Transplantation 1996; 61: 1018–1022.
81. Kobashigawa JA, Kasiske BL. Hyperlipidemia in solid organ transplantation. Transplantation 1997; 63: 331–338.
82. Arnadottir M, Berg A-L. Treatment of hyperlipidemia in renal transplant recipients. Transplantation 1997; 63: 339–345.
83. Bittar AE, Keitel E, Garcia CD et al. Patient non-compliance as a cause of late kidney graft failure. Transplant. Proc. 1992; 24: 2720–2721.

PART EIGHT

Impact of retransplantation on organ allocation

36. Impact of retransplantation on organ allocation in France

YLANA CHALEM, JEAN-LOUIS GOLMARD & DIDIER HOUSSIN

Introduction

In France, organ retransplantation represents a small proportion of all organ transplantations, but becomes a significant difficulty when considering the allocation of a limited number of organs. In fact, the results of organ retransplantations are grosso modo inferior to those of first transplantations. Failures of retransplantations have many causes including surgical complications, immunosuppression, rejection, and often the bad consequences of a long standing disease. Little place is specifically devoted to retransplantation in organ allocation rules. The impact of retransplantation on organ allocation is in fact very largely linked to the medical decision of the transplant team, a decision which certainly would gain to be better analysed.

Practice and results of organ retransplantation in France

As shown in Table 1, 9.8% of all organ transplantations performed since 1985 were retransplantations. The percentage of retansplantations varies according to the type of organ. It did not increase with time during the last 10 years (Table 2) and showed a marked recent decline for the liver (Table 2). Sometimes, retransplantation may take the appearance of a stammer but third retransplantations are rare (15 for the kidney, 6 for the liver, none for thoracic organs) and more than four successive transplantations of the same type of organ were not observed in France during this period.

Table 1. Proportion of retransplantations among all organ transplantations in France from 1985 to 1996

Type of organ	Retransplantations (%)	All transplantations
Kidney	2570 (13)	20,233
Heart	110 (2)	5,678
Heart-lung	23 (4)	499
Lung	10 (1)	740
Liver	550 (9)	6,013
Total	3263 (9.8)	33,163

J.L. Touraine et al. (eds.), Retransplantation, 291–294.

Table 2. Evolution of the proportion of retransplantations among all organ transplantations in France between 1985 and 1996

Type of organ	Percentage of retransplantation											
	1985	1986	1987	1988	1989	1990	1991	1992	1993	1994	1995	1996
Kidney	13	11	10	13	13	14	15	14	14	13	12	9
Heart	3	3	1	2	3	2	3	1	3	2	2	1
Heart-lungs	0	0	0	0	1	3	6	7	13	14	0	0
Lung	0	0	0	5	0	1	2	3	2	1	0	0
Liver	7	8	6	10	11	12	11	10	11	9	7	3

Table 3. Outcome of the patients registered for liver transplantation in 1995 and 1996 in the super-urgent category because of a need for retransplantation less than seven days after a first graft, according to the number of days on the list

	Outcome					
	Transplantation		Death before transplantation		Removed from the list	
Number of days on the list	1995	1996	1995	1996	1995	1996
1	3	4	1	1	0	0
2	11	6	1	3	3	0
3	3	2	0	0	3	0
≥4	1	1	0	0	1	2

As shown in Figures 1–3, cumulative survival rates of organ retransplantations are less than those observed with first transplantations, for the patients grafted between December 1, 1985 and December 31, 1996. It seems that the negative impact of iteration on the results of transplantation is as less important as the overall results of transplantation are good.

Retransplantation and organ allocation rules

In the French organ allocation rules, a secific mention of retransplantation is made in only one case: patients who require urgent retransplantation, less than one week after a first liver transplantation can be placed in a full priority category. This prioritization is of significant efficacy, as shown in Table 3.

Except for this situation, mention of retransplantation is not made specifically but can be considered as indirect through the attention given to patients, either highly immunized or requiring an urgent transplantation. During the process which, between 1995 and 1997, led to the fabrication of organ allocation rules, arguments for and against giving a priority for patients in need for retransplantation were advanced but little room was in the end given to retransplantation in these rules. The prevailing opinion was that the decision of attribution of an organ for a retransplantation should not, in general, be considered as rules-related and should remain the exclusive privilege of the transplant team. It is clear, however, that there is a specific context for retransplantation as a medical decision within the transplant team.

Retransplantation as a medical decision

Facing the prospect of a retransplantation, the transplant team is torn between two types of feelings: on one side, the sense of a failure, of a wastage of organs and efforts, sometimes aggravated by some resentment towards the patient if rejection is due to overt non-compliance with medical treatment; on the other

Table 4. Mean waiting time (months; in parentheses) before heart, heart-lung, lung or liver transplantation or retransplantation between 1995 and 1996.

Type of graft	First transplantation	Retransplantation
Heart	9 (8–10)	6.9 (5.2–8.6)
Heart-lung	18 (16.3–19.7)	9.3 (7.1–11.5)
Lung	15.2 (13.5–16.9)	8.7 (6.3–11.1)
Liver	8.7 (7.5–9.9)	5.8 (3.9–7.7)
Kidney	21 (20–22)	35.3 (33.8–36.8)

side, the engagement that the medical team has taken with its initial decision of transplantation, and to which it tends, consciously or unconsciously, to adhere. As shown by recent psychosociological experimental studies, adherence to the initial decision is increased if the initial decision was a collective one [1–4]. In fact, decision-making in transplant teams is often of the collective type. Therefore, in spite of all individual reticences and objective arguments against it,the patient is usually placed on the waiting list for retransplantation. As if to rapidly solve the problem and the tension created by this medical decision, retransplantation is frequently considered urgent due to the condition of the patient and it is often made on short notice, as soon as a suitable graft is proposed. Analysis of the waiting list showed in fact that the mean duration time on the waiting list tented to be shorter for patients waiting for a heart, heart-lung, lung or liver retransplantation, than for those waiting for a first transplantation (Table 4).

Organ retransplantation is an example of the pecularities of a collective medical decision-making. Its meaning should certainly be further analysed given the context of scarce ressources in which it evolves and its consequences for patients awaiting for a first transplantation.

Acknowledgements

Data presented in this article were given by all the French organ transplant teams.

References

1. Lewin K. Group decision and social change. In: Newcomb T, Hartley E. (eds.), Readings and Social Psychology. New York: Holt, 1947.
2. Staw BM. Knee-deep in the big muddy: a study of escalating commitment to a chosen course of action. Org. Behav. Hum. Perf. 1976; 16: 27–44.
3. Teger AI. Too much invested to quit. New York: Pergamon, 1979.
4. Doise W. Les relations entre groupes. In: S. Moscovici (ed.), Psychologie Sociale. Paris: Presses Universitaires de France, 1984.

37. Influence of retransplantation on organ allocation

BLANCA MIRANDA, FELIX J. LACOMA & JOSE MANUEL GONZALEZ-POSADA

Introduction

In spite of continuous improvement in transplant techniques and patient management there are still a significant number of graft failures affecting every kind of solid organ transplantation. Graft failure after kidney transplantation makes more demanding to find another compatible organ for that patient. More dramatic, primary failure of heart or liver graft is a medical emergency that jeopardizes the patient's life. Retransplantation has been associated with a decreased patient and graft survival for each type of transplant considered [1–4], and significantly increases the cost of the overall process [5, 6]. The inclusion on waiting list (WL) of patients considered for retransplantation might carry a decreased chance of getting an organ for those awaiting a primary graft. Given the shortage of transplantable organs, some authors have advocated that previous transplant history should be taken in account when setting the criteria for organ allocation as it is done with ABO blood group matching [5, 7]. Other have been willing to limit the number of organs available for retransplantation [8] and even completely to ban retransplantation procedures [9] as the way to preserve fairness and justice in the transplantation process.

Spain has an intense activity in organ transplantation, including the world highest rate in liver and kidney transplants. There are national WL for liver, heart and lung transplant. For renal transplant, each transplant team keeps its own list and only hyperimmunized candidates are listed nationally regardless their previous transplant history. Organ allocation and distribution are carried out using clinical and geographical criteria previously convened by representatives of transplant teams, health administration, and the 'Organización Nacional de Trasplantes' (ONT). Overall, this system has given good results and seems to provide a fair distribution of available organs to the different WL. Next, we will describe the organ allocation criteria used in Spain for emergency and elective liver, heart, lung, and kidney retransplantation and how these may influence the different WL.

Liver transplantation

Clinical criteria for liver transplantation in Spain distinguish between elective and urgent situations. Zero urgency (0) includes acute hepatic failure in absence

J.L. Touraine et al. (eds.), Retransplantation, 295–304.

Table 1. Liver retransplantation activity in Spain

	1992	1993	1994	1995	1996
Waiting list (WL)[a]	692	743	971	1031	1164
Transplants performed[b]	468	495	614	698	700
WL for retransplantation (%)[c]					
0 urgency	3.6	1.9	2.6	2.2	2.1
Elective	5.6	3.9	4.9	7.5	7.5
Transplants as retransplantation (%)[d]					
0 urgency	3.8	2.4	3.1	2.4	2.7
Elective	4.7	2.4	4.9	7.4	7.1
Mortality while on WL (%)[e]	6	4	6	4	8

[a] Total number of patients entering the liver transplant waiting list in Spain each year.
[b] Total number of liver transplants performed in Spain each year.
[c] Waiting list for liver retransplantation, as percentage of the total WL, for both 0 urgency and elective listings.
[d] Retransplantations, as percentage of the total liver transplants performed, for urgent and elective indications.
[e] Mortality while on waiting list for liver transplant, as percentage of the total waiting list.

of previous liver disease and primary graft failure within the first seven days after transplantation. Patients considered as 0 urgencies are given national priority, the possibility of waiting for a compatible liver – ABO blood group and weight – and a maximum three-day stay in this code, although a longer period can be allowed if justified by the transplant team. Recurrence of the primary disease, mostly viral hepatitis, needs to be ruled out on those considered for elective retransplantation before admitting them to the WL. Patients awaiting for an elective retransplantation are managed, as for organ allocation and distribution criteria, exactly in the same way that those awaiting for their first graft. Next we will describe the status of liver retransplantation in Spain during the last five years (Table 1 and Figure 1).

From 1992 to 1996, patients admitted each year as 0 urgency because of retransplantation have comprised $2.5 \pm 0.7\%$ of those included on the WL. Of these, $77 \pm 5.4\%$ were finally retransplanted, this being $2.9 \pm 0.6\%$ of the total number of livers that were transplanted yearly. Most of these urgent retransplants were carried out within the first 2 days of the patients' admission to the WL. Recently, early (within 3 days) regraft in acute retransplantation has been associated with better survival [10]. Patients included electively for retransplantation were $5.9 \pm 1.6\%$ of the total WL and, of the total number of liver transplants performed each year, only $5.3 \pm 2\%$ were done due to elective retransplantation. Overall, during each of the last five years, the total number of liver retransplanted patients in Spain, both urgently and electively, has been below 10% of the total number of the performed liver transplants. Considering this five-year period, 64% of those patients listed for retransplantation were

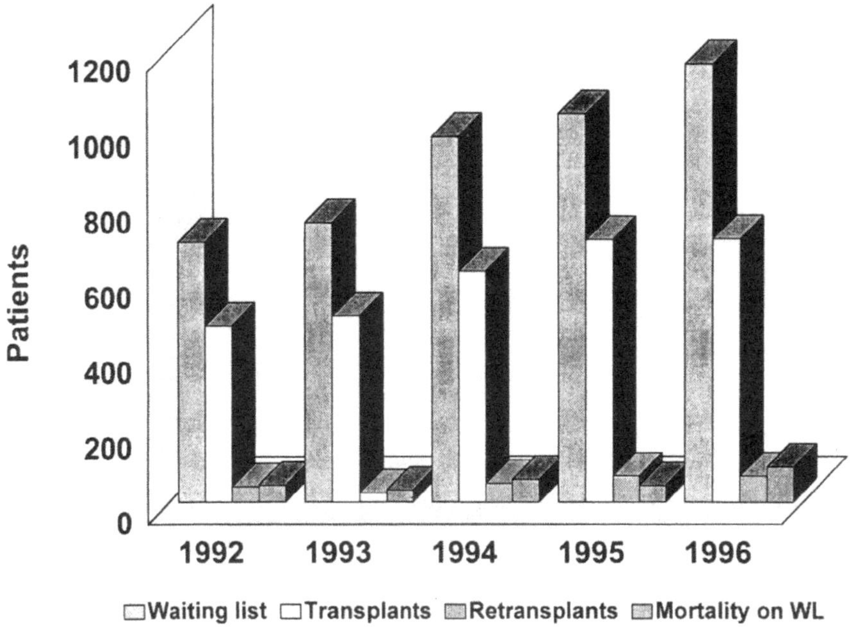

Fig. 1. Liver transplantation in Spain (1992–1996). Waiting list, transplants, retransplants, and mortality while on waiting list expressed as number of patients.

finally regrafted (Figure 2). The distribution between urgent and elective liver retransplantations can be seen in Figure 3.

Mortality rate while on the WL has varied each year, for the total WL, between 4 and 8% ($5.6 \pm 1.7\%$ for the five years considered) and 69% of those awaiting for a liver transplant received their grafts within three months of their listing. Other sources have published hepatic retransplantation rates from 11 to 14.5% [1, 6] with also higher mortality while on WL. Longer waiting time and similar mortality on WL than ours have been recently reported by the United Network for Organ Sharing (UNOS; [11]).

Heart transplantation

Spanish clinical criteria for heart transplant also specify a 0 urgency situation that includes patients with cardiogenic shock, otherwise suitable for transplant, and patients suffering a primary graft failure within the first 48 h after transplantation. This urgent condition has national priority, with organs being offered based on ABO blood group compatibility and with a weight mismatch between donor and receptor lower than 25%. The maximum time allowed for a patient to be on cardiac 0 urgency is 3 days, expandable if the transplant team makes a direct request.

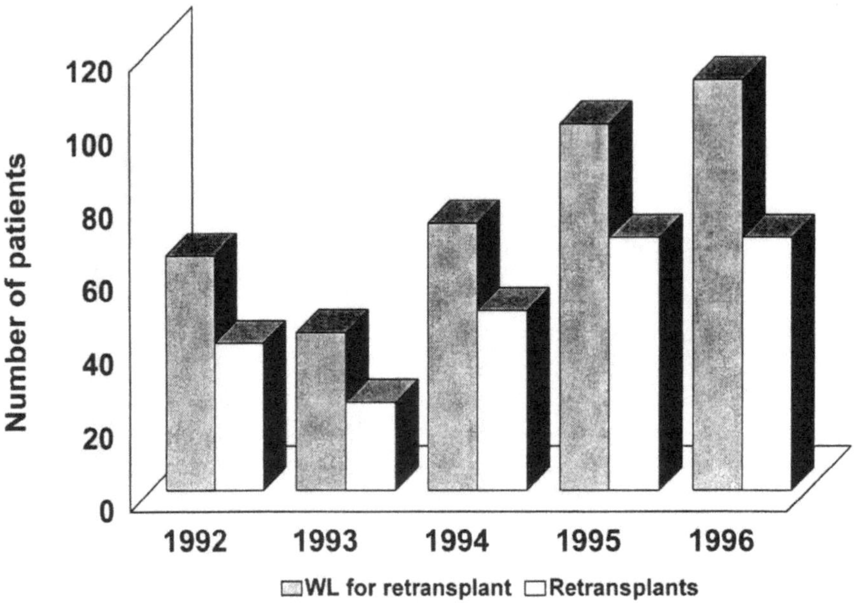

Fig. 2. Liver retransplantation in Spain (1992–1996). Patients admitted to the waiting list for hepatic retransplantation and patients retransplanted per year.

The progress of cardiac retransplantation in Spain can be followed in Table 2 and Figure 4.

Of the total number of patients included on the Spanish heart transplantation waiting list, from 1992 to 1996, $1.8 \pm 0.3\%$ each year were admitted as 0 urgency because of retransplantation. Each year, a wide proportion of these were finally retransplanted, from 28 to 66%, accounting for $0.9 \pm 0.6\%$ of the total number of heart transplants performed. Inclusion on the WL for elective retransplantation oscillated between 0.7 and 2.1% of the total of patients admitted, also with a wide percentage of retransplantations ($71 \pm 42\%$) and comprising only $1.2 \pm 0.8\%$ of the total number of heart transplants done in Spain from 1992 to 1996. Retransplantations, both emergent and elective, have accounted during each of the last five years for less than 4% of the heart transplants done in our country, a similar figure to that reported from Germany by Pasic et al. [12]. During the last five years, half of those admitted to the WL for retransplantation were finally regrafted (Figure 5). The distribution of urgent versus elective cardiac retransplantations can be seen in Figure 6.

Overall mortality while on the waiting list has varied between 5 and 9% during the same period. Of the total of potential receptors listed for a heart transplant, 64% received their grafts within two months of their inclusion on the WL.

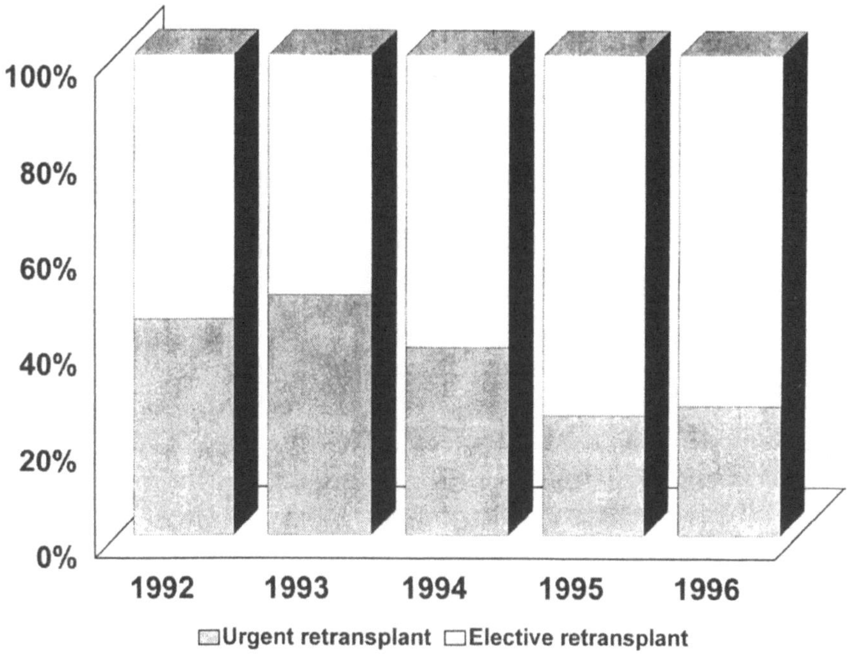

Fig. 3. Liver retransplantation in Spain (1992–1996). Urgent vs. elective liver retransplantation per year.

Table 2. Heart retransplantation activity in Spain

	1992	1993	1994	1995	1996
Waiting list (WL)[a]	326	371	403	392	440
Transplants performed[b]	254	287	292	278	282
WL for retransplantation (%)[c]					
0 urgency	1.8	1.9	2.2	1.3	1.8
Elective	2.1	1.6	0.7	0.7	0.7
Transplants as retransplantation (%)[d]					
0 urgency	1.6	0.7	1	1.1	0
Elective	2.3	1.4	1	0	1.1
Mortality while on WL (%)[e]	5.2	6.2	9.4	6.4	9.3

[a] Total number of patients entering the heart transplant waiting list in Spain each year.
[b] Total number of heart transplants performed in Spain each year.
[c] Waiting list for heart retransplantation, as percentage of the total WL, for both 0 urgency and elective listings.
[d] Retransplantations, as percentage of the total heart transplants performed, for urgent and elective indications.
[e] Mortality while on waiting list for heart transplant, as percentage of the total waiting list.

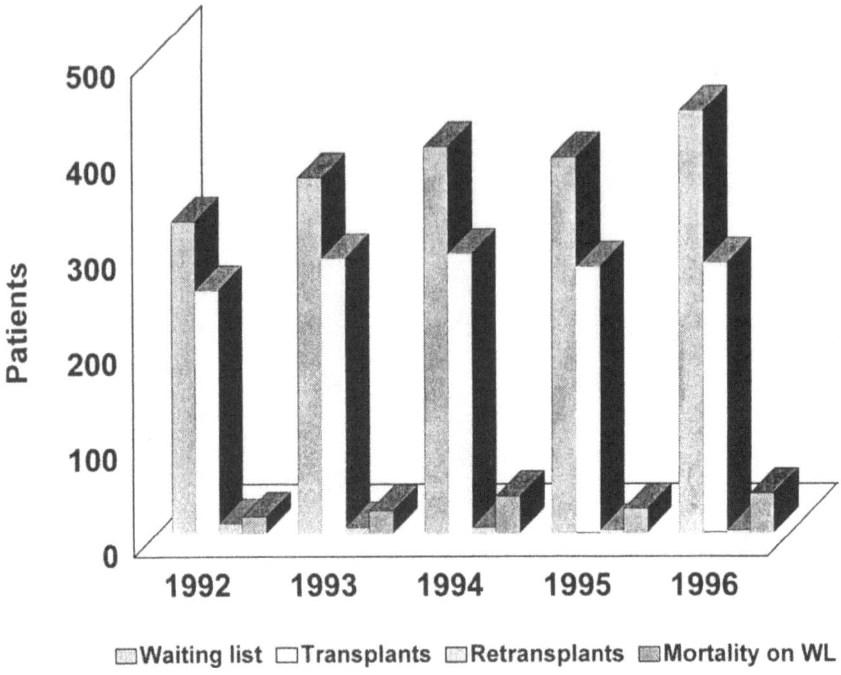

Fig. 4. Heart transplantation in Spain (1992–1996). Waiting list, transplants, retransplants, and mortality while on waiting list expressed as number of patients.

Lung transplantation

Since the first isolated lung transplantation was done in Spain in 1990, a total of 193 procedures has been performed, including both single and bilateral lung transplants, until the end of 1996. During this period, eleven patients were included on the WL for retransplantation accounting for a global 2.8% of the WL. While others have reported a retransplantation rate of 10% [13], ours has been way below this figure with lung retransplantations being only 2.1% of the total activity. Mortality while on the WL for lung transplantation has been about 5.5% during 1995 and 1996 and 67% of transplants were performed within six months of inclusion on the WL. Almost every indication for lung retransplantation was done acutely. Late retransplantation has not been a significant issue so far given the low reported rate of chronic rejection/obliterative bronchiolitis in our country although this situation may change in the future as the number of lung transplanted patients increases. In spite of previous discouraging experience with late and elective lung retransplantation [14], more recent data suggest better results [13, 15, 16]. Although the number of lung transplantations is exponentially increasing in

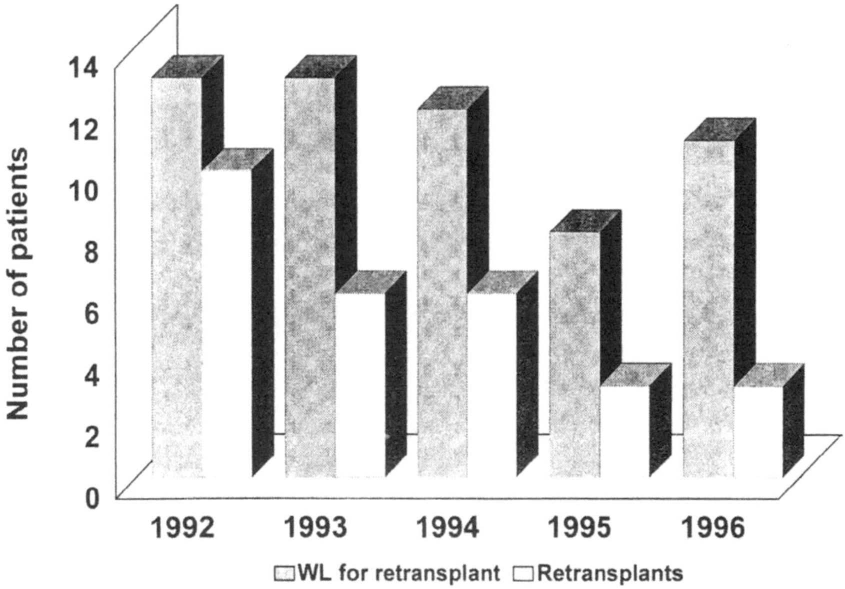

Fig. 5. Heart retransplantation in Spain (1992–1996). Patients admitted to the waiting list for cardiac retransplantation and patients retransplanted per year.

Spain, the WL is also growing probably related with a better knowledge of this procedure and a higher rate of patient referral for transplant. From the data above, retransplantation is clearly not a factor contributing to the increasing WL and efforts should be directed to other perceived problems like improving detection of potential lung donors. Lung retransplantation progress in Spain for the last five years can be seen in Figure 7.

Kidney transplantation

Kidney transplantation in Spain is managed directly by the different transplant teams and only hyperimmunized patients are referred to a centralized national WL. There is an extremely high variability in how many patients wait for retransplantation and how many of them are finally grafted. This is due to several factors that may include the variable experience and length of the different kidney transplant programs, the different medical criteria for entering the WL and retransplantation between programs, and the diverse activity of the transplant teams.

Although partial, data obtained from kidney transplantation teams from three different Autonomous Communities (political and administrative subdivisions of the Spanish State) show that 24–30% of patients included in the WL are waiting for a retransplantation and between 5.1 and 14.6% of the

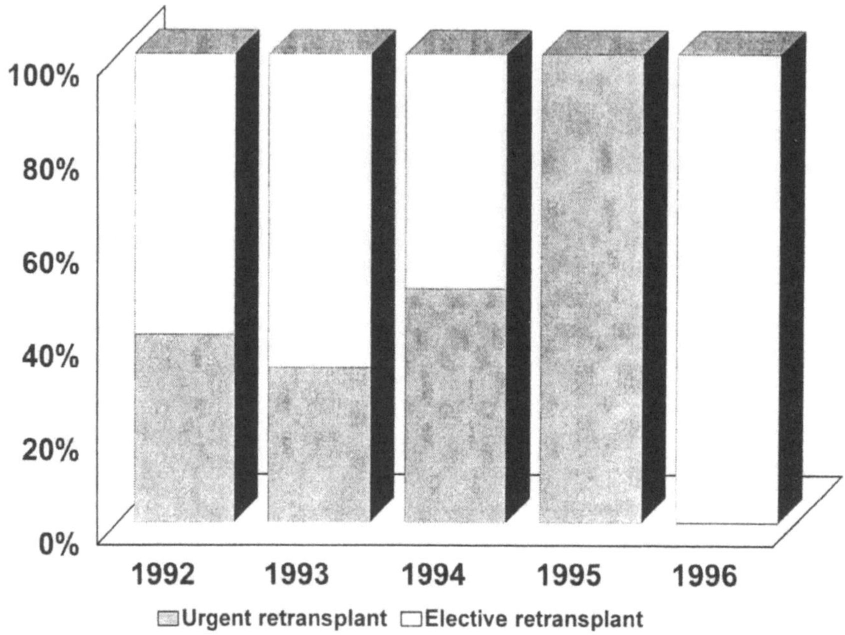

Fig. 6. Heart retransplantation in Spain (1992–1996). Urgent vs. elective cardiac retransplantation per year.

kidney transplants performed are retransplantations. Data previously reported from Spain offered a higher rate of retransplantation, up to 19.1% [17]. Renal retransplantation has been associated with a worse prognosis with compared with first grafts [3], but more recent reports have provided evidence of better results [18, 19] and have shown a retransplantation rate of about 15% [18, 20]. Most important, although Spanish retransplantation rates have remained similar to those reported from other areas, our WL for renal transplant shows a slow but constant decrement over the last few years.

Conclusion

Retransplantation rates in Spain during the last five years have been similar to those reported from other countries and transplant networks for kidney, heart, and liver transplants. Lung transplant, the most recent solid organ transplant activity in our country, still has a low retransplantation rate when compared with more established programs. Clinical and geographical allocation criteria have been jointly developed by all involved agents – transplantation teams, administration, and the ONT – allowing the implementation of a trustworthy network that assures the distribution of available organs to those who need them most. In case of liver and heart retransplantation, only those that

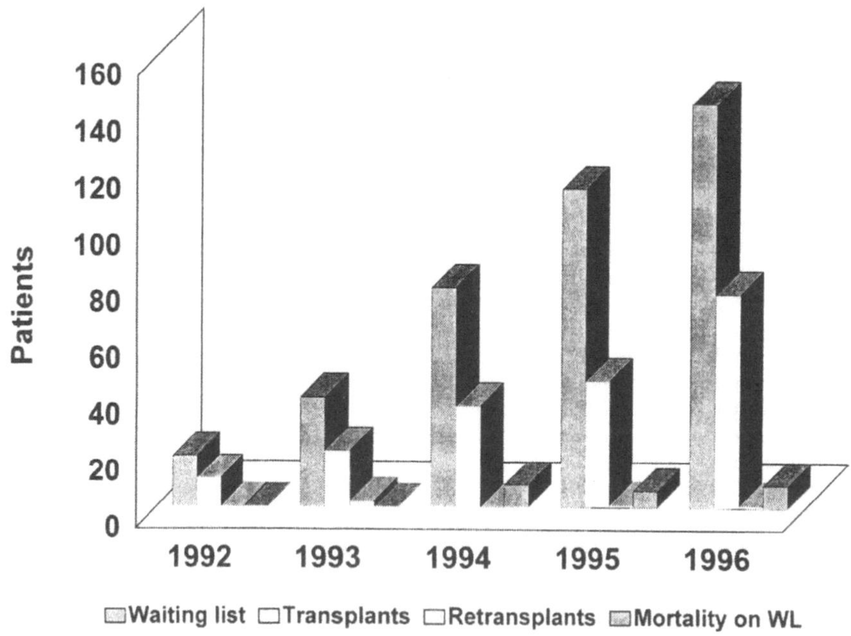

Fig. 7. Lung transplantation in Spain (1992–1996). Waiting list, transplants, retransplants, and mortality while on waiting list expressed as number of patients.

meet some specific criteria are given priority. Patients with a history of failed renal graft, if considered hyperimmunized, are listed in a centralized, national WL thus improving their chance of obtaining compatible match for retransplantation.

Overall, although WL for heart, liver, and lung transplantation have been slightly increasing in Spain over the last few years, retransplantation per se is not perceived as a significant casual factor. The WL for kidney transplantation is, in fact, decreasing in spite of a high retransplantation rate. Based in our experience, solutions for organ shortage should include those oriented to enhance the donor pool (detection, maintenance, improvement of family refusal rates, non-heart-beating donor programs, etc.) and, in our case, a tight regulation of retransplantation does not seem justifiable at this time.

References

1. Powelson JA, Cosimi AB, Lewis WD et al. Hepatic retransplantation in New England – a regional experience and survival model. Transplantation 1993; 55: 802–806.
2. Smith JA, Ribakove GH, Hunt SA et al. Heart retransplantation: the 25-year experience at a single institution. J. Heart Lung Transplant. 1995; 14: 832–839.
3. Perez RV, Matas AJ, Gillingham KJ et al. Lessons learned and future hopes: three thousand renal transplants at the University of Minnesota. Clin. Transplant. 1990; 4: 217–231.

4. Karwande SV, Ensley RD, Renlund DG et al. Cardiac retransplantation: a viable option? The Registry of the International Society for Heart and Lung Transplantation. Ann. Thorac. Surg. 1992; 54: 840–844.
5. Evans RW. Organ transplantation and the inevitable debate as to what constitutes a basic health care benefit. Clin Transplant. 1993; 7: 359–391.
6. D'Alessandro AM, Ploeg RJ, Knechtle SJ et al. retransplantation of the liver – a seven-year experience. Transplantation 1993; 55: 1083–1087.
7. Ubel PA, Arnold RM, Caplan AL. Rationing failure. The ethical lessons of the retransplantation of scarce vital organs. JAMA 1993; 270: 2469–2474.
8. Mentzer SJ, Reilly JJ Jr, Caplan AL, Sugarbaker DJ. Ethical considerations in lung retransplantation. J. Heart Lung Transplant. 1994; 13: 56–58.
9. Collins EG, Mozdzierz GJ. Cardiac retransplantation: determining limits. Heart Lung 1993; 22: 206–212.
10. Washburn WK, Bradley J, Cosimi AB et al. A regional experience with emergency liver transplantation. Transplantation 1996; 61: 235–239.
11. 1995 Annual report of the U.S. Scientific Registry of Transplant Recipients and the Organ Procurement and Transplantation Network – transplant data: 1988–1994. Richmond, Va.: United Network for Organ Sharing, 1995.
12. Pasic M, Loebe M, Hummel M et al. Heart transplantation: a single-center experience. Ann. Thorac. Surg. 1996; 62: 1685–1690.
13. Schafers HJ, Hausen B, Wahlers T, Fieguth HG, Jurmann M, Borst HG. Retransplantation of the lung. A single center experience. Eur. J. Cardiothorac. Surg. 1995; 9: 291–295.
14. Novick RJ, Kaye MP, Patterson A et al. Redo lung transplantation: A North American–European Experience. J. Heart Lung Transplant. 1993; 12: 5–16.
15. Wekerle T, Klepetko W, Wisser W et al. Lung retransplantation: institutional report on a series of twenty patients. J. Heart Lung Transplant. 1996; 15: 182–189.
16. Novick RJ, Schafers HJ, Stitt L et al. Recurrence of obliterative bronchiolitis and determinants of outcome in 139 pulmonary retransplant recipients. J. Thorac. Cardiovasc. Surg. 1995; 110: 1402–'413.
17. Correas Gomez MA, Portillo Martin JA, Gutierrez Banos JL, Monge Mirallas JM, Roca Edreira A. Retrasplante renal. Estudio de 91 casos. Actas. Urol. Esp. 1993; 17: 430–433.
18. Hirata M, Terasaki PI. Renal retransplantation. Clin. Transplant. 1994; 8: 419–433.
19. Mitsuishi Y, Cecka JM. Recent improvements in cadaver-donor kidney retransplantation. Clin. Transplant. 1991; 5: 281–291.
20. Imagawa DK, Cecka JM. Renal regrafts. Clin. Transplant. 1988; 2: 387–398.

PART NINE

Oral communications

RESULTS OF SECOND RENAL TRANSPLANTATION IN PEDIATRIC PATIENTS

M. Charbit, M.F. Gagnadoux, G. Guest, P. Niaudet, D. Beurton, Y. Révillon, M. Broyer
Néphrologie Pédiatrique, Hôpital Necker-Enfants Malades, 149 rue de Sèvres, 75743 Paris Cedex 15, France.

In order to assess the factors that influence the prognosis of pediatric kidney retransplantation, we studied the outcome of 119 second transplantations performed in our pediatric transplantation unit. Between 1972 and 1995, 819 first grafts and 119 second grafts were performed in 716 adolescents and children. The 119 retransplant recipients were 3 years 9 months to 22 years old at the time of the second graft. One hundred and three patients received a cadaveric kidney (CK) and 16 a kidney from a living related donor (LRD). For the analysis of the outcome, we divided the patients into 3 groups according to the cause of first graft loss: 39 patients had had a non-immunological first graft loss (vascular thrombosis, urological problems, non-viable kidney), (group I). In 78 patients graft loss was due to rejection: within the first year in 31 patients (group II) and after 1 year in 47 patients (group III). Two patients were excluded because of uncertain etiology of graft loss. The percentage of patients with cytotoxic antibodies was 59% in group I (mean level 24%), 81% in group II (mean level 42%) and 53% in group III (mean level 19%). As a rule, no more than 2 HLA mismatches were accepted for the second graft when the first graft had been lost from rejection. The mean number of class I and class II mismatches were respectively 1.92 and 0.63 in group I, 1.26 and 0.71 in group II, 1.56 and 0.49 in group III. The immunosuppressive treatment was not different from that of first graft: conventional (prednisone + azathioprine) in 22 patients up to September 1984, thereafter associated induction therapy (antilymphocyte globulin in 65 patients and OKT3 in 22 patients) and cyclosporin from day 6 in all patients. Three patients received tacrolimus as rescue therapy.

Results: Graft survival rates for second transplants at 1, 2, 5 and 10 years were 77, 74, 61 and 54%, respectively compared with 82, 77, 64 and 47% for first transplants. However, it was clear that graft survival rates were better in groups I and III (85, 82, 70 and 61%, respectively at 1, 2, 5, 10 years in group I and 77, 77, 67 and 67% in group III) than in group II (68, 61, 50 and 36%). In group II, the cause of second graft loss was exclusively immunological. The results of retransplantation with LRD were clearly better than with CK, even in the group II patients (losses 2/6 with LRD vs 17/25 with CK). The results did not differ according to induction therapy (antilymphocyte globulin or OKT3). Tacrolimus rescued 2 of the 3 treated grafts. Ten patients had repeated mismatches (6 patients in class I, 3 patients in class II, and 1 patient in class I and II; 3 of these lost their graft.

Conclusion: Graft survival rates for second transplantation as a whole were comparable to those for first transplantation; in particular, survival rates for LRD second graft were excellent. However, when first graft loss was due to early rejection, the outcome of second graft remained relatively poor, and these results raise the question of more potent immunosuppressive protocol for such patients.

PAEDIATRIC RENAL RETRANSPLANTATION

G. N. Fernando

Introduction

While the results of renal transplantation in adults and children have improved over the past decade, there still remains a cohort of patients in whom primary graft failure is inevitable. Early failure results not only from technical and surgical complications but immunological reasons still account for the persistent failure of grafts and an inevitable reduction in graft survival. While in adults the return to haemodialysis or peritoneal dialysis seems to offer a temporary solution, in the paediatric group, the continuation of these modalities of treatment does not offer a viable solution to children who require to grow and develop into near normal adolescent and adult life. The problem of failure has been compounded by the serious problem of non-compliance and even meticulous supervision does not resolve the dangers related in this select group of patients. Most transplant centres have a 15% retransplantation rate.

There are numerous factors which affect the outcome in retransplantation, including donor age and recipient age, HLA/DR mismatching, panel reactive/panel reactive antibodies, cold ischaemia time and also, to some extent, warm ischaemia time, immunosuppression, particularly with regard to the use of induction therapy, incidence of recurrent disease in children, non-compliance, and surgical problems. The best data with regard to the outcome of retransplantation is from the North American Paediatric Renal Transplant Co-operative study and I would like to give the results published in *Transplantation*, September 1996.

The overall graft survival of these patients for a primary transplant over 6, 12, 24, 36 and 60 months was 88, 85, 80, 76 and 69% as opposed to a second transplant which had a graft survival of 81, 77, 71, 64 and 52% with a P value of <0.05. If one then broke this down into cadaver and live related donor transplant, the cadaveric donors showed survival of 83, 79, 74, 69 and 62% compared with the respective values of 79, 74, 68, 60 and 47% for a regraft with a P value of <0.01. The results of live-related donor transplant were almost equal in both groups at 60 months, but the regraft success rate at 6 months was 93 and 88% initially. The UKTSSA data looked at a smaller group of 914 patients during the period 1984–December 1993, 914 first graft and 250 regrafts. The 1 year survival was 75% for the first grafts and the 5 year survival 61% but the regraft rate of success was 73 and 60%.

I would now like to look at the various factors that account for this outcome.

Immunological problems related to retransplantation

While we have noted that graft survival of renal allografts have improved steadily and these improvements have been related to the use of the newer immunosuppressive agents, i.e. Cyclosporin A and FK506, there has also been a better understanding of the other immunosuppressive agents. In terms of quantity, this has meant an overall 15% increase in one year survival of first grafts but there has been an even more striking improvement in the case of regrafts.

Some groups have claimed that HLA matching has no impact on graft survival. However, the larger groups of the collaborative transplant study, the European Transplant Service, UNOS and UKTSSA have also shown a clear benefit of HLA and particularly DR matching. Indeed, detailed analysis of matching for HLA shows a correlation not only with HLA matching but also with the number of rejection episodes. This increase in the number of rejection episodes has naturally resulted in an increase in hospital stay with higher three month serum creatinine levels. This effect is of course more marked in retransplantation patients in the paediatric sector. The clinical course therefore closely follows not only the donor and recipient criteria but also there is a correlation with HLA and DR matching.

Transplant failure was the most immunogenic factor resulting in a high degree of sensitization followed by transfusion and then pregnancy. A recognition of the immunogenic affect of transfusion has resulted in a drop in the transfusion rate from about 80% in 1987 to 52% in 1993.

Assessment and recognition of the titre and identity of panel reactive antibodies is important in the preparatory period prior to retransplantation. A critical identification of HLA specificities to which the patient is sensitive allows efficient selection of donors. Monthly analyses of alloantibody reactivity will give an indication of a particularly sensitized recipients availability for exposure to a compatible donor.

A further factor in the genesis of antibodies is a graft nephrectomy. Several papers have pointed out that primary graft nephrectomy causes a rise in antibody titre. Many centres now reserve graft nephrectomy for patients who develop pyrexia, graft tenderness, haematuria or any symptoms related to the graft.

The development of sensitive crossmatch techniques has prevented hyper-acute rejection in renal transplantation. Flow cytometry, FAC-cell crossmatch and crossmatch by antiglobulin techniques appears to be gaining more widespread acceptance.

There is some conflict and dispute on whether patients with historically positive crossmatches should proceed to transplantation. The question of whether one can transplant patients who have a historically positive crossmatch and have an antigen to which they have been exposed, presents an ethical dilemma. Our practice with regard to historically positive crossmatches has been that we will do it provided there is no antigen to which the recipient has been exposed before. Clearly the selection of well-matched kidneys for regrafting along with the combination of assessment of the antibody status will reduce the risk of immunological failure.

HLA identical living related donor transplant have been used successfully and a report by Laufer et al. have shown the experience of five such children with HLA identical retransplants, following previous failure of one or more cadaveric grafts. The reported success rate of this series makes living related donation in this difficult group a worthwhile experience.

Recurrence and retransplantation

Recurrent disease and *de novo* nephritis may destroy many transplants and for the same reasons that we have discussed earlier, retransplantation is highly desirable even in this group of patients.

A recurrence rate which varies widely from 15 to 100% has been described in relation to focal segmental glomerulosclerosis (FSGS). However this does not necessarily spell loss of kidney. A rapid progression of focal sclerosis from diagnosis to end stage renal failure correlated with the high incidence of the recurrent disease and indeed, graft loss from recurrent FSGS was higher in patients that had lost their graft within a year of transplantation as a result of FSGS. Cameron showed that an increased incidence of recurrence correlated with a younger age group and also with recurrent FSGS in the retransplant kidney. Children below the age of six had a significantly increased risk of recurrence. However if FSGS patients lose a kidney for other reasons, retransplants are inevitably free from recurrent FSGS.

Additional risk factors are a superimposition of mesangio proliferation on the pathologic lesions of FSGS, the age of onset of the disease and the interval from diagnosis of FSGS to end stage failure. If the risk of recurrent disease is deemed to be high, live related donor transplantation is contra-indicated and cadaver transplantation is recommended.

Membranoproliferative disease

This again has a variable recurrent rate and clearly the rapidity of destruction of a graft from this disorder spells a bad prognosis for the retransplant group. If this disorder occurs in the regraft, unfortunately dialysis seems the only path to follow.

Oxalosis

Kidney transplantation is beset with the problem that calcium oxalate crystals deposit in the transplant kidney and there is an inevitable loss of transplant. In these instances, ideally a liver and kidney transplant will yield good results. In fact, most centres now treat patients with end stage failure as a result of oxalosis with combined liver and kidney transplantation.

Cystinosis

While the kidney itself is not affected by cystinosis, the kidney function gradually deteriorates and these patients, who do suffer poor growth, may require retransplantation.

Immunosuppression

Immunosuppression has undergone a radical change over the last 2 decades. The trend has been that all primary grafts have received triple therapy as standard regimen. This has allowed the minimization of side-effects and nephrotoxicity and has allowed vastly improved graft and patient survival. While some centres may utilize monotherapy, there are undoubted risks associated with its use in the active immune system of paediatric patients.

Secondary grafts have been given a combination of triple therapy but induction therapy with ATG or ALG or the monoclonals such as OKT3 have been used as standard practice. In fact, primary dysfunction is often better managed by a reduction or stopping of cyclosporin A followed by the administration of a polyclonal antibody. Episodes of rejection were treated in the regular manner, i.e. with methyl prednisolone, while accurate and critical immune assessment remains the crucial factor in retransplantation. The use or indeed the over use, of immunosuppression is debatable. Our centre routinely uses induction therapy especially in the face of primary non-function.

Patients with antibodies have on occasion been given pre-conditioning plasma exchange with a view to reducing the antibody level. Therapy with intravenous immunoglobulin has also been attempted with varying degrees of success. While there have been a few successful reports, the practice has not achieved universal acceptance. The strategy therefore must be to obtain good matching but to use immunosuppression to the best advantage, i.e. reducing nephrotoxicity yet keeping a critical balance so that the active immune system of children, especially those below the age of 6 years, could be controlled. In all events, the reduction of steroids remains a desirable goal.

Surgical problems

I have discussed the question of graft nephrectomy. If the graft is lost due to technical problems, retransplantation will not prove to be a major problem. However the question of graft nephrectomy for acute or chronic rejection is problematic in that there is a significant rise in PRA. A primary graft nephrectomy is indicated if the patient develops fever, haematuria or graft tenderness, but it is possible to carry out a graft nephrectomy at the time of retransplantation.

In very small children, the placement of a large kidney, say from a parent or a live-related donor, may cause problems because of size incompatibility. Excellent surgical skills are demanded if good results are to be achieved. The use of prophylactic anticoagulation is mandatory. Patients who have bladder problems which have resulted in end stage renal failure may have had multiple surgeries with the result that there may be a scarred, adherent and non-compliant bladder, often with a Mitraffanoff ureterostomy. Much care and planning is required in the handling of surgical manipulation of these patients. At the Hospital for Sick Children we have utilized a multidisciplinary team approach with the utilization of skilled urological surgeons, the use of trained nurses to help with bladder compliance etc. is important.

It is often the practice in small children to anastomose the blood vessels to the aorta and cava. This may necessitate an intra-abdominal operation and these children may often be hampered by multiple adhesions in the peritoneal cavity. While an extra-peritoneal approach is desirable, it may not always be achieved. There is no doubt that the results of regrafting in regard to surgical problems have a definite centre effect and where the skills are developed to the maximum advantage, the results are always better.

Ethical issues and socioeconomic factors

It is extremely important to consider carefully the outcome of retransplantation as one raises the question of appropriate use of scarce donor resources. It is clear from my previous comments that regrafts have a 5 year survival of 69%, if one defines graft failure as a return to dialysis or death. While all the factors that I have discussed may help contribute to averting rejection and graft failure, retransplantation remains the challenge to the management of the patients. Certainly the cost of retransplantation is higher as also is the use of induction therapy. The number of readmissions in both primary and secondary grafts, was roughly similar.

Recurrent non-compliant patients form a special group in paediatric recipients. While psycho-therapy and rehabilitation may play an important role in keeping a retransplant kidney in place, there still remains a cohort who are habitually non-compliant, in which it is ethically unjustified to retransplant. In fact, the question may be raised, is it ethically justified or acceptable to divert the scarce resources of cadaver donor kidneys away from the primary transplant patients who might be expected to have a better rate of success. A decision not to perform retransplants would in fact pose an ethical dilemma, not only for the transplant physician but also for recipients. All the studies support a policy of equal access for both primary and secondary candidates and as the results of secondary transplantation improve there is a compelling case to encourage live-related donor transplantation to retransplant candidates.

Retransplantation in tumor

The penalty of prolonged and heavy immunosuppression in young patients is that they may develop malignancies. Post-transplant lymphoproliferative disorder (PTLD) remains the main malignancy. We have seen problems related to Kaposi sarcoma and other blastogenic tumors such as ovarian granulosa cell tumors.

PTLD responds to chemotherapy and a cessation of immunosuppression, while loss of the graft is not inevitable, the graft may last many years and eventually return to dialysis may occur. Retransplantation in these patients calls for the use of minimal immunosuppression and in fact, their immune system may be so reduced that hardly any immunosuppression is required. Successful outcomes in retransplantation can certainly be achieved after a period of dialysis. Kalposi cell sarcoma has been seen in some of our patients and we have not embarked on retransplantation. I can find no record of retransplantation in regard to this tumor. Other tumors are rare but again a tumor-free period of 5 years would seem to be highly desirable. This clearly would have an impact on the management of these patients but good renal function is sometimes achieved in the face of little or no immunosuppression.

Pre-emptive retransplantation and the timing of retransplantation

Continued dialysis results in poor growth and the social and educational problems of paediatric patients. Should a related donor who is compatible be available, all the evidence points to a more successful outcome in pre-emptive renal transplantation. In addition, while the background of chronic immunosuppression would be useful to prepare the patient, it will of course be possible with a live-related donor, to use the optimum immunosuppression and have all the advantages of living donation, i.e. short ischaemia, etc. which would benefit the outcome. Unfortunately the literature only reports small groups of such patients as the identical siblings of paediatric renal transplant are below the age of consent and therefore cannot offer to undergo a major surgical procedure. If however, after a period, the donor is of the age of consent, an ideal live related donor would be a better option than waiting for a high-urgency donor or a mismatched cadaver donor. Retransplantation in patients with stable but chronically rejecting allografts prior to dialysis to be highly desirable.

Summary

There is growing evidence that the results of retransplantation are not significantly different to those of primary transplants. The cost benefits of transplantation will eventually provide a savings benefit equivalent to life-long dialysis. In the paediatric group this translates to a much improved lifestyle, increased growth, education opportunities and greater rehabilitation. The various aspects such as selection of the best donor, the optimum time and ideal immunosuppression will yield undoubted success. It is therefore unethical to deny retransplantation to all except the habitually non-compliant and the defined recurrent disease recipient. The comparable cost outcome and rehabilitation following retransplantation supports the continued equitable allocation of these resources to these candidates for renal retransplantation.

RISK FACTORS AND RESULTS OF SECOND RENAL ALLOGRAFTS

L. Martins, J. Queirós, A. Henriques, A. Sarmento, S. Guimãres, M. Pereira
Serviço de Nefrología, Unidade de Transplante Renal, HGSA, Porto

Between August 83 and April 97, 8% of 746 kidney transplants (KT) were retransplants. We analysed the prognostic factors of the regraft survival and compared the results with the corresponding pairs. Sixty patients with 36 ± 11 years old were retransplanted with cadaveric kidney, 28.8 ± 23 months after the loss of the first graft. The immunosuppression used was: quadruple ($n = 45$), ATG ($n = 7$) cyclosporine ($n = 6$), triple ($n = 1$), Aza ($n = 1$). We could find no influence of the studied variables (cause of first graft failure, duration of primary graft function, time between primary graft failure and retransplant, immunosuppression schedule, last PRA, nephrectomy of the first graft, sex and donor age) on regraft survival. Peak PRA > 30% or less than 4 AB matching statistically decrease second graft survival ($p = 0.05$). The actuarial graft and patient survival in the first year were 73.1 and 93% and at 5 years 55.4 and 83.9%, respectively. The graft pair's survival at 1 and 5 years was 86.8 and 75.7%, respectively ($p = 0.06$).

Conclusions: 1. Peak PRA and less than 4 matching were risk factors for regraft. 2. Although regraft survival was lower, the results are good.

RETRANSPLANTATION OF THE LIVER GRAFT: INDICATION AND RESULTS IN A SINGLE-CENTER EXPERIENCE

L. De Carlis, C.V. Sansalone, G. Colella, P. Aseni, A.O. Slim, V. Pirotta, K. Arcieri, F. Di Benedetto, G.F. Rondinara, D. Forti
Dept. of Surgery and Abdominal Transplantation, Niguarda Hospital, Milan, Italy

Background: Retransplantation of the liver (ReOLtx) is an outstanding challenge for both the patient and the surgeon. While acute ReOLTx, often a consequence of a primary graft non-function (PGNF) or a vascular accident, is a simple and rapid operation, the clinical conditions of the patients are generally critical and results of the procedure may be poor. On the other hand, ReOltx performed long after the first grafting, has commonly indications such as chronic rejection or recurrence of the initial disease (viral cirrhosis, PBC and others); in these cases the operation may be very difficult, time-consuming and bloody. Anyway, the results of ReOLTX are often unsatisfying and concern exist upon its wide application.

Materials and methods: Over a 10-year period at our Institution, 30 ReOLTx were performed in 25 patients out of a series of 350 primary OLTx (8.5%): 5 patients had a third graft: 4 in the first month after OLTx and 1 3 years after the first ReOLTx. 21 (70%) were a consequence of acute failure of the graft (7 vascular thrombosis, 13 PGNF, 1 acute rejection). 9 (30%) were done between 3 months to 7 years from the primary transplantation due to chronic rejection (5 cases), recurrence of viral cirrhosis (3 cases) or late arterial thrombosis with multiple biliary stenoses and dilatations (1 case).

Results: 7 patients out of the 21 (33.3%) who had ReOLTx for acute reasons survived the operation and are currently alive or died long after for different reasons (2 cases). Intraoperative blood losses were 2.1 ± 3.1 vs 2.7 ± 2.4 l in primary OLTx (p: NS). Causes of deaths were MOF (11 patients) and irreversible brain damage (3 patients). In the second group, 6 patients (66.6%) are alive and well after ReOLTx (mean follow-up 3.6 years range 2 months to 9 years) without relapse of the original disease. Intraoperative blood losses were 18 ± 12 vs 2.7 ± 2.4 liters in primary OLTx ($p < 0.05$). Causes of death were MOF (1 patient), irreversible brain damage (1 patient) and intraoperative hemorrhage (1 patient).

Conclusions: ReOLTx was a therapeutic option only in 8.5% of our entire series. Acute ReOltx had in our experience bad results and this can reflect the fact that these patients are nearly anhepatic and need emergent reoperation: the lack of donors in Italy, in fact, is especially critical in urgent situations. Late ReOLTx is a more complex operation but results were more satisfactory and comparable with primary grafting in complicated patients. Chronic rejection is the indication of choice as sensitization of the patient seem not to play any role in their outcome. In recurrent viral cirrhosis the risk of further relapse is not well established but more and more patients will require a ReOLTx when 10 years of follow up are reached: studies on viral genomas and a wider use of new antiviral agents will be effectual in this field.

EARLY AND LATE LIVER RETRANSPLANTATION

U. Maggi, G. Rossi, A. Lucianetti, L. Caccamo, S. Gatti, L.R. Fassati
Centro Trapianti Fegato, Ospedale Maggiore Policlinico IRCCS, Milano, Italy

Introduction: Retransplantation (RETX) has worse results on graft survival if compared with 1st Liver transplantation (OLT). Recent data (6/1996) about 1st OLT from European Registry (ELTR) report 1 and 5 years survival rates of 70 and 59% respectively, compared to 47, 44, 39% and 39, 33, 32% at 1 and 5 years after 1st, 2nd and 3rd RETX respectively. As long survival after transplantation is achieved, the rate of RETX long time after the 1st OLT is increasing. We reviewed the results of RETX in our patients (patients).

Patients and methods: Since 6/1983 through 3/1997, 308 patients underwent 345 OLT. 32 patients (10.3%, 23 males, 11 females; mean age 32.3 ± 16.1 years, median 35, range 1–54) underwent 37 RETX. 31 patients were retransplanted once, 3 patients twice. In detail, 14 RETX were performed within 30 days from OLT, 12 between 1 and 6 months, 2 between 6 months and 1 year, 2 between 1 and 2 years, 4 between 3 and 4 years (Figure 1).

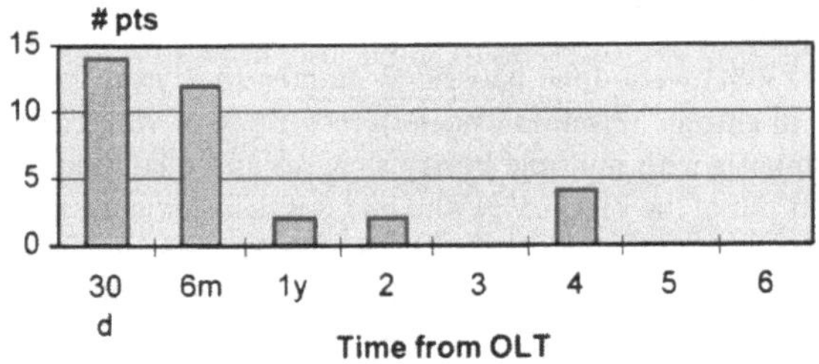

Fig. 1.

28 patients underwent RETX within 1 year from OLT: the ethiology was acute rejection ($n = 10$), primary non function ($n = 8$), hepatic artery thrombosis (HAT) ($n = 3$), liver failure ($n = 2$), chronic rejection ($n = 1$), others ($n = 4$).

6 patients underwent RETX beyond 1 year from OLT: ethiology was HAT ($n = 2$) with a concomitant C-hepatitis in 1, B recurrent hepatitis ($n = 1$), recurrent PBC ($n = 1$), sclerosing cholangitis post biliary stenosis ($n = 1$), biliary cirrhosis with portal vein thrombosis ($n = 1$).

Results: At 30 days, 1, 2, 3, 4, 5, 6, 7 years, graft actuarial survival in 28 RETX performed within 1 year from OLT was respectively 53.6%, 37.7% (1–6 years), 12.6% at 7 years, compared to 66.7% at 30 days, and 50% (1–7 years) in RETX performed beyond 1 year after 1st OLT (Figure 2).

At 30 days, 1, 2, 3, 4, 5, 6, 7 years, patient actuarial survival in 6 RETX performed within 1 year from OLT, was respectively 85.7%, 37.3% (1–6 years), 12.4% at 7 years, compared to 100% at 30 days and 1 year, 83.3% at 2 and 3 years, and 66.7% thereafter in patients who underwent RETX beyond 1 year after 1st OLT.

Global patients survival in 28 RETX performed within 1 year from OLT was 35% with a mean follow-up of 19 (27 months (median 5.5, range 0.5–83) while in patients retransplanted beyond 1 year was 66.7%, with a mean follow-up of 75 (38 months (median 74, range 23–127).

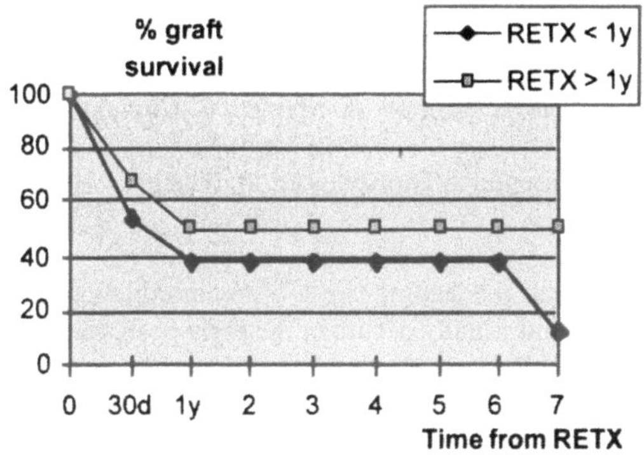

Fig. 2.

Discussion and conclusion: In our retrospective study, RETX performed 1 year after the 1st OLT had better graft survival than RETX performed within 1 year. Late RETX are probably performed in not so urgent conditions compared with early RETX. They are 'elective' RETX. So results of late RETX are worse than after 1st OLT, but better than early RETX: this should be considered in the decision to perform or not late RETX in patients with late hepatic failure.

EARLY PANCREAS RETRANSPLANTION FOR VASCULAR THROMBOSIS IN SIMULTANEOUS PANCREAS-KIDNEY TRANSPLANTS

C.V. Sansalone, G. Colella, L. De Carlis, P. Aseni, A.O. Slim, F. Di Benedetto, G.F. Rondinara, P. Goglia, C. Brunati, A. Meroni, R. Confalonieri, M.L. Follini, G. Civati, D. Forti
Dept. of Surgery and Abdominal Transplantation, Niguarda Hospital, Milan, Italy

Vascular thrombosis is still the leading cause of nonimmunologic, technical pancreatic transplant graft failures and usually occurs in the early postoperative period. Little data exist regarding the issue of pancreas retransplantation although it has been described for chronic rejection in pancreas transplant alone with poor results. From October 1993 to December 1996, 16 patients with type I diabetes mellitus and end-stage renal disease underwent to SPK at our Dept. of General Surgery and Adominal Organ Transplantation. Twelve were males and 4 females with a mean age of 36.8 (range 25 to 56). Therteen had bladder drainage (BD) and 3 enteric drainage (ED). One patient in the BD group and 1 patient in the ED group had vascular thrombosis of their pancreas graft 7 and 3 days after SPK respectively. Both patients presented hematuria, abdominal tenderness, pain and oedema of the ipsilateral lower limb. At operation, hemorragic necrosis involving the whole pancreas with thrombosis of portal vein extended in the external and common iliac veins was seen. Pancreasectomy and thrombectomy associated to pancreas retransplantion was performed in 1 patient in the same time while in the other, pancreas retransplant was performed 1 day later. The postoperative course was uneventful and both patients were discharged 16 and 23 days p.o. They are alive and well 6 and 11 months with functioning grafts.

Conclusion: Reported results of pancreas retransplantation are, in general, inferior to those achieved with primary transplantation. However, based on this initial experience, we believe that pancreas retransplantation is a challenging but safe procedure with results comparable to primary PT. The excellent results in these two patients justifies an aggressive policy of retransplantation in the diabetic with a failed allograft due to early vascular thrombosis.

LIVER TRANSPLANTATION (OLT) FOR ALCOHOLIC CIRRHOSIS WITH RESPECT TO RECIDIVISM

D. Mioni, M. De Bona, U. Cillo, G. Malandrino, S. Targhetta, A. Graziotto, S. Fagiuoli, M. Salvagnini, P. Burra
Gastroenterology and Surgery Depts, University of Study, Padova, Italy

OLT is an effective therapeutic option for end-stage liver disease and survival rates are encouraging. Disagreement however exists as to whether OLT should be provided to patients with alcoholic cirrhosis. The aim of the study was to evaluate long-term results (recidivism to alcohol consumption, incidence of acute rejection, survival) in patients transplanted for ALD.

Thirty-four patients (26 M, 8 F, median age 46 years; range 30–60 years) who underwent OLT for ALD (8 = HCV +; 1 = HBsAg +) were studied and compared with 92 patients (56 M, 36 F; median age 43 years, range 24–61 years) who underwent OLT for non-ALD.

Recidivism in ALD patients or alcohol consumption in non-ALD patients were proved by a semi-structured intereview and self-rating questionnaires to assess physical and psychiatric morbidity, depression and neurosis, social functioning and alcohol dependence of patients before and after OLT, abnormal liver function tests and liver biopsy. Acute rejection was diagnosed using stablished histologic criteria. Patient survival was estimated using Kaplan–Meier methodology.

Recidivism occured in 5/26 (19%) ALD patients and alcohol consumption was declared by 5/71 (7%) of non-ALD patients between 3–13 months after OLT. The incidence of acute rejection was lower in ALD than in non-ALD patients (48% vs 63%). While awaiting OLT, 15% of ALD compared to 4% of non-ALD patients died within the first 6 months. Patient survival at 1, 3 and 5 years after OLT was respectively 70%, 70% and 70% in the ALD group and 69%, 65% and 63% in non-ALD group.

In conclusion: recidivism occurs in 20% of our alcoholic patients, whereas alcohol consumption in non-ALD patients is relatively low; the incidence of acute rejection is lower in ALD compared with non-ALD patients; in patients listed for OLT mortality rate is higher in ALD than in non-ALD group and short-and long-term survival after OLT are similar in the two groups.

ANTI-CLASS I HLA ANTIBODIES IN POTENTIAL KIDNEY TRANSPLANT RECIPIENTS: DIFFERENT CREG PHENOTYPES IN PATIENTS AWAITING A SECOND TRANSPLANT WITH RESPECT TO NON-TRANSPLANTED PATIENTS

G. Fernández-Fresnedo[1], J.M. Pastor[2], J.C. Ruiz[1], J.G. Cotorruelo[1], M. Setién[1], M. López-Hoyos[3], M. Arias[1]
[1]Nephrology, [2]Haematology and Haemotherapy and [3]Immunology Units, University Hospital 'Marqués de Valdecilla', Santander 39008, Spain

Objective: To determine whether there is any difference in the repertoire of cross-reactive groups (CREG) antibodies (Ab) in potential kidney transplant recipients, comparing those who have already lost one kidney with those who have never received one.

Material and methods: A total of 5292 sera from 570 patients awaiting kidney transplantation were screened for the presence of HLA antibodies between 1992 and 1996. 467 patients were awaiting their first transplant whereas 103 had lost a previous allograft. In those sera containing Abs against class I HLA, a specificity was considered when a significant correlation coefficient was observed (r, obtained after 2×2 table analysis; software package: One Lambda 4.02): $r > 0.7$ for monospecific and $r > 0.8$ for polispecific sera were considered in the case of only one positive serum sample per patient, and $r > 0.65$ and $r > 0.7$, respectively, when more than one positive samples appeared.

Ab specificities were converted to the major CREGS each specificity belonged to and compared to the CREGS phenotypes the HLA alleles of the patients and graft donors belonged to. The following CREGS phenotypes were considered: 1C (A1, 3, 10, 11, 19, 36), 2C (A2, 9, 28), 5C (B5, 15, 17, 18, 35, 70), 7C (B7, 22, 27, 40, 73), 8C (B8, 14, 16, 67), 12C (B12, 13, 21, 37).

Results: Thirty-six patients developed Abs not related to transplantation (AbNRT). Seven of them (19%) showed Abs to specificities included into their own CREG. Interestingly, these Abs were specific only for CREG 1C. Twenty-nine patients with AbNRT (81%) developed Abs to specificities included into different CREGS (15% 1C, 34% 2C, 6% 5C, 9% 7C, 9% 8C and 25% 12C). A significantly greater proportion of these patients had Abs specific to an unique CREG (89%).

Twenty-one patients had sera containing Abs related to transplantation (AbRT). Eleven of them (52%) were Abs to specificities included into their own CREGS ($p = 0.009$ compared with patients with AbNRT): 50% 1C, 25% 2C, 16% 5C and 9% 8C. Ninety-one percent of patients with those Abs had Abs directed to an unique CREG, and 2 patients (18%) had also Abs against different CREGS (5C y 2C). Among the remaining patients, ten patients with AbRT (48%) showed Abs against different CREGS (50% 2C, 10% 7C, 40% 12C).

Conclusions: Failed solid grafts seems to be able to induce a stronger immune response than other sources of sensitization. This is manifested by a significantly higher frequency of Antibodies to specificities included in the same CREGS than the receptor alleles.

The development of Abs to specificities included into CREG 1C in subjects with AbNRT suggests that this CREG is highly heterogeneous.

COMPARATIVE INFLUENCE OF HLA IN THE SURVIVAL OF THE FIRST AND SECOND RENAL GRAFTS

J.L. Garnier, L. Gebuhrer, S. Daoud, N. Lefrançois, A. Guérard, M.C. Bonnet, J. Carrie, J.M. Dubernard, J.L. Touraine
Hôpital Edouard Herriot, Pav P, Lyon, France

In a retrospective study, we have analysed the outcome of the first and the second graft according to HLA compatibility and duration of the first graft.

Between January 1990 and December 1995, 96 consecutive second or third renal grafts (6) have been performed in our institution. Have been excluded from this study, patients receiving a liver or heart transplant combined with the kidney graft, 3 patients who had a first graft which failed for vascular obstruction within 2 days after the transplant, and patients whose follow-up did not reach 6 months (6 who died of cancer, infection or heart attack). 80 patients received a second kidney and details are presented in the table below.

Conclusions: HLA compatibility has improved for the second graft in all groups; it does not influence the survival of this graft in patients who lost rapidly a first graft. In patients who had a first graft for a longer period, a better match is observed in patients who had a functioning second graft at the time of analysis.

	Duration of first graft							
% patients	< 12 months 35		12 months–5 years 26		5–10 years 21		> 10 years 18	
	Function of the second graft (loss due to rejection)							
	lost	retained	lost	retained	lost	retained	lost	retained
% patients	5.2	28.7 26% CR 10% rec.	13.5	12.5 60% CR (1 rec.)	4	17 40% CR 10% rec.	1.5	16.5 20% CR
1st graft duration (months)	1.4	2.5	31	32.6	100	89	120	154
HLA								
A:	1	0.6	0.7	0.8	0.6	0.85	1	0.76
B:	0.8	0.57	0.33	2.2	0.3	0.5	2	0.76
DR:	0.6	0.6	0.33	0.7	0.3	0.6	1	0.8
≥3 ident	40%	28%	0	20%	30%	36%	100%	46%
2nd graft: HLA ab								
> 50%	20%	52%	54%	50%	100%	21%	100%	8%
< 50%	40%	39%	36%	40%		65%		46%
0	40%	4%	9%	10%		14%		46%

Continued.

duration (months)	42.8	56.8	11.8	54.6	15	45	2	46
HLA								
A:	1.2	1	0.7	0.9	1.2	1	0.7	0.9
B:	1.2	0.86	1.3	1.2	1.2	0.86	1.3	1.2
DR:	1	1.04	0.44	1.4	1	1.04	0.44	1.4
$\geq$3 ident	100%	60%	36%	70%	100%	60%	36%	70%

CR: chronic rejection; rec: recurrence of the original disease on the transplanted kidney.
HLA ab: panel reactive anti-HLA antibodies.

A PRETRANSPLANT 'BOOSTER' DOSE OF AN ANTI-T-ACTIVATED RATG (ANTI-JURKAT) INDUCES MASSIVE ENDOGENOUS IL-10 RELEASE WITH TRANSIENT DRASTIC LYMPHOCYTE DEPLETION AT THE PRIMING TIME OF ANTIGEN PRESENTATION WITH 100% OF PATIENTS AND GRAFT SURVIVAL AT A MEAN OF 30 MONTHS IN 17 KIDNEY RETRANSPLANTATIONS.

Y. Saint-Hillier, V. Fournier, E. Racadot, B. Hory, C. Bresson-Vautrin, M. Jamali, D. Ducloux, H. Bittard, J.M. Chalopin
Dept of Nephrology, CHU St Jacques and Blood Transfusion Center, 25030, Besançon, France.

Experimentally manipulation of cytokine networks is a realistic opportunity for tolerance induction in transplantation but graft tolerance is also influenced by the timing of immunosuppression, the degree of blockade of costimulatory signals and adhesion molecules, production of IL-10, Th1/Th2 ratio and T-cell depletion. The purpose of this study was to evaluate a new induction protocol using a pretransplant 'booster' dose of an anti-T-activated rabbit polyclonal antibody (ATG, Fresenius) anti-Jurkat, given pre- and intraoperatively in order to achieve maximal immunosuppression at the priming time of antigen presentation. ATG-F contains specificities against adhesion molecules (LFA-1, ICAM-1, CD2), and important costimulatory signals (CD28) and many others, stimulates IL-10 production, induces T-cell depletion and has a long half-life of more than 15 days.

Between June 93 and Dec 96, 17 patients received a cadaveric renal retransplant. All were treated with an induction protocol using a single 'booster' dose of ATG-F (9 mg/ kg), 3 times the recommended dose, infused over 3–4 hours pre and intraoperatively after 500 mg of methylprednisolone and subsequently a dose of 3 mg/kg/day for a short period of 4 days only (to avoid overimmunosuppression). Other immunosuppressants included prednisone, azathioprine and CyA at low dosage. Patients, 10M and 7F were aged 22–61 years (average 44). 14 were second and 3 were third transplants 4 (22%) had a positive B Facs cross-match. All patients have lost their first graft for immunological reasons but two after arterial thrombosis. Cold ischemic time was at 1389 ± 717 mn and mean HLA ABDR MM at 2.25 with only one pt with a repeat MM. ATG-F were very well tolerated without cytokine release syndrome. Initial IL-10 level were at 15 ± 28 pg/ml. They rose during and after ATG-F infusion reaching a peak 660 ± 798 pg/ml (range 66–2150) at the time of reperfusion of the transplant and returned to low level at 24 hr in the 6 tested patients. The Th1 cytokines IL-2 and IFN-γ were inhibited simultaneously. There was synergisticaly a marked but transient T cell depletion of CD3+ lymphocytes count at $12 \pm 15/\text{mm}^3$ at the time of graft, which returned to more than 50 at day 1 to reach more than $150/\text{mm}^3$ at day 5. Only five patients (29%) had an acute reversible rejection during the follow-up (mean$\geqslant$30, range 45–4 months) treated only by 1 g of methylprednisolone for three days, without the need of OKT3 rescue therapy.

Actual patient and graft survival was 100%, despite the fact that this group were high risk patients and the mean last creatinine was at 145 ± 41 μmol/l. This uncontrolled study suggests that a pretransplant 'booster' dose of ATG-F, given at the time of transplantation is well tolerated, cheap, induces IL-10 production, T cell depletion, simultaneous blockade of multiple T cell coreceptors and improves graft survival without inducing overimmunosuppression.

KIDNEY RETRANSPLANTATION IN SENSITIZED PATIENTS: EXPERIENCE WITH A NEW IMMUNOSUPPRESSIVE PROTOCOL

J.V. Woellwarth, M. Behrend, H.J. Schlitt, K.J. Oldhafer, B. Nashan, V. Kliem, R. Brunkhorst, R. Pichlmayr
Abteilung für Abdominal- und Transplantationschirurgie, Klinik für Nephrologie, Medizinische Hochschule Hannover, 30623 Hannover, Germany

The results of retransplantation in those patients with high panel reactive antibodies (PRA) are worse than in other recipients. Nevertheless the number of retransplantations and the number of sensitized patients on the waiting list are increasing. To improve the results we used a new immunosuppressive strategy with a single shot of intraoperative ATG followed by a high dose mycophenolate mofetil maintenance immunosuppression. The working mechanism of mycophenolate mofetil with lymphocyte suppression is likely to improve the results in those patients, especially in conjunction with an intraoperative ATG bolus.

Methods: Immunological high risk patients were defined as follows: historical or latest PRA levels > 30%, graft loss of a previous transplant by rejection or more than one previous transplantation. The immunosuppression consisted of an intraoperative ATG bolus of 2 mg/kg bw, cyclosporine A 10 mg/kg bw, mycophenolate mofetil 3 g/day and an intraoperative steroid bolus of 500 mg followed by an oral steroid taper to 7.5 mg/day.

Patients: We report on 19 patients treated with this new protocol. 5 patients received a first kidney transplant, 6 a second, 6 a third and 2 a fourth. Two patients had PRA levels of 0–30%, 7 patients had PRA of 30–70%, and 10 patients had PRA of more than 70%. 13/19 patients had specific antibodies. Mismatches were 0 in 5 patients, 1–2 in 8 patients, 3–4 in 4 patients and 6 in two patients.

Results: 10/19 (52.6%) patients developed no clinical sign of rejection within the first 3 months after transplantation. 9/19 (47.3%) developed a histological proven rejection. 4/9 responded well to a single steroid bolus therapy. 2/9 responded after conversion to FK 506, 1/9 with a child kidney as third graft has a marginal function after conversion to FK 506, 2/7 grafts were lost. The last two showed never a renal function after transplantation. The mean creatinine of the 17 surviving organs was 130 μmol/l ($\pm$39) at 3 months and 149 μmol/l ($\pm$55) at 6 months.

Summary: The rejection rate of 47% is extraordinarily low for sensitized patients with high panel reactive antibodies. The graft survival rate is actually 89%. The overall results in this high risk patient population are promising to continue with this immunosuppressive protocol. The strategy to combine a single shot of an antilymphocyte preparation given intraoperatively with a lymphocyte specific maintenance immunosuppression is superior to earlier results in this patient.

MEDICAL COMPLICATIONS AFTER LIVER TRANSPLANTATION (OLT): IMPACT ON QUALITY OF LIFE (QOL)

M. De Bona, F. Foti*, E. Favero*, R.M. Jemmolo†, P. Boccagni‡, S. Fagiuoli, D. Mioni, M. Ermani, G.P. Rupolo*, P. Burra
Gastroenterology, †Internal Medicine, ‡Surgery and *Psychiatric Depts, University of Padua, Italy

OLT is indicated as a procedure for patients with end-stage liver disease to restore not only liver function, but also a good QOL. Few data assessing correlation between medical complications and QOL after OLT are available. The aim of this cross-sectional study was to evaluate the effect of OLT on QOL in adult liver transplant recipients.

Ninety-three patients were evaluated: Group A = 19 patients, pre-OLT (14 M, 5 F; mean age 49.1 years, range 26–61); Group B = 33 patients, first year post-OLT (26 M, 7 F; 43.9 years, 22–65); Group C = 41 patients, 1 to 5 year post-OLT (27 M, 14 F; 47.7 years, 26–64). They were asked to complete the Brief Symptom Inventory (BSI, 49 items grouped by 9 categories), LEIPAD Quality of Life Scale (25 items, 6 categories) and Mini Mental State Examination (MMSE, 10 items), when listed for OLT and at 3, 6, 12 months and then yearly after OLT. Numerical scores were assigned to each question and added to derive scores on categories (mean ± SD, Mann-Whitney U test). Group B patients underwent assessment of liver function tests (LFTs), cyclosporine blood levels (CyA). At one year after OLT, infections, hypertension, renal failure, osteoporosis, gingival hyperplasia, cephalea, tremors, and recurrence of the original liver disease (RLD) were assessed.

In the BSI scale, Somatization scores were significantly worse in Group A than in Group B (6/1 ± 5/4 vs 2.7 ± 3.2; $p = 0.029$) but also in C than in B (3.7 ± 2.9; $p = 0.043$). In the LEIPAD scale, Physical Functioning (B vs A 4.3 ± 2.4 vs 7.4 ± 3.9, $p = 0.004$; C 5.3 ± 2.3 vs A, $p = 0.036$) and Life Satisfaction (B vs A 2.9 ± 1.4 vs 5.5 ± 2.7; $p =$ 0.0006, C vs A 3.6 ± 1.9; $p = 0.01$) improved after OLT; Depression and Anxiety improved 1 year after OLT (B vs A 3.6 ± 2.5 vs 2.0 ± 2.3, $p = 0.01$) but worsened later (2.8 ± 2.2, $p = 0.05$). The MMSE scores were similar in the pre- and post-OLT groups. LFTs and CyA did not correlate with any area of QOL, whereas among medical complications RLD correlated with Depression and Anxiety categories ($p < 0.05$).

In conclusion: OLT improves most of the domains of QOL by the end of the first post-transplant year, though these results do not all persist in the long-term, but does not change cognitive functioning. Depression and anxiety worse in patients with RLD.

SAME PROGNOSIS FOR FIRST AND SECOND KIDNEY TRANSPLANTATION: WHAT IS THE PRICE TO PAY?

M. Hazzan, F. Dufosse, F. Bourdon, F.R. Pruvot, M. Dracon, G. Lelièvre, C. Noël
CHRU Lille, France

The number of patients waiting for a second graft is increasing each year due to the fear of failure imbalanced with the hope of improving new immunosuppression treatments. To ascertain the most important prognostic variables up to 5 years post transplantation, we analysed 570 patients, 512 receiving first and 58 second kidney grafts from cadaver donors, between January 1, 1986 and December 31 1995. During this period, the immunosuppression was not modified and consisted of induction with lymphoglobulin for the first grafts and thymoglobulin for the second grafts. Tritherapy was systematic for the second grafts (AZA-CsA-PRED) but AZA was stopped for the first grafts in the absence of rejection episode or delayed graft function (DGF). We applied a good matching policy in MHC class II in the second grafts (0 HLA-DR mismatch: 60% in the group of the second grafts, vs 27% in the group of first grafts, $p < 0.001$). Second graft patients were younger at the time of retransplantation than first graft patients (34 ± 8 years vs 39 ± 11 years, $p < 0.01$) but there was no other differences in pretransplant characteristics. DGF was more frequent with the second grafts (41% vs 24%, $p < 0.005$) but the incidence of rejection episodes and infectious complications was the same. In spite of these two bad prognostic factors (recipient's age <50 years and DGF), actuarial patient and graft survival rates were not different between the 2 groups.

Multivariate analysis (Cox model) showed a significant relationship between graft survival and the occurrence of a rejection episode in the 2 groups (relative risk: 3.82 and 10.94 for first and second grafts respectively, $p < 0.05$). Recipient's age less than 50 years was an independant risk factor for graft lost in first graft patients (relative risk: 2.57, $p < 0.01$). Because only one retransplanted patient was higher than 50 years old, this factor was not significant in the second graft group. The main risk factor for graft lost in the regrafted patients was the duration of the first graft survival: relative risk 16.11 when the first graft failure occurred during the first year ($p < 0.05$).

In conclusion, kidney retransplantation is generally associated with a diminished overall graft survival but however, it is not the case in our experience. We think that our policy of good HLA-DR matching and the use of thymoglobulin could be the explanation but the trade off is the higher cost due to the use of thymoglobulin in retransplantation (antilymphocyte globulins: 18609 FF vs 21834 FF per patient for first and second grafts respectively), and the increase of the waiting time before retransplantation.

SHORT OKT3 INDUCTION FOR KIDNEY RETRANSPLANTATION

J. Pascual, R. Marcén, G.F. Juárez, L. Orofino, T. Cano, T. Tenorio, F.J. Burgos, F. Liaño, C. Quereda, J. Ortuño
Servicios de Nefrología y Urología, Hospital Ramón y Cajal, Madrid, Spain

The short term results of renal retransplantation are probably related to the efficacious prevention of severe acute rejection episodes. Similarly, long term results could be related with the development of chronic rejection, one of which most important determinants is probably the number and severity of acute rejection episodes. There is not adequate evidence supporting aggressive induction protocols including monoclonal antibodies for first cadaveric renal transplantation. The results of such attempts in retransplantation are even more scarce.

In an open label way, between January 1995 and December 1996 we have performed 8 kidney retransplantations including a short period of initial induction with monoclonal antibodies (OKT3 5 days, 5 mg iv each day) with cyclosporine introduction (8 mg/kg/day po) at 4th day independently of graft function. Seven patients underwent their second transplantation and one his third procedure. All donors were cadavers and the recipients were 5 males and 3 females aged 40 ± 11 years. Six of them had glomerulonephritis as the underlying nephropathy, one interstitial nephritis and one nephroangiosclerosis. The cause of first renal allograft loss was: acute rejection ($n = 4$), vascular thrombosis ($n = 2$), chronic rejection ($n = 2$). In this small group of patients we observed an unexpectedly high percentage of delayed graft function (6/8, 75%; 40% in our overall series of 670 kidney transplants). No immediate or medium term complications related to OKT3 treatment could be identified. Two patients (20%) developed acute rejection episodes: one of them was resolved after 9 moderate steroid pulses and the other one was steroid-resistant and required 5 additional OKT3 boluses of 5 mg each to be controlled. One patient developed linfocele and another one an ureteral leak that required surgical reconstruction. Only two patients presented infections: both were mild urinary tract bacterial ones. After a mean follow-up of 13 ± 8 months the grafts are functioning (mean serum creatinine 1.8 ± 0.4 mg/dl) without ongoing complications (100% of patient and graft survival).

Our results with this short series of kidney cadaveric retransplantations support short OKT3 induction in these patients. Low incidence of acute rejections and very low rate of infections constitute the most important combination of features with this protocol.

HEPATOCYTE GROWTH FACTOR ON CsA-INDUCED NEPHROPATHY

R. Yoshimura, S. Ksai, K. Sugimura, A. Ohyama, T. Nakatani, K. Yamamoto, T. Kishimoto
Department of Urology, Osaka City University Medical School, 1-5-7, Asahimachi Abeno-ku, Osaka 545, Japan

Cyclosporine (CsA) has several side effects, the most serious being nephrotoxicity. CsA-induced nephropathy is diagnosed by clinical data, including BUN, Cre, urine volume. However, if we can detect the drug-induced nephropathy before clinical data change, nephropathy treatment will be easier. To address this problem, we have examined the effects of CsA treatment on hepatocyte growth factor (HGF) levels in rats. HGF, originally identified as a potent mitogen for mature hepatocytes, is a stromal-derived polypeptied that targets a wide variety of cells, predominantly epithelial and endothelial cells. Exogeneous HGF remarkably stimulated mitogenesis of renal tubular cells and induced rapid reconstruction of normal renal tissue structure after acute renal failure and after unilateral nephrectomy.

Methods: Male Lewis rats weighting 200–250 g were used. Group A ($n = 5$) received daily 0.1 ml of olive oil by intramuscular (im) administration for 10 days: Group B ($n = 5$) received 30 mg/kg/day of CsA for 10 days: and Group C ($n = 5$) received 3 mg/kg/day of FK-506 for 15 days.

Results: In the control rats, BUN and S-Cr levels were 15.5 mg/dl and 0.5 mg/dl, respectively. In group A and C, no elevation of BUN and S-Cr were observed after treatment until day 10. On the other hand, in group B, after treatment with CsA, BUN was elevated to 18.6, 31.0 and 58.8 mg/dl, and S-Cr was elevated to 0.55, 0.65 and 2.1 mg/dl on the 5th, 7th and 10th day, respectively. BUN and S-Cr levels started to be elevated on day 7. The level of HGF in the untreated normal Lewis rat was 0.301 + 0.038 ng/ml. In group A, the HGF levels were not increased on the 7th and 10th day (0.320, 0.328 ng/ml). However, after treatment with CsA, the level of HGF was elevated 0.508 ng/ml and 0.857 ng/ml on the 5th and 7th day in group B, respectively. The level of HGF was elevated on day 5, 2 days earlier than BUN and S-Cr levels in CsA-induced nephropathy. However, on the 10th day, the HGF level was going back to the normal range (0.316 ng/ml). In group C, the HGF level increased on the 9th, 11th and 15th day (0.280, 0.444, 0.783 ng/ml).

Conclusion: The level of HGF was elevated earlier than BUN and S-Cr levels on CsA-induced nephropathy. Those data suggested that HGF might be induced in rats model to protect to the CsA-induced nephropathy. Moreover, the results presented herein might contribute to the diagnosis of CsA-induced nephropathy earlier than by another clinical data.

PART TEN

Posters

EXPERIENCE WITH FOURTH TIME KIDNEY TRANSPLANTATION

M. Behrend, J.v. Woellwarth, K.J. Oldhafer, H.J. Schlitt, B. Nashan, V. Kliem*, R. Brunkhorst*, R. Pichlmayr
Abteilung für Abdominal- und Transplantationschirurgie, *Klinik für Nephrologie, Medizinische Hochschule Hannover, 30623 Hannover, Germany

Between December 68 and February 97, 2991 kidney transplantations were performed in our unit: 2514 were first transplants, 297 were second transplants, 63 third transplants, 15 fourth transplants and 2 fifth transplants. We report our experience with 10 fourth transplants in adult recipients performed in our unit between October 80 and October 96.

Patient	Fourth transplant	Reason for graft loss of previous transplant			Mismatch			PPA %	Current result with fourth graft
		first	second	third	A	H	DR		
1	10/80	acute	acute	chronic	–	–	–	–	lost by chronic rejection
2	12/83	acute	chronic	chronic	2	0	0	60	function
3	09/84	acute	acute	acute	0	0	0	90	lost by acute rejection
4	10/87	acute	acute	acute	0	1	0	99	lost by acute rejection
5	07/88	acute	recurrence	recurrence	1	1	1	83	lost by chronic rejection, function for 4 years
6	12/88	acute	chronic	technical	1	1	0	92	function
7	01/92	acute	acute	acute	1	1	0	65	lost by acute rejection
8	09/93	technical	technical	chronic	1	0	1	38	function
9	10/96	chronic	acute	chronic	0	0	0	83	function
10	03/96	chronic	chronic	chronic	1	2	0	0	function
11	04/96	acute	acute	acute	1	0	1	45	lost by acute rejection

Patients: Details about the actual and previous transplants are shown in the table:

Immunosuppression: The first three patients were treated with cyclosporin A, steroids and ALG, the next 4 patients were treated with cylosporin A, steroids, ATG and azathioprine, two patients with hemolytic-uremic-syndrome were treated without cyclosporin. Two patients were treated under a new protocol with single shot ATG, cyclosporin A, mycophenolate mofetil and steroids.

Results: It is difficult to summarize the result in such a heterogeneous patient population and over this time span into a short report. Six of the 11 patients reached a significant renal function, and five are currently living with a sufficient renal function without dialysis. Those who never reached any significant function all lost more than one graft by acute rejection.

Summary: The results of a fourth kidney transplantation are, of course, worse than the results of other groups. Nevertheless 45% (5/11) of the patients are currently living with their graft without dialysis. It is difficult to draw conclusions from such a small and heterogeneous patient population, but those who lost more than one previous graft by acute rejection have a worse outcome. The individual match and the panel reactive antibodies play a less significant role.

RETRANSPLANTATION OF HLA IDENTICAL SIBLING'S KIDNEY IN ONE PATIENT: THE 'ROYAL' WAY FOR A HAPPY FEW

B. Branger[1], G. Mourad[2], F. Iborra[2], J. Seignalet[2]
Nephrology departments, University Hospitals of [1]Nimes, and [2]Montpellier

M.B.Z. presented a chronic renal failure (CRF) secondary to a familial tubulo-interstitial nephritis. Immunological screening of the five other siblings of the family showed two of them with complete HLA A2, A24; B7, B62; DR 14, DR15; Dq5, Dd6 identity. No renal abnormalities were found in these two potential donors. The first transplantation was performed with a sister's kidney on November 19 1979. Outcome was excellent but local infection of the wound, followed by CMV infection led to a 3 month stay in the nephrology department. Progressively, the patient completely recovered and worked full time. Seven years later the patient spontaneously stopped his immunosuppressive drugs (imuran 100 mg/day, prednisolone 15 mg alternate days) without refering to the staff: one reason could be the normal health feeling and the absence of any problem during these seven years. Eight months later, after a dental infection episode, acute rejection occured with only partial response to methylprednisolone pulse therapy and addition of cyclosporin A. The transplant biopsy showed chronic cellular rejection with major interstitial fibrohyalinosis. 17 years after this first graft, terminal renal failure was present. The decision was taken to perform a second kidney graft from his HLA identical brother. The retransplantation was performed on November 13 1996, with no dialysis and the first graft still present. A uretero-ureteral anastomosis was performed because of the short ureta from his living donor. Outcome was excellent and within 10 days the patient was back home. This observation underlines the feasability of retransplantion from identical siblings. This allows dialysis prior to the second graft to be avoided. No anti-HLA antibody was discovered since late in the first graft rejection. Furthermore, immunosuppression was stable and cyclosporin A level constant.

This royal way of retransplantion still exists and has to be used as much as possible in CRF patients.

COMPARISON OF ECHODOPPLER AND CLEARANCE METHOD FOR THE EVALUATION OF RENAL VASCULAR RESISTANCES

S. Daoud, D. Poix, J.L. Garnier, A. Guerard, N. Lefrançois, J.L. Touraine, A. Hadj-Aïssa
Service de Transplantation et Immunologie Clinique, Service de Radiologie, Service d'Exploration Fonctionnelle Rénale Hôpital E. Herriot et Université Claude Bernard, Lyon, France

Patients: We studied 104 patients – 45 females, 59 males – aged 20 to 64 years (mean = 42.4 ± 11.5 years). All patients were recipients of cadaveric kidney transplants. They received conventional immunosuppressive therapy (prednisolone, ciclosporine, azathioprine).

Methods: The measurement of the Index of Resistance (IR) and of the Renal Vascular Resistance (RVR) was carried out by:

The Echodoppler method: The Index of Resistance (IR) was estimated using an echograph associated with a Doppler unit (probe of 3.5–5 mHz). The IR was calculated by the following formula:

$$\text{Index of Resistance} = \frac{\text{maximum systolic speed–end diastolic speed}}{\text{maximum systolic speed}}$$

The Clearance method: The PAH clearance was measured, as an estimation of Renal Plasma Flow (RPF), by standard continuous infusion technique and urine collection. The RPF was corrected with hematocrit measure to calculate the Renal Blood Flow (RBF). The RVR were then calculated by the following formula:

$$\text{RVR (mmHg/ml/min)} = \frac{\text{mean arterial pressure}}{\text{RBF}}$$

These measurements were performed at the end of the first year, the second year and the third year after renal transaction.

Results and discussion: Table 1 shows a significant increase in mAP form the first year to the third year ($p < 0.001$: ANOVA for repeated measures). The RVR did not show a significant increase because of wide dispersion of individual RBF. There was no significant correlation between the RVR and the IR. Two methods have been used to evaluate RVR: (a) echography associated with the doppler, and (b) measures of mean arterial blood pressure and PAH clearance. No satisfactory correlation has been found in transplant patients, probably because each of the methods has limits and pitfalls:

- The echography method is an indirect estimation of resistance and it is dependent on blood velocity within the vessel;

Table 1. Measures of various parameters over 3 years after transplantation (mean ± S.D.)

	1 year	2 years	3 years
IR	0.65 ± 0.05	0.65 ± 0.05	0.65 ± 0.05
mAP (mmHg)	95 ± 12	96 ± 12	99 ± 14
RBF (ml/min/1.73 m^2)	477 ± 177	498 ± 178	491 ± 173
RVR (mmHg/ml/min/1.73 m^2)	0.24 ± 0.15	0.24 ± 0.16	0.25 ± 0.18

- The PAH clearance method is accurate but it cannot measure the renal plasma flow with precision in case of renal insufficiency.

Further improvement in these methods will provide more accurate measures of RVR, an important parameter to follow in transplant patients, whether the renal function is satisfactory or poor.

CHRONIC LUNG GRAFT DYSFUNCTION: IS OXYGEN DEPENDENCE A RELEVANT CRITERIA FOR RETRANSPLANTATION?

N. Declerck, T. Perez, S. Jaillard, D. Roumilhac, J. Dupont, M.C. Copin, C.H. Marquette, A. Wurtz, A.B. Tonnel, F.R. Pruvot
Division of Surgery and Transplantation, Pulmonary Medecine, Hopital Calmette, 59037-Lille, France

Backgrounds: Lung retransplantation (LRT) has become a recognized option for chronic lung graft failure. However, besides scarcity of organs or technical problems, retransplantation may be hazardous for patients on the waiting list (WL). In this study we analyzed the course of chronic lung graft failure in 5 patients and the ultimate evolution to death or LRT.

Patients and methods: From August 1993 to December 1996, five lung transplanted patients (mean age: 44.8 years) experienced chronic graft failure. Indications for lung transplantation (LT) were emphysema ($n = 3$), cystic fibrosis ($n = 1$), pulmonary fibrosis ($n = 1$). All patients returned home after LT. Retransplantation was considered for secondary respiratory failure in absence of infection or curable bronchial complication. Patients were put on the WL in the context of Oxygen (O_2) dependence. LRT was performed by unilateral procedure. Immunosuppression for LRT was initiated as for the first LT.

Results: Bi-weekly surveillance detected a decrease in FEV_1 less than 1 year after LT in 4 patients (Table 1). Mean FEV_1 value fell to $35 \pm$ %. Obliterative bronchiolitis (OB) was confirmed by transbronchial biopsies in only 1 case. Enhanced immunosuppression failed to improve lung function in all patient. In one patient hypoxemia without change in FEV_1 occurred 2 months after SLT. Three patients were rapidly accepted on the WL for LRT because of early O_2 dependence (1 with isolated hypoxemia, 2 with hypoxemia appearing 2 and 3 months after FEV_1 decrease). The two remaining patients tolerated respiratory failure for a long time (more than 1 year after decrease of FEV_1) until hypoxemia occured. In all patients O_2 requirements regularly increased in the final course. Two patients died from intractable hypoxemia before LRT less than 2 months after inscription on the WL (1 outpatient, 1 in ICU). One patient had LRT 8 months after his first LT, two others could be retransplanted, 2 and 3 months after the onset of O_2 dependence but late after their first LT. In these 3 patients there was no postoperative

Table 1

First LT	FEV_1 after LT (% pred)	FEV_1 or CV decrease (% pred)	FEV_1 or CV decrease[a]	O_2 dependence[a]	Inscription on waiting list[a]	LRT[a]	Follow-up/ status[a]
BLT	81	25	4	7	7	8	alive/32
SLT	55	47	3	2	4	no	died/6
SLT	60	23	6	8	8	no	died/10
SLT	35	24	3	15	15	17	alive/30
SLT	52	18	7	26	26	29	alive/46

[a]Time since first LT in months.

morbidity, examination of explanted lung confirmed OB and survival was good (respectively 24, 13 and 17 months after LRT).

Discussion: LRT may be considered in transplanted patients with chronic graft failure in the absence of contraindications such as infection or poor general status. Most of these patients start lung failure by only reduction of FEV_1 that may be tolerable for a long time. Subsequently, LRT may appear questionnable at that time. Thus, O_2 dependence leads more easily patients and transplant teams to propose reinscription on lung WL. But, regarding the scarcity of lung donors, this critical event may occur too late to attempt LRT.

TREATMENT OF POST-TRANSPLANT B-CELL LYMPHOMAS WITH MONOCLONAL CHIMERIC ANTI-B-CELL ANTIBODIES

J.L. Garnier*, D. Glotz, J. Dantal, E. Alamartine, Y. Lebranchu, P. Deteix, G.T. Stevenson†
*Hôpital Edouard Herriot, Pav P, Lyon, France; †Tenovus Laboratory, Southampton Hospital, UK

Treatment of post-transplant B-cell lymphomas has proved to be difficult because the decrease of the immunosuppressive therapy can lead to rejection and chemotherapy is hazardous. Anti-CD21/24 monoclonal antibody therapy has previously offered the advantages of a good tolerance and efficiency on oligoclonal lymphomas. With a better knowledge of the phenotype of post-transplant lymphomas, we tried to develop chimeric monoclonal antibodies (mAb) that could be more efficient on the lymphomas and could permit to keep the immunosuppression in order to avoid graft loss.

Monoclonal chimeric antibodies are prepared by biochemical methods: 2 or 4 human, Fc are linked to 2 mouse Fab of the same CD19, CD22 or CD20 specificity or 2 different CD20, CD37 or CD38 specificities. The presence of human Fc can prolong the half-life of antibodies and increase the recruitment of human killer cells and complement to kill the tumor cells. CD20 is a pan-B-cell marker, but it is only present in 70% of post-transplant lymphomas, when CD38 is expressed on all tumor cells. Both anit-CD20 and anti-CD38 are able to prevent the development of EBV-positive human B-cell lymphomas in the Scid/hu mice model.

Eleven patients have been treated for a B-cell lymphomas developing after kidney graft (7), liver graft (1), heart (1), kidney-heart (1), heart-lung (1). B-cell lymphoma has been diagnosed 36 ± 47 months after graft (4–120 months). Six patients presented with enlarged nodes; liver was involved in 5 patients; other sites were hilum of the renal graft (3), lung (2), digestive tract (1), spleen (1). Clonality could be proved in 5 cases, and EBV was present in 8 tumors.

Two patients received anti-CD37 or anti-CD38 Fab Fc_2 mAb; 4 patients received anti-CD20 combined with anti-CD38 or anti-CD38, or anti-CD37/CD38 Fab_2 Fc_4 mAb; 1 patient received anti-CD19 mAb then anti-CD22 coupled to immunotoxin; 4 patients received anti-CD20 Fab_2 Fc_2 mAb. Treatment was usually performed as 2 weekly infusions over 2 to 3 weeks.

Complete remission has been obtained in four patients of whom 3 had monoclonal lymphomas; two patients are currently under treatment. Three patients with heart or liver graft died during treatment because of the progression of lymphoma in 2, because rejection in 1 patient. Treatment was inefficient in 1 patient who had relapse of the lymphoma one year after she received chemotherapy. The efficiency of the treatment with mAb is unevaluable in 1 patient who received chemotherapy a few days after the end of the mAb infusions.

Side-effects have been mild in all patients; we have not observed any changes in leucocyte count, nor other biological tests.

Conclusions: Chimeric monoclonal antibody therapy should be offered in more patients since we have proven it is safe and can be efficient on monoclonal tumors. When the lymphoma is diagnosed too late, it could be combined with a non-aggressive chemotherapy to reduce tumor mass, since we have observed that about 2 weeks can spend before the tumor begin to shrink. We think that the immunosuppressive treatment should be only slightly reduced in order to save the graft because the high risk of relapse will make it very difficult to retransplant these patients after they have presented a B-cell lymphoma during a previous transplantation.

RENAL RETRANSPLANTATION IN THAILAND

Sopon Jirasiritham, M.D.
Faculty of Medical School, Ramathibodi Hospital, Mahidol University, Bangkok, Thailand

Since the graft and patient survival rates in renal retransplantation have much improved recently in most reports, we retrospectively studied the factors affecting retransplantation from our experience in Thailand.

Between February 1986 and January 1997, 490 ESRD patients received a renal transplant in Ramathibodi Hospital Medical School and Pra Ram 9 Hospital, which are the two biggest centers of renal transplantation in Bangkok. Among these patients, 23 cases were retransplantation, including 14 females and 9 males, age from 23 to 48 years with the average age of 38.7 years. The causes of their first graft loss were: 13 intractable severe acute rejections, 7 chronic rejections, 2 renal infarct, 1 renal sepsis. Most of the graft loss from acute rejection followed transplantation abroad. 17 transplant nephrectomies were performed with the main indication as irreversible acute rejection. The interval between the first graft loss and the retransplantation ranged from 3 to 28 months with the average period of 14 months. The pattern of donor was different between the first and second transplantation. In the first graft, there were 21 cadaveric and only 2 living related donors while in the second one, there were 8 cadaveric and 15 living related donors.

Immunosuppression in the induction phase was mostly triple drug regimen, composed of 12 ATG + CyA + Pred, with 2 CyA + Pred + Aza, 2 CyA + Pred + MMF and 7 double drug regimen-CyA + Pred. The maintenance immunosuppression were mainly double drug regimen, i.e. Cya + Pred.

Patients who experienced acute rejection received triple drug immunosuppression, either Cya + Pred + Aza or Cya + Pred + MMF. There were 5 episodes of acute rejection in 4 patients. All responded to steroid pulse therapy except one which needed monoclonal antibody to rescue the graft. The complications included: 5 herpes infections, 2 perianal abscess, 2 infected lymphoceles, 1 acute pyelonephritis and 1 post-operative hemorrhage. There was one death, with still functioning graft, due to intracerebral hemorrhage 2 months after retransplantation. The rest of the grafts have been functioning from 3 months to 4 years. The 2 year graft and patient acturial survival rate was 95%.

Conclusion: The results of renal retransplantation in this study was as good as those of the graft. These could be due to:

1. The use of more living related donors than cadavers in renal retransplantation.
2. Use of the antilymphocyte antibody in the induction phase of immunosuppression.
3. More selection of patients for renal retransplantation.

KIDNEY TRANSPLANTATION
C. Mouquet*, C. Sylla, E. Chartier-Kastler, H. Benalia, S. Ourahma*, P. Coriat*, M.O. Bitker
Kidney Transplant Unit and *Department of Anesthesiology, Pitié Salpêtrière Hospital, Paris, France

Background: Patients undergoing retransplantation after surgical or immunological failure of a first kidney transplant have been considered at high risk [1, 2]. Some recent studies have shown, with a short follow up, that retransplantation could be performed with good results [3]. The aim of this study is to relate our experience in retransplantation.

Patients and methods: From October 1987 until February 1997, 51 patients (Grp1) had a second kidney transplantation in our Unit. Two of them received later a third graft. Grp 1 was compared to 96 patients (Grp2) having received a first kidney during the same period. Groups were paired for age, sex, and date of transplantation. Type of nephropathy, duration of dialysis, sensitization rate, immuno-suppressive regimen, cause of first allograft failure, incidence of acute rejection, mean creatinine plasma level for patients with a functionnal graft were studied. Data analysis were compared with χ^2 test, patients and grafts survival rate were studied with the Kaplan Meier method and compared with a Logrank test. In both groups, mean age of patients was 41 ± 10 years, (range: 19–66) and mean follow up was 44 ± 32 months. Both groups were similar before transplantation for etiology of nephropathy. Mean duration of dialysis before the first graft was 28.9 ± 36.4 months in Grp1 vs 29.4 ± 31.2 months in Grp2. Duration

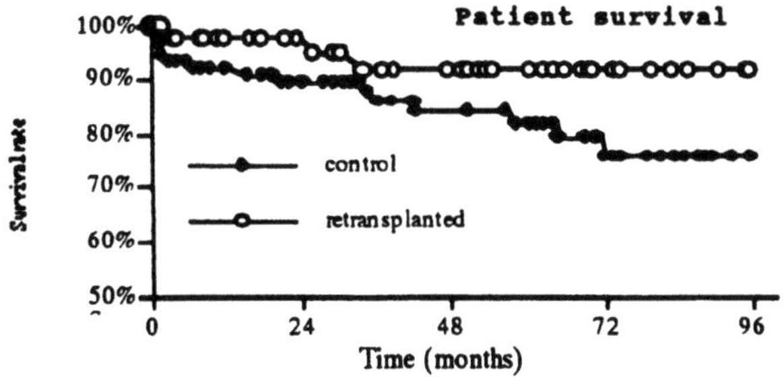

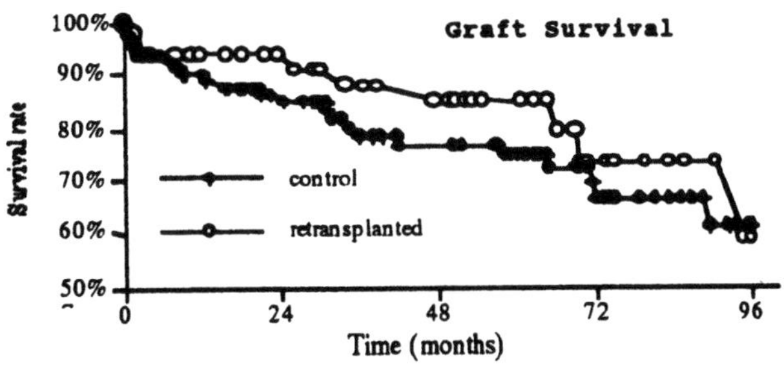

of dialysis before the second graft in Grp1 was 52.5 ± 54.2 months. In Grp1, reason of graft loss was immunological in 34 cases, surgical in 8, medical in 3, recurrence of initial disease in 2 cases and de novo glomerular disease in 1 case. Interruption of treatment was responsible of 5 grafts loss. HLA mismatching for the class I antigens was 1.4 ± 1.0 in Grp1 vs 2.2 ± 1.0 in Grp2 and for the class II 0.7 ± 0.8 vs 0.9 ± 0.7. Highly sensitized patients are more numerous in Grp1, 29.4% vs 5.2%, $p < 0.01$. Immunosuppressive regimen was the same in both groups, but cyclosporine was used more frequently in Grp1: 64.7% vs 44.8%, $p < 0.05$.

Results: Incidence of acute rejection was not statistically different in the 2 groups, 33.3% in Grp 1 vs 47.9% in Grp 2. With a mean follow up of 44 months, mean creatinine plasma levels were identical: 140.2 ± 51.0 μmol/l vs 139.5 ± 65.1 μmol/l. Survival rate were not statistically different respectively: 92% vs 82% at 5 years and 92% vs 76% at 8 years for patients and 85% vs 75% at 5 years and 59% vs 61% at 8 years for grafts.

Conclusion: The loss of a first or second kidney transplant, either for surgical or immunological reason, may not be a resignation for dialysis since this study confirms that kidney retransplantation, despite a higher pretransplant sensitization, gives similar long term results [4].

References:

1. Rosenthal JT et al. J. Urol. 1984; 131: 17–18.
2. Howard RJ et al. Arch. Surg. 1984; 119: 796–799.
3. Jackson CL et al. J. Urol. 1991; 142: 694–696.
4. Bitker MO et al. Sémin. Uro-Néphrol. 1995; XXI; 403–408.

INCIDENCE OF SPECIFIC CLASS II ANTIBODIES AFTER KIDNEY GRAFT LOSS

A. Parissiadis[1], M.L. Woehl-Jaegle[2], C. Meyer[2], P. Wolf[2], M.M. Tongio[1]
[1]Etablissement de Transfusion Sanguine de Strasbourg
[2]Unité de transplantation de l'Hôpital de Strasbourg Hautepierre

A group of 80 kidney graft recipients was studied for HLA immunization after loss of graft function. Sera were screened (1) by the classical lymphocytotoxicity technique using PBMC, CLL cells and normal B cells isolated with magnetic beads, with and without DTT and before and after platelet adsorption to remove class I antibodies and (2) by ELISA techniques.

A total of 49 (61%) recipients had developed donor specific class II antibodies. Among these, 19 (39%) had class II antibodies only while 30 (61%) had class I and class II antibodies. A total of 14 (17.5%) recipients had developed donor specific class I antibodies only. The specificity of the class II antibodies was directed against DR antigen(s) of the donor in 18 cases, against DQ antigen(s) in 27 cases and against DR and DQ antigens in 4 cases. These results were compared with those for 76 patients awaiting a first kidney graft. Among these, 12 (16%) had HLA class I antibodies and only 2 (2.5%) HLA class I and class II antibodies.

KIDNEY RETRANSPLANTATION AFTER RECURRENT GLOMERULONEPHRITIS

J. Pascual, R. Marcén, G.F. Juárez, L. Orofino, T. Cano, M. Crespo, F.J. Burgos, F. Liaño, C. Quereda, J. Ortuño
Servicios de Nefrología y Urología, Hospital Ramón y Cajal, Madrid, Spain

Since 1979 we have performed 669 kidney transplantations (KT) in our unit, 613 first and 56 retransplantations (KRT). Among the causes of graft loss in our first graft group, recurrence of glomerulonephritis (GN) was the fifth in importance (4%) after death with functioning graft, chronic and acute rejections and vascular thrombosis. Thus, ten patients lost their grafts after recurrent glomerulopathy: focal segmental glomerulosclerosis (FSGS) ($n = 3$), membranoproliferative ($n = 3$), IgA ($n = 2$) and membranous ($n = 2$), after a post-KT period variable from some weeks to 15 years. We have attempted KRT for three of them.

The first KRT was performed in a male patient with membranoproliferative GN in 1987. Six months later he developed acute rejection and recurrence of the GN in the renal biopsy and lost the graft. A female patient with FSGS underwent cadaveric KRT in 1990; she had lost the first graft in 1980 (azathioprine-steroids) some weeks after recurrence of the disease was noted. She received cyclosporine and steroids, and gross proteinuria and nephrotic syndrome immediately developed again. Despite immunoadsorptive therapy, graft nephrectomy was necessary for the management of intractable nephrotic syndrome 5 months post-KRT. Finally, a 36-year-old male patient with recurrence of membranous GN in his first renal allograft underwent KRT in 1992. Chronic graft dysfunction due to chronic rejection was detected in 1994, but he has now a stable functioning graft on triple therapy with azatioprine, cyclosporine and steroids.

KRT can be accomplished in patients who lost their grafts after recurrence of their GN. In our small experience, the risk of a new recurrence, particularly in FSGS, is high and individual adaptation of the immunosuppressive strategy remains speculative.

KIDNEY RETRANSPLANTATION IN CYCLOSPORINE TREATED PATIENTS

J. Pascual, G.F. Juárez, J. Herruzo, T. Cano, R. Marcén, L. Orofino, F.J. Burgos, F. Liaто, C. Quereda, J. Ortuто
Servicios de Nefrología y Urología, Hospital Ramón y Cajal, Madrid, Spain

Renal retransplantation (RRTx) has a worse short and long term prognosis than first renal transplantation. It is associated to a higher incidence of medical and surgical complications. Except for the Collaborative Transplant Study, most of the published series include recipients with conventional and cyclosporine-A (CyA) basal immunosuppression, and the real information about prognosis and complications of RRTx in the CyA era is not extense.

During the last ten years we have performed 450 cadaveric renal transplantations with a standard immunosuppressive protocol including CyA and steroids. Four hundred and four of them were first transplants and 46 RRTx. The induction protocol for the RRTx patients included four iv boluses of 6-methylprednisolone of 250 mg each (days 0–3) while first transplants received only one on day 0. An additional difference is that since 1995, the RRTx recipients ($n = 8$) received an induction of 5 boluses of OKT3 with introduction of CyA at fourth day, while first transplant recipients received only CyA and steroids from day 0.

Mean age and sex distribution were similar in both groups. Demographic data of the donors were also similar. HLA-DR matching, cold and warm isquemia times, percentages of delayed graft function and length of hospitalization were similar. Acute rejection episodes developed in 49% of first renal transplants and in 50% of RRTx (NS). Treatment requirements were not different. Actuarial survival rates are depicted and compared in the table.

The incidence of complications arising from the surgical wound, the linfoceles, urinary leaks or urinary tract stenosis was not different. RRTx recipients had a higher incidence of vascular thrombosis, but the difference did not reach statistical significance (6.8% vs 15.1%, $p = 0.11$). The distribution of causes of graft loss was different between the two groups. No RRTx recipients lost the graft as a consequence of acute rejection, while 21 first transplants did (0 vs 17%, $p = 0.13$). Graft loss secondary to chronic rejection was similar (28 vs 25%). The most frequent cause of graft RRTx loss was vascular thrombosis (39% of all losses had this origin). Mean serum creatinine at one year and thereafter was similar in functioning first transplants and functioning RRTx.

Our data support RRTx in patients immunosuppressed with cyclosporine and steroids. Long-term patient survival is excellent. Short term graft survival is slightly worse than in first transplants probably due to a higher incidence of vascular complications.

	1 year	*3 year*	*Log-rank test*	
Patient	*First*	*97%*	*94%*	
	RRTx	*96%*	*93%*	$p = 0.47$
Graft	First	83%	76%	
	RTx	71%	65%	$p = 0.08$

BEST SURVIVAL OF CORNEAL RETRANSPLANTATION USING SYSTEMIC IMMUNOSSUPRESSION

Maria Cristina Ribeiro de Castro, Tadeu Cvintal
Instituto Tadeu Cvintal de Oftalmologia, São Paulo, Brasil

In all domains of organ transplantation, retransplants are a major immunological concern. First corneal grafts are usually not rejected, but further grafts show the same rate of rejection than solid organs. In our experience 50% of corneal retransplants have never attained good function. With the aim to improve corneal retransplants survival and function, 18 patients received a corneal retransplant using immunossupression. Ten patients were female, median age was 58 years old (ranging from 25 to 81 years old), the majority received a secondary graft. Thirteen received triple therapy (cyclosporin A: 5 mg/kg/day; azathioprine: 2 mg/kg/day; prednisone: 1 mg/kg/day, as initial doses from the day of grafting), and 5 received no prednisone because of concurrent diseases or advanced age. Severe clinical assessment, performed before surgery, and a frequent clinical surveillance posttransplantation avoided major complications. Reactivity against T lymphocytes was tested by a panel reactivity assay (PRA) in 8 patients and was positive in only one (13% of reactivity). One year follow-up shows 77% of patients with good function and no rejection. Fifteen percent of them lost the graft because of non-immunological problems, mainly glaucoma. Only 1 patient has lost the graft because of rejection, probably due to non-compliance. One patient presented one episode of hypertensive emergency and hypervolemia, due to the unintentional association of cyclosporine and a non-steroid anti-inflammatory drug, promptly reversed with the withdrawal of the second one. There was one bacterial pneumonic process in a diabetic patient, one episode of gastritis, one Herpes zoster infection and 2 mild rises in liver enzymes. No death occurred.We concluded that, comparing these, to our previous results using no immunossupression, patients that were submitted to retransplantation using this protocol had better results. A good selection and a rigid clinical evaluation are essential to avoid severe complications. Mechanism of action of these drugs in corneal retransplantation are still to be better identified.

PATHOLOGIC FINDINGS OF GRAFT REJECTION IN FIRST AND SECOND TRANSPLANTS. DIFFERENCES ACCORDING TO BANFF CLASSIFICATION

J.C. Ruiz,[1] A. Garcia-Valtuille,[2] F. Val-Bernal,[2] R. Escallada,[1] E. Rodrigo,[1] M. Arias[1]
[1]Nephrology and [2]Pathology Departments, University Hospital Valdecilla, 39008 Santander, Spain

Second grafts do have poorer outcome than first grafts, although survival rate of regrafts has steadily improved over the last years. Nevertheless no studies comparing pathological analysis of first and second grafts based on the Banff classification have been performed to date.

Objective: The purpose of this study was to compare pathological findings of acute rejection in first and second transplants in order to find differences in the appearance of acute rejection in those patients receiving a retransplant.

Methods: Three-hundred and eleven graft biopsies in 224 renal transplants (193 first and 31 second tx. performed between 1986 and 1996) were analysed and pathologic findings (glomerular, interstitial, tubular and vascular damage) computed according to the Banff classification. Frequency and severity of acute rejection as well as frequency of glomerular, interstitial, tubular and vascular findings were compared between first and second transplants. A selected group of 22 transplants (11 patients with biopsies in two consecutive transplants) was separately analysed (35 biopsies) in order to compare the same factors in the first and second transplant of the same patient.

Results: Acute rejection was diagnosed in 61% of first and 55% of second transplants (pNS). Grade III acute rejection was more frequent in second tx. although that difference was not statistically significant. When the whole group was considered glomerular damage was observed more frequently in second transplants (39.6% vs. 57.9%) but this difference was not significant. Nevertheless when the selected group of two grafts and biopsies in both grafts was analysed a statistically significant difference in glomerular damage was observed, being more frequent in second transplants, 27% (4/15) in first transplants vs. 65% (11/17) in second transplants in the same group of patients ($p < 0.05$). No differences could be observed in any of the other factors studied.

Conclusion: No differences can be demonstrated between first and second transplants with respect to pathologic appearance of acute rejection. Nevertheless glomerular damage seems to be more frequent in acute rejection of second transplants when compared to the first transplant in the same patient.

SECOND RENAL ALLOGRAFT TRANSPLANTS. EXPERIENCE AT A SINGLE INSTITUTION

C.V. Sansalone, G. Colella, P. Aseni, A. Meroni, G.F. Rondinara, L. De Carlis, C. Brunati, B. Brando, E. Minetti, R. Confalonieri, A.O. Slim, P. Goglia, G. Civati, D. Forti
Dept. of Surgery and Abdominal Transplantation, Niguarda Hospital, Milan (Italy)

Registry data of heart and liver retransplantation have revealed a pattern of patient survival that is significantly worse than results achieved by primary transplantation. To verify the trend of graft survival following renal retransplantation, we analyzed the results of 67 patients who received a second renal graft at Niguarda Hospital, Milan. Between March 1, 1984 and December 31, 1996, 67 second renal transplants (64 from cadaveric and 3 from living related donors) have been performed in 67 adult recipients (male 37) of mean age of 39 years. This series represented 8.5% of the 787 total renal transplants performed at our institution during the same period after the introduction of routine cyclosporine immunosuppression. In 51 (76.1%) of 67 patients, the cause of their primary renal graft failure was rejection (graft failure was defined by patient death or a return to dialysis). Nine of these 51 primary renal grafts were lost within 6 months of transplantation. Forty-nine (73.1%) had good function until after 5 years. The only contraindication to second transplantation was non-compliance with the medical regimen following a primary transplantation. Primary and second renal transplant patients received quadruple drug therapy (cyclosporine, azathioprine, anti-thymocyte globulin, steroids). Episodes of acute rejection were treated with methylprednisone boluses.

With a median follow-up of 61 months following retransplantation (range, 5–128 months), 46 (68.6%) of the 67 patients had functioning grafts. The 1-, 3-, and 5-year actuarial survival rates for all 67 patients was 83, 71 and 68%, respectively, which was not significantly different when compared to the outcome of primary renal graft transplants. In this group, rejection remained the most common cause of failure in 12 (57.1%) of 21 patients. Only 3 (4.4%) of the 67 recipients experienced both primary and second transplant rejection failure within 6 months of transplantation. In conclusion, in our experience second renal graft survival is comparable to primary renal graft survival. In both groups, rejection is the main cause of graft loss.

ANATOMICAL COMPORTMENT OF THE MEDIAL SEGMENT OF THE LIVER IN THE PROCUREMENT OF THE LEFT LOBE GRAFT FROM LIVING DONORS. AN EXPERIMENTAL STUDY ON DOG

Trinh van Minh, Lê dĩnh Roanh, Nguyễn van Mão, Nguỹen van Uóc,
Vũ công Dũng, Nguyễn van Thiêng, Nguyễn van Hà, Nguyễn van Tuòng et al.
Hanoi Medical College

The partition of right and left lobes, as well as the procurement of the left lobe from a living donor, keeping the medial segment totally interrupted of portal supply in continuity with the right hemiliver, is to be forbidden by some authors (Couinaud and Houssin), because of the risk of 'immediate lethal necrosis' of this segment.

In an experimental study on dogs, such procurement of the double left lobe graft (II + III) from living donors (and auto-reimplantation in one of them) showed, after 4 and 26 days, no necrosis, but functional elimination of the medial segment (IV), with light atrophy, darker coloration, and microscopically portal and sinusoidal congestion and dilatation, with some tendency to venous thrombosis, arteriolar proliferation, hepatocytes hydropic change, enlargement and inflammatory infiltration of some portal spaces, even micro abscess in one case, biliary stasis, and neoformation of biliary canaliculus.

Macroscopic anatomical observations on corrosion casts (with fine colored injections of different intrahepatic structures) revealed complete interruption of the portal, arterial and biliary pedicles of the medial segment in 2 dogs, residual arterial and biliary twigs on the third one, and a compensative development of collateral arterial system in all of them, with a trans-scissural arteriolar plexus coming from the right hemiliver (developed in early stage: even 4 days post operative, and constant in all cases observed), a trans-parenchymatous arteriolar development from the cystic artery, and a local arteriolar hyperdevelopment from a preserved arterial twig around a preserved biliary duct.

Conclusion: The operation, simple for the transplant surgeon, seems not to be dangerous for the living donor, although not functionally economic in parenchymatous mass.

RENAL RETRANSPLANTATIONS – RESULTS AND SURGICAL ASPECTS

M. Zelić, P. Orlić, D. Dimec, G. Velčić, M. Uravić, M. Fučak, S. Rački
Rijeka, Croatia

From January 30 1971 to January 30 1997, 625 renal transplants and 4 simultaneous pancreas and kidney transplants were performed at Clinical Hospital Center in Rijeka, Croatia. There were 28 kidney retransplantations in 27 patients because one patient received the third transplant. The majority, 22 patients were males and only 5 patients were females. Fifteen patients received their first graft from a living related donor and 12 patients received a kidney from a cadaver. Vascular complication in 5 patients, two nonviable kidneys, and chronic rejection in 20 patients was cause for graft loss.

Kidney for retransplantation was provided from a living related donor in 10 patients, a living unrelated donor (free kidney) in one patient and from a cadaver in 17 patients. Eight patients who had undergone renal transplantation before 1984 (group A) received conventional immunosuppression and 20 patients after that (group B) received cyclosporine and prednisone.

In group A, 3 patients received a kidney from a living related donor, one patient from a living unrelated donor and 4 patients from a cadaver. Patient survival in group A after one and five years was 88% and graft survival was 50% and 13%, respectively. One patient with functioning graft died from pneumonia. Two kidneys were nonviable, others were rejected from a month to 12 years after transplant.

In group B, 8 patients received a kidney from a living related donor and 12 from a cadaver. Patient survival in group B was 80% after one year and 69% after 5 years. Graft survival was 75% and 54% after one and five years, respectively. Three patients died from cardiac reason: two patients first postoperative day and one patient four years after transplant. One patient died a month after transplant from CMV infection. The other patient died 18 months after transplant from lymphoma. A kidney with spontaneous rupture was saved with suture.

Conclusion: Retransplantations accounted for 4.48% of our renal transplantation activity. The only surgical challenge was the transplantation of a free ectopic pelvic kidney of an unrelated living donor with multiple vessels and a third transplantation. Results of survival after retransplantation are worse in comparison with results of first graft, but acceptable with cyclosporine immunosuppression. The shortage of organs for transplantation diminishes chances for retransplantation to many suitable patients.

Name index

J.L. Touraine et al. (eds.), Retransplantation, 349–352.

MIX
Papier aus verantwortungsvollen Quellen
Paper from responsible sources
FSC® C105338

If you have any concerns about our products,
you can contact us on
ProductSafety@springernature.com

In case Publisher is established outside the EU,
the EU authorized representative is:
Springer Nature Customer Service Center GmbH
Europaplatz 3, 69115 Heidelberg, Germany

Printed by Libri Plureos GmbH
in Hamburg, Germany